THE CIPP EVALUATION MODEL

THE CIPP EVALUATION MODEL

How to Evaluate for Improvement and Accountability

Daniel L. Stufflebeam
Guili Zhang

THE GUILFORD PRESS
New York   London

Library of Congress Cataloging-in-Publication Data is available from the publisher.

ISBN 978-1-4625-2923-0 (paperback)
ISBN 978-1-4625-2924-7 (hardcover)

Preface

This book is an up-to-date, practical rendition of the CIPP (Context, Input, Process, Product) Evaluation Model. The book is intended for use wherever programs are evaluated, including all disciplines and service areas across the world. Intended users include evaluators, administrators, practitioners, professors, students, and community groups. The book offers a well-developed evaluation framework, illustrations of how the model has been applied, practical procedures, evaluation tools, references to relevant computer programs, and aids to teaching the model. Fundamental themes are that evaluations should assist program improvement, provide documentation for program accountability, meaningfully engage stakeholders, draw upon the full range of applicable qualitative and quantitative methods, meet professional standards for evaluations, and be suitable for metaevaluation.

The CIPP Evaluation Model originated in the 1960s as a guide for evaluating programs launched in connection with Lyndon Johnson's War on Poverty. In contrast to the then prevalent evaluation approaches, the new CIPP Model stressed ongoing evaluation for continuous improvement and accountability; and it provided for assessing not only a program's outcomes but also the needs of targeted beneficiaries plus program plans, costs, and operations. Although the model was initially tailored to evaluate programs in U.S. schools and colleges, over the years it has been applied in virtually every discipline and service area across the globe. While the model's users have been assisted by a range of pertinent journal articles and book chapters, a full-length book that delineates the model—especially in consideration of its many and varied applications—has been lacking. This book has built on what has been learned from many applications of the CIPP Model and is focused on providing both evaluation specialists and lay users of evaluation with guidance they can use to get the best service from their evaluations.

Coverage

The book's 12 chapters provide background on how and why the CIPP Model was developed; a detailed presentation of the model; an explanation of the key role of an evaluation-oriented leader who can decide what and when to evaluate; detailed presentations on evaluation design, budgeting, and contracting; procedures and tools for collecting, analyzing, and reporting evaluation information; and procedures for conducting standards-based metaevaluations (evaluations of evaluations).

These topics are interspersed with illustrative evaluation cases in such areas as education, housing, and military personnel evaluation. To help guide discrete evaluation tasks, the chapters include many helpful charts, checklists, and references to relevant computer programs. To support its use as a textbook, each chapter concludes with a set of review questions. The Appendix provides detailed information on the model's uses in many fields and different countries. The book is supported by suggested supplementary readings, a detailed glossary, and extensive author and subject indexes.

The Book's Organization

Chapters 1 and 2 provide background information on why and how the model was developed, as well as the detailed, current version of the model. The next nine chapters follow the typical sequence in planning, conducting, and reporting an evaluation. Chapter 12 lays out a standards-based approach to conducting formative and summative metaevaluations. Basically, we advise instructors who teach evaluation courses to have students work through the 12 chapters in the sequence in which the book presents them. Of course, those instructors may teach a workshop or short course should select chapters that are especially responsive to the assessed needs of their students.

All readers of the book can gain an appreciation for the CIPP Model's unique contributions by studying both Chapter 1, on the model's background, and the Appendix, on the model's uses in various disciplines and countries and in a wide range of doctoral dissertations. All readers definitely should study Chapter 2 to gain an in-depth understanding of the model's main concepts and its theoretical, philosophical, and professional underpinnings. Evaluators and their clients may selectively study Chapters 3–11 to obtain guidance for specific evaluation tasks—that is, design, budgeting, contracting, data collection, analysis, and reporting. Those who are charged to evaluate an evaluation will find detailed guidance in Chapter 12.

Students who plan to use the CIPP Model to guide their doctoral dissertation or master's thesis will find the book's Appendix to contain a rich set of information about completed dissertations that used the CIPP Model. In general, the book has been organized to help users grasp and make efficient use of the model's key principles.

Pedagogical Features

We have sought to make the book as understandable and user friendly as possible. Key features in this regard are as follows:

- *Chapter introduction boxes* provide succinct overviews of each chapter's contents.
- *Key terms*, when first introduced, are highlighted in **boldface**, with their definitions appearing in the end-of-book Glossary.
- *Within-chapter boxes* contain comments and references to relevant evaluations to help illustrate the applicability of the preceding content.
- *Computer programs* that provide efficient data analysis tools are referenced in Chapter 10.
- *End-of-chapter review questions* provide readers with both a summary of some of the chapter's most important lessons and a means to test one's mastery of the chapter's content.
- *End-of-chapter suggestions for further reading* offer both evaluators and evaluation students leads to sources of information to enhance their grasp of certain concepts or procedures.

Supplementary Online Materials

The book's product page on The Guilford Press website contains information and tools to support use of the book. In particular, the website houses a highly specific CIPP Evaluation Model Checklist, which provides step-by-step guidance for planning, conducting, and reporting CIPP Model–based evaluations, and a Program Evaluation Metaevaluation Checklist, which provides step-by-step guidance for assessing a program evaluation's design and implementation and, ultimately, for judging its final report.

Acknowledgments

We are indebted to C. Deborah Laughton, Senior Editor at The Guilford Press, for her excellent guidance and support throughout the process of writing this book. We also wish to thank Dr. Gary Wegenke (former school district superintendent in Des Moines, Iowa, and

Dean of the Western Michigan College of Education) for his detailed, critical review of a previous draft of the book. We also are grateful to David M. Miller, Department of Educational Psychology, University of Florida; Mina Singh, School of Nursing, York University; and Zandra Gratz, School of Psychology, Kean University, for their incisive critiques of drafts of the book's first three chapters. Our writing of the book benefited greatly from their highly professional and competent input.

DANIEL L. STUFFLEBEAM
GUILI ZHANG

Brief Contents

Chapter 8   **Contracting Evaluations**   163

Chapter 9   **Collecting Evaluative Information**   175

Chapter 10   **Analyzing and Synthesizing Information**   214

Chapter 11   **Reporting Evaluation Findings**   250

Chapter 12   **Metaevaluation: Evaluating Evaluations**   288

Appendix   **The CIPP Model in Perspective: Evaluation's Ubiquitous Nature,**   317
             the Need for Systematic Program Evaluations,
             and the CIPP Model's Wide Range of Applications

             Glossary   337

             References   355

             Author Index   365

             Subject Index   370

             About the Authors   384

Extended Contents

Chapter 3   **A Case Illustrating Application of the CIPP Model**   57
to Evaluate a Self-Help Housing Project

Chapter 4   **Evaluation-Oriented Leadership in Launching and Supporting**   76
Effective Evaluations

Chapter 11   Reporting Evaluation Findings   250

Chapter 12   Metaevaluation: Evaluating Evaluations   288

CHAPTER 1

Introduction

This chapter introduces the book's central focus—the CIPP (Context, Input, Process, Product) Evaluation Model. The book is intended for use especially by those individuals and groups who, possibly having considered several alternative evaluation approaches, have chosen to apply the CIPP Model. A wide diversity of such users have applied the model to a wide range of needs for evaluation. The chapter explains why and how the model was developed and identifies its key features. The model is presented in the context of basic definitions of program evaluation and formative and summative uses of evaluation. Overall, this chapter foreshadows the remaining chapters, which together provide the concepts, illustrations, procedures, checklists, and standards that evaluators and their clients need to plan, budget, contract, staff, carry out, report, apply, and defend evaluations.

Overview

Sound evaluation is essential to effective programming in all sectors of a society. Evaluation is part and parcel of every other discipline and of the wide range of service areas. It is inconceivable that professionals in any field would conduct their work without evaluating its essential elements, for example, research designs and instruments, resources, equipment, manufacturing processes, staff qualifications, staff performance, **credibility** to constituents, community relations, completed products, success of services, or draft research manuscripts. In any field systematic, defensible evaluation is essential for assessing the relevance and quality of policies, plans, budgets, processes, products, outcomes, and other entities; pointing the way to needed improvements in both assessed programs and the organizations that house them; assessing the costs, **safety, fairness, impacts,** success, and **importance** of improvement efforts; and holding developers, researchers, and service providers accountable for fulfilling responsibilities, making appropriate use of resources, and producing valuable results.

Evaluations typically are collaborative ventures that engage, at one level or another, the full range of persons whose effective involvements are required to assure that an evaluation is properly focused and funded; competently planned, executed, and reported; appropriately examined and judged; and effectively used. Cleary, all persons with responsibilities for sound conduct or use of programs or **program evaluations** need a valid concept of evaluation, as well as the knowledge, skills, and tools required to carry out their particular roles in applying the **principles of sound evaluation.** To perform in the real world of evaluation, evaluation participants need a theoretically sound, user-friendly, standards-based, practical approach by which they can communicate efficiently and collaborate effectively to meet their common and individual evaluation responsibilities.

Evaluation specialists bear a heavy responsibility for effectively engaging stakeholders in the entire process of evaluation. Such stakeholders include evaluation clients, program funders when different from the client, program administrators and staffs, program **beneficiaries,** research and development personnel in the subject program's content area, and perhaps others. In the context of evaluations, the term **stakeholders** denotes those who are the intended users of an evaluation's findings, others who may be affected by the evaluation, and those expected to contribute to the evaluation. These persons are appropriately engaged in helping affirm foundational values, define evaluation questions, clarify **evaluative criteria,** contribute needed information, interpret findings, assess evaluation reports, and make use of findings. Lead **evaluators** should identify a representative group of stakeholders, including those requesting feedback from the evaluation; orient them to the overall evaluation plan; obtain their reactions to drafts of evaluation questions and data collection plans; secure their assistance in collecting needed information; obtain their reviews of draft interim and final evaluation reports; assist them to make sound, effective uses of findings; and, as appropriate, secure their assistance in disseminating the findings.

Program Evaluation Defined

At its most general level, program evaluation is the assessment of a program's value. Specifically, a program evaluation is the systematic process of delineating, obtaining, reporting, and applying descriptive and judgmental information about a program's quality, **cost-effectiveness,** feasibility, safety, **legality, sustainability, transferability,** fairness, importance, and the like. The result of an evaluation process is an evaluation as product—that is, an evaluation report for intended uses by intended users.

A program evaluation's **conclusions** should be grounded in relevant, valid information and succinctly address the questions that guided the evaluation. Key questions addressed by sound program evaluations are:

- *Needs*—What needs should the program target and meet?
- *Solution*—What is the best way to meet the assessed needs?

- *Implementation*—Is (or was) the solution effectively executed?
- *Outcomes*—Were the targeted needs met, and what are the full range of outcomes?

Typically, program evaluations will employ both quantitative and qualitative research procedures. Among the relevant procedures are print media reviews, **surveys,** interviews, observations, photography, **logic models, rating scales,** focus groups, laboratory tests, field experiments, correlational studies, **trend analysis,** simulation studies, **significance tests,** cost analysis, data mining, and document analysis.

The main uses of program evaluations are to guide and strengthen programs, issue accountability reports, help disseminate effective practices, contribute to the relevant knowledge base, and make **decision makers,** stakeholders, and consumers aware of projects that succeeded and those that proved unworthy of further investment and use.

Program evaluation is a ubiquitous process that applies across organizational areas and levels, national boundaries, and all disciplines and service areas.

Choosing an Evaluation Model

The **CIPP Evaluation Model** is one of a number of legitimate approaches to evaluation. The term *evaluation approach* refers to any of a broad array of different ways to design, conduct, and report evaluations. This term is intended to cover all the ways employed to conduct evaluations, be they very general or quite specific or legitimate or corrupt. We have reserved the label *evaluation model* for those approaches that are designed to convey valid **descriptions** and **judgments** of a program or other entity.

Some evaluation approaches are illegitimate, as in the *psuedoevaluations* identified and assessed by Stufflebeam and Coryn (2014, pp. 117–127). These include the following biased approaches:

- *Public relations studies* that present positive findings, while downplaying or failing to report negative results.
- *Politically controlled studies* that produce valid findings but conceal them from a segment of the right-to-know evaluation audience.
- *Pandering evaluations* that—in an evaluator's

hope of winning future **evaluation contracts**—tell the client group what they want to hear, instead of giving them a valid assessment of a program's strengths and weaknesses.

- *Evaluation by pretext,* in which the evaluation is oriented, designed, conducted, and reported to confirm a client group's advance, desired evaluative findings.
- *Empowerment under the guise of evaluation,* in which an outside evaluator cedes authority to an evaluation client group to reach and report their own conclusions and to claim that the evaluation was conducted by the independent evaluator.
- *Selectively reported customer reviews* that include only positive reviews or even fictitious testimonials.

In contrast to pseudoevaluations, legitimate evaluation approaches are sufficiently credible and vetted against standards of sound inquiry to merit consideration for use by evaluators and evaluation clients. Such evaluation approaches fit our concept of evaluation models. Among others, such evaluation models include the CIPP Evaluation Model (Stufflebeam, 1983), experimental and quasi-experimental design (Campbell & Stanley, 1963), deliberative democratic evaluation (House & Howe, 2000), discrepancy evaluation (Provus, 1969), educational connoisseurship and criticism (Eisner, 1983), EPIC evaluation (Hammond, 1972), goal-free evaluation (Scriven, 1973), the key evaluation checklist (Scriven, 2007), naturalistic evaluation (Guba, 1978), responsive evaluation (Stake, 1976), the success case method (Brinkerhoff, 2003), and utilization-focused evaluation (Patton, 2008). Because of their quality, we refer to all of these approaches as evaluation models.

Table 1.1 is an example of the preliminary assessment of alternative evaluation models that an evaluator might have conducted in the process of choosing one of them for application. The evaluation models across the top are only a few of the options that might be considered. The row headings comprise a quite extensive set of the aspects of an evaluation model that a person or group might take into account in their process of choosing an evaluation model. In general, we see this list of aspects as what should be addressed in a fully functional evaluation model.

The different labels that authors assign to their evaluation approaches, as illustrated in Table 1.1, mainly reflect the authors' preferences. In general, we see evaluation approaches that are well articulated, technically sound, and grounded in the evaluation field's standards to qualify for the label evaluation model. In our view, an evaluation model should stipulate, define, and illustrate the following aspects:

- The types of evaluation purposes served.
- The general sequence of steps for conducting a sound evaluation.
- The approach's orientation to grounding evaluations in explicit values.
- The sources of evaluation questions to be addressed.
- Key foci for collecting data.
- The recommended extent and nature of stakeholder engagement.
- Main inquiry designs and data collection and analysis methods.
- The appropriate means and schedule for reporting evaluation findings.
- The model's underlying epistemology.
- Core qualifications for lead evaluators.

As is seen in the remainder of this book, the CIPP Evaluation Model includes considerable detail concerning the above referenced aspects of a sound evaluation model. Before leaving the discussion of evaluation models that are alternatives to the CIPP Model, we stress that we judge several such models as strong in meeting the requirements of an extensively articulated evaluation model. Among others, such useful evaluation models include Robert Stake's (1976) responsive evaluation, the **experimental design** approach, Michael Scriven's (2007) consumer-oriented approach, and Michael Patton's (2008) **utilization**-focused evaluation.

This book is addressed to evaluators, evaluation clients, and others who have decided to apply, or are considering applying, the CIPP Evaluation Model. Users of the CIPP Evaluation Model are many and diverse, as we have documented in this book's appendix[1] This book is designed to guide persons and groups—from across disciplines, service areas, and national contexts—in making proper and useful applications of the CIPP Evaluation Model.

TABLE 1.1. Example Framework for Choosing an Evaluation Model

Comparison Factors	CIPP Evaluation Model	Consumer-Oriented Evaluation	Discrepancy Evaluation Model	Experimental Design	Responsive Evaluation	Utilization-Focused Evaluation
Purposes	Improvement and accountability	Judge merit, worth of the evaluand, and help consumers choose wisely	Stabilize a project and assess and assist goal achievement	Establish causal links between a fixed treatment and defined outcomes	Respond usefully to the evaluative questions of a program's stakeholders	Foster use of findings
Evaluation process	Delineate, obtain, report, and apply evaluation findings	Cycle through an extensive set of checkpoints required to reach an evaluation conclusion	Process to identify and remove discrepancies between designed and actual program processes and outcomes	Operationalize, carry out, and report findings from a controlled, randomized, comparative experiment	Assess program antecedents, transactions, and outcomes and continually respond to stakeholder concerns	Identify and address the evolving evaluation questions of intended evaluation users and assist application of findings
Values orientation	Democratic values of a free society	Theory of democracy	Developer's objectives	Value neutral	Pluralistic values	Values of intended users of findings
Sources of questions	Stakeholders and relevant values	Criteria of interest to targeted consumers	The program's objectives	The program treatment design and defined dependent variable(s)	Stakeholders and relevant experts	Intended users
Key foci for collecting data	Needs, plans, processes, outcomes	Needs, full range of outcomes	Program objectives, design, implementation, and outcomes	Independent and dependent variables	Program background, transactions, and outcomes	Intended uses of findings
Stakeholder engagement	Extensive and sustained	Very little	Extensive involvement of a representative set of stakeholders	Very little, viewed as a threat to validity	Extensive and continuous	Continuous engagement of intended users
Main inquiry methods	Multiple qualitative and quantitative methods	Key Evaluation Checklist, goal-free evaluation, needs assessment, cost analysis	Tests, focus groups	Randomized, variable manipulating, controlled design	Case study	Multiple quantitative and qualitative methods as needed
Reports	Formative and Summative	Mainly summative	Succession of interim reports aimed at reducing discrepancies between actualities and intentions	Summative, at the end	Ongoing, mainly formative	Mainly oral and may not include written reports

(continued)

TABLE 1.1. *(continued)*

Comparison Factors	CIPP Evaluation Model	Consumer-Oriented Evaluation	Discrepancy Evaluation Model	Experimental Design	Responsive Evaluation	Utilization-Focused Evaluation
Standards for judging the evaluation	Utility, feasibility, propriety, accuracy, accountability	Generally referenced to standards of scientific research and not much to utility	Reliability and validity	Internal and external validity	Values of stakeholders, avoids use of published standards	Utility, feasibility, propriety, accuracy, and accountability
Epistemological orientation	Objectivist	Objectivist	Value-free orientation to a developer's objectives	Scientific method/logical positivism	Relativism	Eclectic
Core qualifications for lead evaluators	Expertise in communication, qualitative and quantitative methods, and management plus credibility to stakeholders	Expert in philosophical analysis, critical thinking, and mixed methods	Expertise in operational objectives, quantitative and qualitative measurement, and statistical analysis	Expertise in experimental and quasi-experimental design and inferential statistics	Case study methods	Sociological inquiry methods and group process
Key strengths	Aids decision making and accountability at all organizational levels, stresses formative and summative metaevaluation, keyed to professional standards for evaluations	Comprehensiveness and independence	Extensive stakeholder engagement, focus on goal achievement	Rigor of design	Searches for side effects, empowers stakeholders to reach their own conclusions and judgments	Heavy orientation to getting findings used
Key weaknesses	Extensive stakeholder engagement introduces opportunities for threatened persons to impede the evaluation	Minimizes opportunities for stakeholder involvement and use of findings; heavily retrospective	Narrow focus, lack of attention to side effects, and prone to bog down in endless succession of meetings to remove discrepancies	Stymies development (by holding treatments constant), reports only narrow results, doesn't search for side effects, often breaks down under real-world conditions and constraints	Overly divergent and often fails to converge on conclusions, leaving judgments to the eyes of the beholder	Vulnerable to turnover and lack of sustained involvement of intended users

The CIPP Evaluation Model

The CIPP Evaluation Model is one of the most widely used and arguably tried and true evaluation approaches. That model embodies and builds on the definition of evaluation presented at the outset of this chapter. Basically, the CIPP Model provides direction for assessing a program's Context, Inputs, Process, and Products. Unlike many other evaluation approaches, the CIPP Model assesses not only an enterprise's outcomes but also its environment, goals, plans, resources, and implementation. Its orientation is proactive in guiding **needs assessments,** goal setting, planning, implementation, and **quality assurance,** with an emphasis on continuing improvement. It is also retrospective in looking back on, summing up, and judging the accountability and value of completed programs or other enterprises. It not only guides evaluation specialists to effectively carry out evaluations, but it also provides for meaningful involvement of a program's stakeholders throughout an evaluation's process. The model provides the wide range of evaluation participants with a common framework and language they can use to facilitate their collaborative efforts to secure and use sound evaluation results.

Users of the CIPP Model can be confident in the model's soundness, generalizability, and utility because, over a period of more than 40 years, it has been continually updated and applied successfully in many countries and across a wide range of disciplines and service areas; because it has been extensively researched as seen in the published literature that we document in subsequent chapters and the book's Appendix; because it is keyed to professionally developed standards for sound evaluations—notably the **Joint Committee on Standards for Educational Evaluation** (2011) *Program Evaluation Standards*; because it carries a requirement that evaluations based on the CIPP Model themselves be subjected to systematic evaluation against accredited standards of the **evaluation profession**; because it provides a general framework by which organizations can institutionalize and mainstream sound evaluation services; and because it provides organizational leaders with direction for mining lessons learned from various program evaluations and using the lessons for organizational improvement. The CIPP Model is not an obscure, highly technical approach accessible only to highly skilled research methodologists but a common-sense approach that can be understood and applied by a wide range of evaluation clients, program staffs, and program constituents as well as evaluation specialists. Overall, the CIPP Model is an overarching, comprehensive approach that, when applied correctly, can meet users' full range of evaluation needs.

Purposes of This Book

We wrote this book because many users of the CIPP Model have urged us to produce a comprehensive, definitive presentation on the model. Prior to this book's publication, material on the CIPP Model appeared only in journal articles, professional papers, chapters in evaluation books, and evaluation reports and doctoral dissertations that applied the model. There was no book-length, definitive explanation of the CIPP Model. We believe this up-to-date, selectively illustrated, and practical rendition of the CIPP Model will be of service to a wide range of persons who engage in the various roles involved in systematic program evaluation.

It is important to stress that this book is aimed at general practitioners as well as evaluation students and experts; that its contents apply across the various disciplines and service areas in which programs are evaluated; that it is applicable, not only in North America, but throughout the world; that it is designed for use as a general reference, textbook, and guide to field applications; that it is intended for use in both internal/self-evaluations and independent, external evaluations; and that it is presented in an accessible (rather than highly technical) language. In structuring and writing this book, we have sought to provide users with a conceptual framework within which to plan evaluations, guidelines to follow in proceeding through the entire process of program evaluation from start to finish, cases that illustrate the effective application of the CIPP Model in a variety of fields, checklists to facilitate the correct conduct of the wide range of tasks in program evaluations, and standards and an associated metaevaluation checklist for judging evaluation plans, processes, analyses, and reports based on the model's use.

The CIPP Evaluation Model is one of the most widely applied evaluation approaches. In doing background work for this book, we identified about 500 CIPP-related evaluation studies, journal articles, and doctoral dissertations across nations, disciplines, and service areas. As a service to those users of this book who want to identify and study the model's applications in areas like those in which they work, we have chronicled detailed information about past applications of the model in the book's appendix.

Why the CIPP Model Was Developed

Work on the CIPP Model began in 1965 because U.S. public schools could not meaningfully and feasibly meet requirements for evaluating their federally supported projects in President Lyndon Johnson's War on Poverty.[2] These projects were being conducted in about 26,000 school districts in a nationwide approach to combat poverty and improve the public schools, especially their services to disadvantaged students. Because of the federal government's huge financial investment in the effort, the U.S. Congress, at the insistence of Senator Robert Kennedy (D-NY), required every funded school district to evaluate its federally supported projects. However, it soon became apparent that the project staffs throughout the country were little experienced and underqualified to conduct systematic evaluations. Moreover, even if they had been trained in the then evaluation orthodoxy, it would not have equipped them to conduct credible, useful evaluations of the federally funded projects.

The evaluation technology available in the early 1960s was mainly limited to controlled, variable-manipulating, randomized, comparative experiments; the outcomes-oriented objectives-based approach to determining whether behavioral objectives were achieved; and norms-referenced standardized testing. Attempts to apply these approaches to evaluation of thousands of federally funded, nationwide, evolving, innovative projects in their complex, dynamic school settings proved to be unsatisfying and counterproductive (Cronbach, 1963; Guba, 1966; Scriven, 1967; Stake, 1967; Stufflebeam, 1966a, 1967b; Stufflebeam et al., 1971).

Limitations of the Experimental Design Approach

Experimental designs didn't work in the dynamic world of War on Poverty projects because (1) emergent, developing, innovative projects needed continually to evolve and improve (especially in the early stages), a flexibility that contradicts experimental design's requirement for constancy of treatment throughout a study period; (2) limiting evaluation findings to the collection of posttreatment, dependent variable data and (possibly) pretreatment, dependent variable data

(as required by classical experimental design) stifled staffs' efforts to continually obtain and use process evaluation feedback to both strengthen their project and document its implementation; (3) randomizing groups of students into experimental (assisted) and control (unassisted) groups was neither feasible nor politically acceptable in schools that needed to serve all eligible students, especially the underprivileged students; (4) those experimental design studies that were conducted reported only end-of-project findings and usually concluded with a judgment that the project contributed no significant improvement in dependent variable performance for the project group over that of the **control group** (although disappointing, these unsatisfying outcomes likely were predictable considering that experimental design studies provide project staffs with no improvement-oriented feedback along the way); (5) experimental design studies focused narrowly on pre-established dependent variables and did not search out what often were crucially important, unanticipated **side effects**; and (6) experimental design studies offered no preproject help in setting goals through such means as needs assessments or evaluating draft funding proposals and budgets, although evaluative feedback for these purposes was critically important to help assure a project's relevance and success. Clearly, evaluators of innovative War on Poverty projects needed a much more flexible, responsive, informative, facilitative, and politically viable approach to evaluation than the narrow, procrustean, research laboratory-oriented, experimental design approach.

Limitations of the Objectives-Based Evaluation Approach

The rhetoric of the objectives-based approach of Ralph W. Tyler (Smith & Tyler, 1942) was very popular but proved unsuitable to evaluating the schools' thousands of federally supported projects (Stufflebeam, 1966a, 1967b; Stufflebeam et al., 1971). This approach instructed curriculum developers and evaluators to work through a time-consuming, rigorous process to specify a project's behavioral/operational objectives and subsequently to determine through a variety of outcome measures the extent to which the objectives had been achieved. This approach proved inadequate, even counterproductive, for evaluating the War on Poverty projects of the 1960s and 1970s. Staffs that spent inordinate amounts of time defining behavioral objectives soon discovered that the objectives were largely irrelevant because they weren't grounded in empirical assessments of and responsive to the needs of the targeted students. When a project staff encountered the actual students to be served, it often became apparent that the previously defined objectives were not focused on those students' real and most important academic deficiencies and associated needs. Moreover, by collecting only end-of-project outcome information, objectives-based evaluations failed to examine and provide feedback on the strengths and weaknesses of project processes, including such vital matters as planning, resource allocation, teaching, counseling and other student support services, parent involvement, community support, and project management. Also, the outcome measures that were keyed to preordained objectives failed to look for a program's positive side effects, such as increased involvement in schools of parents and local businesses, or negative side effects, such as unsustainable costs or neglect of the education needs of gifted students. Clearly, the objectives-based approach failed to assist either ongoing project improvement or determination of a project's full range of outcomes; also, its use wasted educators' valuable time by engaging them in a time-consuming, unproductive process of writing behavioral objectives, typically before they had encountered and examined the needs of the particular students to be taught.

Standardized Tests' Limited Localized Validity

The standardized, norms-referenced testing approach also proved inadequate for determining the success of the federally funded War on Poverty projects. Such tests existed across a range of school subjects and had been developed as efficient, multiple-choice devices that produce results with high levels of objectivity, efficiency, **reliability,** and content validity. They were widely used across the United States and generally respected by the public and policymakers. Many such tests on the market were accompanied by national norms for determining how well test scores of students and groups of students compared to the scores of relevant norm groups.

At first blush, standardized tests, with their characteristic rigor, objectivity, efficiency, and credibility with the public, seemed to provide "just the ticket." They had been rigorously developed, provided for objective scoring and analysis, were available for purchase at acceptable costs, employed the efficiencies associated with multiple-choice items and automated scoring, had good

face validity related to various curriculum areas, often were accompanied by carefully developed national and state norms, were widely used in schools, and had the advantage of public familiarity and acceptance.

It soon became clear, however, that these "off-the-shelf" evaluation tools generally were not appropriate for evaluating the wide range of War on Poverty projects. Among the reasons were (1) the contents of published tests often were general and lacked **validity** for assessing specific projects because the tests had not been keyed to the project's objectives and content specifications and, more importantly, the assessed needs of the students to be served; (2) such tests were developed to discriminate between test scores of students of average ability rather than those of either below- or above-average ability and consequently often were neither valid nor reliable for assessing the achievements of a project's targeted disadvantaged students; (3) the process of planning and developing a new standardized test keyed directly to an individual project's objectives typically was not feasible because of the many months and considerable resources required to develop, field-test, norm, and validate a sound test; and (4) even if a new, valid, reliable standardized test could be developed within a project's time frame and resources, it would only assess student outcomes and not produce evaluative feedback on such important project aspects as goals, structure, and implementation. Moreover, inappropriate use of a published standardized test could erroneously brand a project as failed because it showed no gains on scores of a test that was far removed from project objectives and the targeted needs of project beneficiaries. Overall, published standardized tests typically lack sufficient scope and validity for use in evaluating a wide range of different, innovative projects; it is almost never feasible to develop a sound, new test for use within a project's time frame and available resources; and inappropriate use of published standardized tests can unjustly label a project as ineffective.

A Caveat Concerning the Use of Traditional Evaluation Approaches

Before proceeding, we need to state a caveat. Despite the limitations of experimental design, objectives-based evaluation, and standardized testing as stand-alone evaluation approaches, they may be incorporated usefully into broader evaluation approaches under the right circumstances. This is especially so when they are employed not as sufficient evaluation approaches in and of themselves but as specific techniques for use in a relevant, comprehensive, fully functional evaluation approach.

The methodology of experimental design can contribute usefully to an evaluation, especially after a project approach has been successfully developed and stabilized and when it has been determined that it should be rigorously contrasted and compared, under randomized, controlled conditions to the effectiveness of alternative project strategies. Even then, it is desirable that the experiment be embedded in a broader evaluation approach that, for example, assesses the different alternatives' goals, costs, and side effects and that at least documents the implementation of experimental and control conditions.

The quite narrow objectives-based approach can play a useful part in the more comprehensive evaluation approaches. This is especially so when an evaluator reviews and makes selective application of the wide range of qualitative and quantitative methods that users of the objectives-based approach have employed in assessing project outcomes (Madaus & Stufflebeam, 1989; Tyler, 1932). Also, given sufficient time and resources to develop a sound achievement test before launching a project, an evaluator can beneficially apply the technology of test development in producing one or more needed, valid tests.

Overall, as explained below and in Chapter 2, the CIPP Model is not exclusive of other defensible approaches to evaluation or the wide range of available specific inquiry techniques. Instead, it embraces and makes room for selectively and appropriately incorporating the complete pharmacopeia of sound, qualitative and quantitative inquiry methods and tools.

Development of the CIPP Model: Based on Daniel Stufflebeam's Personal Reflections

This book's first author (Stufflebeam) is appropriately qualified to write about the inappropriateness of experimental design, objectives-based, and standardized testing approaches to evaluate War on Poverty school-based projects. Like many other evaluators of the period, he was extensively trained in these approaches and tried and failed to succeed in usefully applying them. Based on these failed attempts, he shortly set out to develop a new approach to evaluation that would work in the context of developing innovative projects in a wide range of real-world settings. Although the CIPP Model retains the option of applying experimental design, objectives-based, and standardized testing approaches to evaluation when circumstances warrant their use, it became clear in early evaluations of War on Poverty projects that each of these approaches is by itself insufficient to conduct a comprehensive evaluation of a project; that each approach rarely has much to offer in evaluating innovative, developing projects; and that, even when applicable, it needs to be applied as one technique within a broader evaluation approach.

Stufflebeam's Entry into the Evaluation Field

At the beginning of President Lyndon Johnson's War on Poverty in 1965, Stufflebeam was only tangentially engaged in educational evaluation. As director of The Ohio State University (OSU) Test Development Center, he was leading the development of standardized tests such as the General Educational Development (GED) and a wide range of college-level achievement tests in different content areas for the U.S. military, as well as conducting research on **psychometrics** and surveys of innovations in Ohio's 500-plus public school districts.

At the same time, the U.S. federal government was offering the nation's public school districts the incentive of billions of dollars to support efforts to improve schools and better serve needy students. For the school districts, the catch was that financial assistance would be forthcoming only if the districts included sound **evaluation designs** in their funding proposals. This evaluation requirement spawned a nationwide crisis. The school districts wanted and needed the federal funds to improve their programs and especially to better serve disadvantaged students; however, most of the districts could not produce the required evaluation designs. Throughout the nation, school districts' boards of education, parent groups, and other stakeholders were concerned at the prospect that their district would miss out on federal funding due to an inability to meet project evaluation requirements. In this respect, Ohio's school districts were no different from those in other states.

Consequently, Dr. John Ramseyer, head of OSU's School of Education, decided that OSU had to help Ohio's schools meet the federal requirements for evaluation. Accordingly, he assigned Professor Stufflebeam to "go into the evaluation business." In clarifying the assignment, Ramseyer explained that the U.S. Office of Education had offered huge school improvement

grants to U.S. school districts under the **Elementary and Secondary Education Act of 1965 (ESEA)**; that Ohio's schools needed such funding to improve their education offerings and especially to improve their services to disadvantaged students; and that, unfortunately, most of the schools could not meet ESEA's evaluation requirements. Dr. Ramseyer stressed that OSU, as Ohio's flagship university, had to help the schools, and he reiterated that it would be Stufflebeam's responsibility to lead OSU's evaluation assistance effort.

Although Stufflebeam had never taken a course labeled evaluation, he was in a good place to start an evaluation career. Ralph Tyler—widely acknowledged as the father of educational evaluation—had created an evaluation reputation for OSU, especially through directing the famous Eight-Year Study of progressive schools (Smith & Tyler, 1942). Perhaps Tyler would assist OSU's evaluation effort, since he frequently visited OSU to see his brother Keith. Stufflebeam's educational background included substantial work in clinical psychology and assessment, psychometrics, experimental design, and statistics. In addition, he was developing many standardized achievement tests; researching matrix sampling (Cook & Stufflebeam, 1967; Owens & Stufflebeam, 1964); field-testing the **Program Evaluation and Review Technique** (PERT; Stufflebeam, 1967a); and surveying innovations in Ohio's public schools. Moreover, he had been trained in experimental design and statistics, during his Purdue University PhD program, by the renowned statistician Benjamin Winer, and had attended the 1965, 8-week University of Wisconsin summer institute on experimental design and statistics that was led by national experts Julian Stanley, Donald Campbell, and Gene Glass.

At first, it seemed that Stufflebeam had the appropriate background to succeed in his new evaluation assignment. He could reference Ralph Tyler's (1942) "General Statement on Evaluation"; use it to help schools write behavioral objectives; select or construct valid and reliable achievement tests; apply the advice of Campbell and Stanley (1963) in assisting schools to conduct comparative experiments; administer selected achievement tests following project cycles; conduct analyses of variance and appropriate a posteriori tests for identifying and investigating statistically significant project outcomes; and help school projects develop defensible evaluation reports.

Although Stufflebeam had been a teacher in rural Iowa and Chicago from 1958 to 1961, by his own account, he had since abandoned the constraints of real school settings in favor of subscribing to theories and procedures learned in graduate school. As this book's coauthor, he acknowledges that, for the time being, he had forgotten that dynamic school settings typically are not amenable to laboratory research controls and that disadvantaged students have widely varying needs and problems that are not sensitively measured by published standardized tests. His initial thinking about evaluating the schools' "War on Poverty" projects was consistent with the conventional thinking about evaluation at the time. As he would discover, however, this perspective would prove relatively useless, even counterproductive, in meeting the real-world, War on Poverty evaluation assignments.

Establishment of The Evaluation Center

Despite his initial unrealistic views about evaluating school projects, Stufflebeam took some steps in his new assignment that over time worked out quite well. Dr. Ramseyer approved his recommendation to start a new evaluation center. The Evaluation Center's mission was then (and 50 years later still remains) to advance the theory and practice of evaluation. Because no center could directly serve the evaluation needs of all Ohio schools, Stufflebeam projected that the new evaluation center would conduct a few representative evaluations; use these as training and research laboratories; produce models, methods, and data collection instruments that schools could select, adapt, and apply; graduate some well-trained evaluation masters and doctoral students; and help establish and staff a few exemplary school-district-based offices of evaluation to serve as demonstration sites.

Evaluations of ESEA Projects in Columbus, Ohio

The Evaluation Center's first project was for the Columbus, Ohio, public schools. In 1965, the 110,000-student district was tentatively entitled to receive $6.6 million for 3-year, ESEA, Title I projects (for service to economically disadvantaged students). However, the superintendent told Stufflebeam that the district had no staff member with the requisite training and background for planning and conducting sound project evaluations. Stufflebeam projected that The Evaluation Center could and would help the district meet the ESEA evaluation requirements but only if the district agreed to meet certain conditions keyed to The Evaluation Center's mission. These conditions included (1) contracting with OSU for 9% of the ESEA project budgets; (2) authorizing OSU to prepare the needed evaluation plans and supervise their execution; (3) collaborating with OSU to select and assign Columbus school district teachers to staff the evaluations; (4) authorizing and supporting OSU to provide these teachers—the school district's evaluators—with graduate degree programs and on-the-job evaluation training in evaluation; (5) committing the school district to fund, staff, and install its own office of evaluation at the end of 3 years; and (6) agreeing that the Evaluation Center could use 2 of the 9% of contracted evaluation funds to document, analyze, and publish findings on the evaluation experience. The school district's superintendent agreed to the basic intent of these conditions but objected to conditions 3, 4, and 5. Stufflebeam responded that the new Center aimed not to provide one-time, terminal evaluation services, but to help the contracted districts to set up and operate, over time, their own systems of evaluation. The Evaluation Center's motivation in this regard was to try to help create institutional models of school-district-based evaluation that other districts could study and possibly replicate. Otherwise, Stufflebeam was convinced that the Center's staff would fail to advance evaluation theory and practice and make little impact on the long-term evaluation capacities of Ohio's districts. The Columbus School District's superintendent reluctantly agreed to Stufflebeam's conditions, and he then proceeded on a well-intentioned but partly misguided effort.

With consultant assistance, Columbus educators had completed essentially fill-in-the-blanks proposals, and Stufflebeam added the evaluation plans. Following funding by the government, Stufflebeam and the school district's deputy superintendent selected school district teachers to serve as the ESEA evaluation team. This team engaged "focus groups" of staff members from each funded project in a time-consuming process to delineate the project's objectives. Subsequently, Stufflebeam intended to engage the evaluation team in selecting or developing the needed achievement tests and other instruments. He and the evaluators soon abandoned the notion of randomly assigning disadvantaged students to the Title I projects and control groups because this clearly was not feasible, was politically untenable, and likely was illegal. In addition, Stufflebeam and the Columbus evaluation team soon found that existing achievement tests were poor matches for the widely varying achievement levels and needs of the students to be served by the ESEA projects. These students could not wait the 2 or more years required to

design, construct, pilot test, revise, norm, and validate new achievement tests.

Into the Schools to See What Was Occurring in the ESEA Projects

Upon becoming bored of watching Columbus evaluators help project committees write behavioral objectives, Stufflebeam decided to visit schools to find out what was happening in the funded projects. He encountered confusion wherever he went. Nothing like the proposals' intended procedures and scheduled activities was occurring. Teachers and other staff members with responsibility for conducting the projects had not helped plan the projects; many had not seen the plan they were supposed to carry out; promised project materials and other resources had not been delivered; and the needs and problems of students and teachers in the involved classrooms often were clearly important, even urgent, but not a focus of the objectives being written by the project planning committees, nor of the procedures that had been specified in the funding proposals. For good reason, the teachers and principals often were upset with the ESEA project scene, and many expressed lack of confidence in the district's approach to programming and evaluation.

Rejection of Orthodox Evaluation Approaches

In this unfortunate project situation, Stufflebeam saw a silver lining as well as a problem. Here was an opportunity to advance evaluation theory, if only to discredit the generally accepted evaluation approaches. The ESEA proposals' evaluation plans were consistent with the existing evaluation orthodoxy that evaluations should employ methods of behavioral objectives, objectives testing, and experimental design to determine whether project objectives had been achieved. However, these designs were wrong for the situations that existed in the involved Columbus classrooms. Execution of these evaluation designs would only confirm the schools' failures to achieve the stated objectives. In any case, those objectives were not reflective of the assessed needs of the students who were to be served by the projects. Evaluations to determine whether the misdirected objectives had been achieved would not help the teachers and other project participants effectively address the needs of their students.

After Stufflebeam had decided to reject the existing evaluation orthodoxy and call for a reconceptualization of evaluation, he was presented with a relevant opportunity. In January 1966, the Michigan Department of Education engaged him to give the keynote address at a statewide conference on evaluation of **ESEA Title I** projects. At the conference, Stufflebeam (1966b) observed that he had learned just enough in his evaluations of such projects to reject most of what he had thought appropriate and necessary for evaluating innovative, educational projects. Behavioral objectives, experimental designs, and standardized tests, he told his startled audience, had little to offer in evaluating ESEA Title 1 projects.

Keying Evaluation to Decision Making

As an alternative to these approaches, he advised educators to focus evaluations on providing information for decision making. The main types of decisions, he said, were those day-to-day choices involved in making projects work, together with the annual decisions about whether to retain, expand, or discontinue a project. For these implementation and recycling decisions, Stufflebeam advised schools to concentrate, respectively, on conducting process and product evaluations and reporting the results to key decision makers, including project staff members, participating teachers, school principals, school district administrators, and officials of the relevant external funding organization.

Overall, the Michigan educators disliked Stufflebeam's message. As staunch supporters of local control of schools, most seemed averse to federally mandated evaluations and (possibly as supporters of the Michigan Wolverines and determined enemies of the Buckeyes from the state to the south) were not receptive to advice from an Ohio State professor. However, three influential people strongly supported his analysis and invited him to assist their evaluation efforts. They were Robert Lankton and Stuart Rankin, the heads of testing and evaluation in the Detroit Public School District, and a representative of the U.S. Office of Education.

An Opportunity to Try Out a New Approach to Evaluation

Shortly after returning from Michigan to Ohio State, Dr. Ramseyer informed Stufflebeam that a U.S. Office of Education official had requested that OSU release him so that he could devote his full time in Washington leading the federal evaluations of **Titles I and**

III of ESEA. (Stufflebeam considered this a dubious request inasmuch as he had stated in the Michigan speech that the evaluation procedures he had been trained in wouldn't work in evaluating school district–based ESEA projects.) Ramseyer told Stufflebeam he had rejected the government's request for him to work full time in Washington, but had committed him to work there for a few years on Mondays and Tuesdays. Thus, for the next 2 years Stufflebeam spent 2 days a week at the U.S. Office of Education in Washington chairing the government committee on evaluation of the ESEA Titles I and III programs (respectively, for strengthening education of disadvantaged children and supporting innovation in schools) and the subsequent 3 days in Columbus directing The Evaluation Center.

A Lesson Regarding Levels of Audiences and Their Different Evaluation Needs

Through the related but different assignments, Stufflebeam gained an appreciation for the problem of keying evaluations to the widely differing information requirements of local, state, and national audiences. Largely to appease school personnel throughout the nation, the U.S. Office of Education had allowed each school district to submit an annual evaluation report addressed to its own evaluation questions, methods, and instruments. The 26,000-plus school districts subsequently flooded the U.S. mail system with tens of thousands of idiosyncratic evaluation reports that were not amenable to storage, retrieval, and reading, let alone data aggregation and summarization. The official charged with reporting on the effectiveness of the ESEA Title I program to Congress futilely attacked the impossible task of pulling the information together to answer the Congress's pointed questions until he suffered a stress-induced heart attack.

This debacle was predictable, considering a key principle of information science: Investigators must specify in advance at each administrative level at which an audience requires answers the questions to be addressed and the associated data requirements. Invariably, the questions and associated information requirements will be different at the different levels (e.g., general at the top level and increasingly specific at the successively lower levels). In the case of the ESEA program, separate evaluations needed to be designed to address the particular questions and information needs of the

Congress, the Office of Education, the participating school districts, and the individual projects. Clearly, the thousands of ESEA project-based reports that were keyed to project-level criteria and questions of local school district audiences did not address the questions and meet the information needs of Congress and other national-level audiences. Also, national-level data and reports keyed to questions dictated by federal clients would not meet the evaluative needs of audiences in individual school districts and projects.

Uncovering the Need for Context Evaluations

Soon after Stufflebeam began his weekly trips to Washington, some OSU faculty members invited him to report on his ESEA evaluation experiences at a university-wide colloquium on evaluating ESEA projects. Attendees readily agreed that laboratory research methods wouldn't work well in school-based development projects. Instead, evaluations should be useful to project staff members, helping them to guide their decisions, and evaluators should assess process as well as product. However, some attendees argued that process and product evaluations were not enough. They stressed that Stufflebeam's new ideas about evaluation were missing the crucially important evaluative act of assessing and judging project goals.

Stufflebeam agreed with these critics, having seen several ESEA projects fail because of their focus on unclear or inappropriate goals. In keeping with his new view that evaluations should inform decisions, he decided that goal setting was a critically important area of decision making and should be guided by what he termed *context evaluations*. He saw context evaluation as including identification and assessments of (1) the needs of targeted students (or other beneficiaries); (2) problems that could hinder a project's efforts to meet the assessed needs; (3) **assets** that could be used to meet the assessed needs; (4) relevant **opportunities,** such as funding, that might be helpful in the project; and (5) social, economic, and political dynamics in the project's environment that should be taken into account.

The CIPP Model Takes Shape

At this point, the CIPP Model's basic structure was nearly complete. It included context evaluation of needs, problems, assets, opportunities, and environ-

mental dynamics to guide goal setting; process evaluation of project activities to guide and document project implementation; and product evaluation of outcomes to assess project success and guide recycling decisions. Subsequently, Stufflebeam added input evaluation—for identifying and assessing alternative approaches to meeting beneficiaries' assessed needs—to aid in planning projects, especially proposal writing (Stufflebeam, 1967b).

An Early Test of the CIPP Model

Following the presentation of the CIPP Model at a national conference in Florida (Stufflebeam, 1968), Edwin Hindsman, then director of the Southwest Educational Laboratory in Austin, Texas, invited him to test the model on one of the lab's major projects. Hindsman's lab had been assigned to evaluate a $10 million project for addressing the educational needs of migrant children. It was agreed that Egon Guba and Robert Hammond would assist Stufflebeam in applying the CIPP Model to help the lab evaluate the migrant education program. Among the lessons learned from this rich experience were that the CIPP Model has to be applied flexibly (e.g., what Robert Stake, 1983, terms *responsively*); active members of the migrant community (including children, parents, teachers, social workers, and employers) provided more cogent information on the needs of migrant children than did experts who had been conducting research on migrant workers and their families; and ongoing face-to-face reporting and exchange with project stakeholders was more effective in addressing their information needs than issuing formal, printed reports.

The Advocate Teams Technique

Based on this test of the CIPP Model, Stufflebeam and his colleagues further developed the concept of and procedures for conducting input evaluations. To guide the needed input evaluation in the Texas case, they invented the **Advocate Teams Technique** (see Reinhard, 1972). In this approach, ideologically oriented teams develop competing proposals for meeting a set of targeted needs (e.g., alternative strategies, plans, and procedures for addressing the assessed and targeted needs of migrant students). Evaluators then assess the **merits** of the alternative proposals on predetermined criteria and report the findings to the decision-making group.

This group may then choose the highest rated proposal or develop a new one by combining the strongest features of the competing proposals.

An advantage of this technique in the Texas migrant project evaluation was that it positively exploited the biases of different groups regarding how best to use $10 million to address the needs of migrant children. For example, one group favored developing residential education centers for migrant children along the northbound routes migrant families followed in harvesting crops, whereas another group proposed spending the money on developing bilingual educational materials that migrant students could study along the migrant routes. In the end, there were nine such proposals. Through use of the Advocate Teams Technique, the nine teams explicated the nine positions, and an independent evaluation team assessed the proposals against preestablished criteria. What at first had appeared to be counterproductive biases had been exploited to eventually present the Texas decision makers with a politically viable input evaluation report that laid out the alternative proposals and comparatively assessed their merits against the criteria that the decision makers had stipulated at the evaluation's outset.

The PDK Book

In 1969, Phi Delta Kappa International (PDK) engaged Stufflebeam to head a national study committee on evaluation, which culminated in the book *Educational Evaluation and Decision Making* (Stufflebeam et al., 1971).[3] In that book, Stufflebeam and his coauthors sharply criticized the traditional views of educational evaluation, analyzed decision makers' needs for evaluative information, explained the CIPP Model, and showed how organizations could use it to institutionalize evaluation. The book also argued that the criteria for judging evaluations should include utility and feasibility as well as technical adequacy. The coauthors noted that evaluations can go very wrong if they are keyed exclusively to criteria of technical adequacy, particularly the requirements for **internal validity** and **external validity** which were then being advocated as the criteria for judging experiments (Campbell & Stanley, 1963). (The PDK book's breakout of criteria for guiding and judging evaluations into relevance, importance, timeliness, clarity, credibility, and technical adequacy was a precursor of the work done by the Joint Committee on Standards for Educational Evaluation [1981]—which Stufflebeam chaired—to identify and define standards for an evaluation's utility, feasibility, propriety, and accuracy.)

Formative and Summative Evaluations

Formative evaluation and summative evaluation refer to the main uses of evaluation. Michael Scriven (1967) coined these terms based on his exchanges with Lee Cronbach. Cronbach had argued that evaluation's most important use is to provide ongoing guidance for strengthening an educational program while being conducted. He saw this use as far more valuable to teachers than its use to judge the program after the fact. Conversely, Scriven, who was devoted to the approach embodied in product evaluations published in *Consumer Reports* magazine, posited that an evaluation's summative judgments of a completed program's accomplishments were far more important to potential adopters of the program than were the interim, formative evaluations that had occurred along the way to help improve the program. (Both positions are defensible, considering that the two "debaters" were interested in serving different audiences—for Cronbach, it was classroom teachers working in a program still under development; for Scriven, it was the potential purchases of a completed program.)

The CIPP Model includes both formative and summative uses of evaluation. These two uses of evaluations do not necessarily reference different types of information. For example, project staffs can make proactive, formative use of reports from context, input, process, and product evaluations to focus, design, and guide their project. After completing the project, the evaluator can synthesize the formative evaluation reports and present the client and interested stakeholders with a summative evaluation of the project's implementation and accomplishments. Nevertheless, in conducting a summative evaluation, it is always appropriate to consider whether the available formative evaluation reports are sufficient to support a sound summative evaluation. If not, the evaluator should collect the additional information that is needed to complete a comprehensive, final evaluation report.

The formal definitions of formative and summative evaluation employed in this book are as follows:

• A **formative evaluation** proactively assesses a program usually from start to finish. Ideally, it regularly issues feedback to assist in formulating goals and priorities; provide direction for planning by assessing alternative courses of action and draft plans; guide project management by assessing and reporting on implementation of plans and interim results; and supply a record of collected formative information and how it was used. A wide range of information is useful for formative purposes, including, for example, needs assessments, proposal critiques, cost analysis, monitoring of activities, and identification and assessment of interim results. Formative evaluations primarily seek to help program staffs improve a project. Often, formative evaluations are conducted by internal evaluators or even the project's staff.

• A **summative evaluation** is a comprehensive evaluation of a project after it has been completed. It draws together and supplements previous evaluative information to provide an overall judgment of the project's value. Such evaluations help interested audiences decide whether a project—refined through development and formative evaluation—achieved its goals, met targeted needs, made a significant contribution in an area of professional and societal interest, and was worth what it cost. Often, summative evaluations are based mainly on information previously collected and used for formative purposes but may include newly collected evidence. Summative evaluations are especially useful to funding organizations, oversight bodies, client groups, and the public and should be keyed to their questions as well as fundamental **values,** such as excellence, equity, feasibility, efficiency, and safety. Ideally, summative evaluations are conducted by independent evaluators but may be conducted by internal evaluators. Having a project's staff conduct its own summative evaluation is not optimal because the evaluation's audience might find such a self-report biased and thus suspect. Sometimes, however, a self-summative evaluation is the only available option and a better one than acquiring no summative evaluation at all. When the summative evaluation is conducted by either an internal evaluator or the project's staff, the evaluation should be subjected to an independent audit—what we term an **independent metaevaluation** (i.e., an evaluation of the evaluation).

As explained above, the original development of the CIPP Model was focused on informing decisions in the process of developing and carrying out emerging, innovative projects. Accordingly, such CIPP Model–based evaluations had a formative role. They were designed

and applied to supply project leaders and staffs with evaluative information for use in setting goals and priorities; planning, budgeting, contracting, and carrying out project activities; and monitoring emerging project outcomes as a basis for adjusting procedures and thereby pursuing continually better results. This formative function was in keeping with the CIPP Model's fundamental **improvement orientation.**

Of course, evaluations also have an accountability role, especially after projects have had sufficient time and opportunity to evolve, mature, stabilize, and meet their intermediate or long-range objectives. Then it is often appropriate to conduct a thorough, retrospective, summative, project evaluation. This is necessary to address the bottom-line questions of project sponsors, oversight boards, beneficiary groups, the public, and other stakeholders.

In the early 1970s, the Western Michigan University Evaluation Center was invited and funded to apply the CIPP Model to conduct a number of summative evaluations. Two examples were evaluations of statewide systems projects (in Delaware and Oregon) for the U.S. National Science Foundation (NSF) aimed at reforming science and mathematics education in the states' public schools, intermediate educational service centers, state education departments, educational research laboratories, and universities. The NSF had invested $5 million in each of these projects, funded them as possible models for widespread replication, and needed summative evaluations to help determine whether it should fund similar projects in other states. Another example was an evaluation—also for the NSF—of the success of a Columbus, Ohio, collaborative effort by city government, public schools, universities, public media, and business and industry to deliver elementary and secondary school services in the context of a citywide, acute shortage of natural gas that occurred during one of the city's most severe winters. Because there was insufficient natural gas to heat school buildings, the collaborators in Columbus conducted what they labeled "school without schools." Educational services were delivered by providing instruction over public radio and television; publishing student assignments in newspapers, delivering instruction in buildings that had sufficient heat (such as bank lobbies, funeral parlors, bus terminals, movie theaters, and museums), and conducting field trips outside the state. Because this unusual, innovative, community-based approach to education might in the future be applicable to emergency situations in other cities, the NSF saw a need and opportunity to document and preserve a comprehensive evaluation of the Columbus experience. Accordingly, The Evaluation Center's evaluators employed the CIPP Model to conduct the needed summative evaluation of this unique educational project (Sanders & Stufflebeam, 1978).

Evaluators have often applied the CIPP Model, not only to address audiences' needs for formative feedback, but also to look back comprehensively on what the subject projects had accomplished. In such evaluations, the concepts of context, input, process, and product evaluation guided the collection of needed information and also provided a framework for issuing judgments of both the overall project and its key parts, that is, its background, goals, plans, budget, execution, costs, main effects, and unanticipated consequences. It also became clear that the feasibility of conducting a comprehensive, summative evaluation was enhanced to the extent that the subject project had, throughout its life, obtained and retained formative evaluation information—keyed to all parts of the CIPP Model.

Experiences in developing and applying the CIPP Model have shown that project staffs and project evaluators should adopt and regularly apply an evaluation framework that includes both formative and summative approaches to evaluating context, input, process, and product. Moreover, the framework should be keyed to an appropriate range of values—not just the program developer's objectives but all the values of concern to the full range of program stakeholders (e.g., the project's **quality,** cost, practicality, **effectiveness,** safety, and probity) and to the possibility of both positive and negative side effects. Chapter 2 presents and explains such a framework in the form of the CIPP Evaluation Model.

In the wake of its humble beginnings and development, the CIPP Model has been extensively developed and widely applied (e.g., Candoli, Cullen, & Stufflebeam, 1997; Gally, 1984; Granger, Grierson, Quirino, & Romano, 1965; Guba & Stufflebeam, 1968; Shinkfield & Stufflebeam, 1995; Stufflebeam, 1968, 1982, 1997, 2003a, 2003b; Stufflebeam et al., 1971; Stufflebeam & Webster, 1988; Webster, 1975; Zhang et al., 2011b). Evaluators, evaluation clients, and evaluation students have often requested information about the CIPP Model's applications. Such persons will find this book's appendix a useful resource for identifying evaluations that have applied the CIPP Model in a wide range of national settings, disciplines, and service areas.

Uses of This Book

This book is designed to serve as a core textbook or supplementary textbook for evaluation courses as well as a handbook for guiding fieldwork in evaluation. As a textbook, it can serve as a primary source in program evaluation courses and continuing education workshops. It can also be used as a supplemental textbook in a wide range of disciplines, including applied sociology, educational administration, public administration, community development, special education, curriculum development, philanthropy, social work, psychology, nursing, continuing medical education, and engineering. Many graduate students may find the book valuable for structuring their evaluation-oriented theses and dissertations. Another main intended use of this book is as a field manual for guiding the planning and execution of evaluations by evaluation specialists, program staff members with responsibilities for evaluation, and evaluation and other students doing practicums. Particularly valuable to practicing evaluators will be the **checklists** presented in subsequent chapters for use in planning and assessing the wide range of tasks in evaluation, such as designing, budgeting, and contracting evaluations; collecting information and reporting findings; and conducting metaevaluations. The full range of intended audiences will find the book useful both as a general reference and as a specific guide to correct application of the CIPP Model. Overall, we have targeted the book for use across disciplines and service areas and in a wide range of countries. Table 1.2 summarizes how we envision different audiences using the book.

In the ensuing chapters, we delineate the model's current configuration, illustrate its application with actual cases, provide direction and procedures for carrying out the steps required to conduct a sound evaluation, and discuss the model's uses in dissertations and publishing journal articles. We conclude the book with a discussion of metaevaluation as a means of employing accepted standards of the evaluation profession to assess both formatively and summatively CIPP Model–based evaluations. At the end of each chapter, we provide a list of review questions. It is our firm desire that this book will help those who commission, conduct, participate in, and use evaluations to apply the CIPP Model in evaluating, strengthening, and meeting the accountability needs of their programs and projects.

TABLE 1.2. Projected Uses of This Book

Intended Uses	Intended Users							
	Practicing evaluators	Students specializing in evaluation	Students in public and educational administration	Students in various disciplines and service areas (e.g., curriculum, special education, applied sociology, and continuing medical education)	Evaluation funders and clients	Program/ project staff members	Libraries	Instructors
Primary textbook		X						X
Supplementary textbook		X	X	X				X
Field manual	X	X	X	X		X		
Guide for theses and dissertations		X	X	X				
General reference	X	X	X	X	X	X	X	X

Summary

This chapter introduces the book's central focus—the CIPP (Context, Input, Process, Product) Evaluation Model—by explaining why and how it was developed and identifying the model's key features. The model is grounded in basic definitions of program evaluation and formative and summative uses of evaluation. We stress that the CIPP Model addresses the evaluative needs of evaluators and their clients, across a wide range of disciplines and countries and in all types of organizations. The model conveys not a narrow, alternative evaluation approach—good only for discrete project evaluations—but an overarching, comprehensive approach that an organization can employ to meet its full range of evaluation needs at policy, management, and operation levels. The model is strongly oriented to engaging stakeholders—including program administrators, staffs, beneficiaries, and sponsors—and to supporting their uses of evaluation for both program improvement and program accountability. The model addresses the need for formative evaluations—of beneficiaries' needs, program plans, activities, and accomplishments—that provide guidance for structuring and implementing programs and also for summa-tive evaluations that document and judge what a program accomplished. The model embodies a common evaluation language and approach that organizations can adopt and employ in grounding ongoing organizational improvement in areas such as strategic planning, policy development, staffing and training, budgeting, communication, and accreditation. The CIPP Model is keyed directly to meeting professionally defined standards for evaluations of utility, feasibility, propriety, accuracy, and accountability. In its operationalized form, the model is supported by a wide range of techniques and checklists related to the tasks required to conduct and report sound and useful evaluations. Overall, this chapter foreshadows the remaining chapters, which together provide the concepts, illustrations, procedures, checklists, and standards that evaluators and their clients need to plan, budget, contract, staff, carry out, report, apply, and defend evaluations.

REVIEW QUESTIONS • • • • • • • • •

1. What main historical events and needs led to the development of the CIPP Evaluation Model, and how did the model respond to the events and needs?

2. React to the statement that the CIPP Model is designed mainly for use by evaluation specialists in North America.

3. Do you agree that the book's authors have targeted this book for users with sophisticated skills developed through graduate courses in research design, statistics, psychometrics, and information technology? Why or why not?

4. What reasons does this chapter give for stating that experimental design is an inadequate general approach to evaluating programs?

5. What is this chapter's position concerning the applicability of the objectives-based approach to evaluating programs?

6. For what reasons does this chapter conclude that standardized testing is an insufficient approach to program evaluation?

7. Is it enough that evaluations meet requirements for reliability and internal and external validity? Why or why not? If yes, do you think that evaluation and research are essentially the same? If not, what other criteria should a sound program evaluation meet?

8. To give your characterization of the CIPP Evaluation Model's main components, state summary questions that could be used to represent each of its four main parts.

9. Having read this chapter, how would you explain the meaning of program evaluation to an evaluation client group?

10. How would you respond to the same client group's request that you define, contrast, and illustrate the concepts of formative and summative evaluation?

11. Explain and illustrate what is meant by the claim that the CIPP Model provides for evaluations that are both formative and summative.

12. React to the statements that (a) the CIPP Model is not distinct or exclusive from other ways of evaluating, such as experiments, objectives-based studies, and uses of standardized tests, but (b) it is overarching and encompasses other approaches.

13. What is this book's rationale for advising evaluators to identify an evaluation's stakeholders and give them opportunities to engage in all stages of an evaluation? What's in such a practice for the stakeholders? What's in it for the evaluator?

14. What is the Advocate Teams Technique, what is its use in the context of the CIPP Model, and what is the basis for the claim that the technique helps a client and evaluator positively exploit the biases of different interest groups regarding how best to meet a project's objectives?

15. Identify a program with which you are familiar that you might evaluate. List the types of stakeholders you would seek to involve in the evaluation. Under the assumption that you are holding a first meeting with a group of these stakeholders, (a) briefly explain the role you want them to play in the evaluation, (b) identify at least three main activities in which they likely would be involved, and (c) summarize the benefits they should expect to derive from their involvement.

NOTES

1. This book's appendix apprises readers of the extensive array of organizations, disciplines, nations, and types of professionals and technicians that have applied the CIPP Model. We think that extensive documentation should be useful to potential users of the CIPP Model who might want to study actual applications of the model that are relevant to their situations and needs for evaluation. Especially, the appendix of CIPP Model applications makes a compelling case that the CIPP Evaluation Model is responsive and applicable to addressing evaluation needs in all sectors of society.

2. We believe it is important to recount the CIPP Model's history, because its creation was integral to the development of the evaluation field as we know it today. In the 1960s, the CIPP Model was one of several innovative approaches to evaluation that emerged in response to the new federal requirements for evaluation that appeared in the War on Poverty's Elementary and Secondary Education Act (ESEA) of 1965. That Act's evaluation requirements awakened education and the broader society to the needs to find effective ways to make large federal funding programs accountable for producing needed outcomes. Before 1965, systematic program evaluations were almost unknown and there was no semblance of an evaluation profession. Educators' responses to the federal evaluation requirements of 1965 revealed an almost total inadequacy within education to evaluate and be accountable for programs. Although progress was subsequently slow and difficult, the evaluation models, training programs,

competent evaluations, literature, standards, evaluation companies, and professional societies that we see today largely emerged over the past 50 years and grew into the substantial evaluation profession we see today. The CIPP Model was one significant product of that evolutionary development.

3. Members of the Phi Delta Kappa Study Committee included Howard Merriman (director of the Columbus, Ohio School District evaluation office), Egon Guba (Indiana University expert in statistics, experimental design, and naturalistic inquiry), Malcolm Provus (director of evaluation in the Pittsburgh Public School District), Walter Foley (University of Iowa expert in information technology), Robert Hammond (Arizona University creator of the EPIC Evaluation Model), William Gephart (director of research at Phi Delta Kappa International), and Daniel Stufflebeam (Director of The Evaluation Center at The Ohio State University) as chairman.

CHAPTER 2

· ·

The CIPP Evaluation Model

A Framework for Improvement- and Accountability-Oriented Evaluations

"Evaluation's most important purpose is not to prove but to improve."

This chapter explains the CIPP Model, including its concepts of context, input, process, and product evaluation; improvement orientation; grounding in values; keying to professional standards; requirement for advanced evaluation contracting; objectivist epistemology; configuration in a problem-solving logic model; imperative of stakeholder engagement; advocacy and support for **evaluation-oriented leaders**; employment of multiple methods; uses for formative and summative purposes; requirement for metaevaluation; and guidance to organizations for institutionalizing and mainstreaming systematic program evaluation. The chapter concludes with a checklist for planning and guiding evaluations based on the CIPP Model.

Overview

· ·

Chapter 1 chronicled the development of the CIPP Model as a process of incrementally adding components—based on its wide-ranging applications over a period of more than 40 years—until the model took on its present-day form. This chapter presents an up-to-date, comprehensive version of the CIPP Model.

As explained in Chapter 1, the model's development originally was undertaken because the existing evaluation approaches of objectives-based evaluation, standardized testing, and experimental design had proved inadequate to meet the evaluation needs of the 1960s- and 1970s-era War on Poverty projects that were

aimed at reforming the United States' public schools. In that context, the objective for developing the CIPP Model was to provide educational organizations and government agencies with a credible, practical approach that would meet educators' needs for program improvement-oriented evaluation and the government funding agencies' needs for credible public accountability reports. As documented in this book's Appendix, over the years the model has been continually applied and updated based on applications in a wide range of disciplines and across many national settings. The result of the ongoing model development work is the comprehensive approach that we describe in this chapter.

The CIPP Model in General

Basically, the CIPP Model provides for systematic, principled evaluation of a program's context, inputs, process, and products. Essentially, these four types of evaluation address four fundamental questions:

1. What needs to be done?
2. How should it be done?
3. Is it being done?
4. Did it succeed?

Reports from the four types of evaluation serve both formative and summative purposes. Formatively, the reports are to be configured and delivered in a timely manner to help a program's personnel effectively focus, plan, guide, and sum up their program's value. At the program's end, the formative reports are to be combined and supplemented to provide the program's funders, beneficiaries, and other interested parties with a credible, comprehensive, summative program accountability report.

The model's primary orientation is to foster and assist program improvement through continuous, proactive, decision-oriented assessments. The model is also designed to meet a program's needs for accountability. Regarding program accountability, the final report should be compiled to help the evaluation's audience understand why and how the program was conducted, what it cost, what it accomplished, what side effects it may have produced, whether its successes are likely to be sustained, and whether it shows promise for dissemination to and effective utilization in other settings.

To address issues of complex, dynamic conditions that are part and parcel of most field-based evaluations, the model advises evaluators to employ multiple information collection methods, both quantitative and qualitative. Interpretation of findings is to be rooted in clearly defined values of the program's parent organization, and such values are to be consistent with the principles of democracy, especially freedom and equality of opportunity. Also, evaluations based on the model should be conducted pursuant to advance, written agreements. The model calls for interpreting findings in terms of an **objectivist** rather than **relativist epistemology.** In this respect, evaluators are advised to seek conclusions that are beyond a reasonable doubt. Because of the frequent presence of many uncontrolled, possibly confounding variables, the CIPP Model also cautions evaluators to be circumspect in reporting conclusions, especially conclusions about the causes of observed outcomes and their generalizability to other settings.

Given the model's emphasis on getting findings used, it requires evaluators to meaningfully engage intended users of the findings throughout the evaluation process in essential tasks such as clarifying the values for use in interpreting findings, helping define evaluation questions, facilitating data collection, reviewing draft reports, and making principled, informed **uses** of the findings. The model stresses the key role of the **evaluation-oriented client** and advises the evaluator to engender and support her or his **evaluation-oriented leadership** throughout the evaluation. In that vein, the model directs the evaluator to thoroughly acquaint the client and a panel of selected stakeholders with the CIPP Model's concepts and activities, needs for their participation in carrying out selected activities, how they are asked to implement those activities, and, overall, how they can best contribute to the evaluation's success.

The model is grounded in professional standards that require evaluations to be useful, feasible, ethical, accurate, and accountable. Commensurately, the model requires that the evaluations themselves be evaluated through internal/**formative metaevaluations** and external/**summative metaevaluations,** both of which should assess and report the evaluation's adherence to the guiding **evaluation standards.**

It is recommended that the final evaluation reports be divided into three subreports: (1) a description of the program's background and why the evaluation was initiated; (2) an objective description of the program's **design,** actual operation, and costs; and (3) the evaluation design, the context, input, process, and product findings, and the conclusions about the program's quality and worth. Additionally, the final report should be supplemented by an appendix or separate **technical report** that documents the evaluation's staffing, technical details, costs, and metaevaluation findings.

A Common-Sense Example of a CIPP Model Evaluation

At its most elementary level, the CIPP Model is a common-sense approach. Its logic is such that it can guide teams of highly trained specialists to conduct complex, multi-million-dollar evaluations. At modest levels, laypersons with little or no training in evaluation can also use the model to meet their evaluation needs.

In the case of the layperson, a home owner could use the CIPP Model to guide and assess a home remodeling project. He or she could employ context evaluation to assess the home's adequacy for meeting the family's housing requirements and to identify and delineate other needs requiring attention (such as needs for landscaping, painting, replacement shingles, new flooring, added insulation, energy efficient windows, rewiring, new plumbing lines, and termite eradication and protection) and then deciding on which improvements to pursue. The home owner would use input evaluation to guide her or his planning of the rehabilitation project; to identify and assess the quality and costs of alternative house improvement products and services; and to contract and budget for the selected products and services. Through process evaluation, the home owner (often with support from licensed inspectors) would monitor and take steps to assure quality solutions, safety, cost containment, on-time performance, and adequate clean-up and follow-up. Before paying the bill(s), the home owner would assess the results of the remodeling project and obtain any required inspections to assure compliance with relevant codes and laws.

Main Concepts Related to the CIPP Model

As the above example illustrates, the CIPP Model is a common-sense approach to assuring cost-effectiveness in starting, planning, carrying through, completing, and assessing the results of needed improvement efforts. The model is applicable to one's day-to-day decisions and actions as well as to complex, long-term enterprises operated by private and public organizations. It lays out a systematic process for helping to hold service providers accountable for delivering cost-effective services. Moreover, it is applicable to guiding and conducting creative, innovative projects that seek new and better responses to targeted needs. The CIPP Model is grounded in general and operational definitions of evaluation. It identifies and addresses the main uses of evaluations, and it is constituted to meet professional standards for guiding and judging evaluations.

Evaluation Defined

Generally, an **evaluation** is a systematic investigation of some object's value. Operationally, evaluation is the process of delineating, obtaining, reporting, and applying descriptive and judgmental information about some object's value—for example, its quality, **worth,** probity, equity, feasibility, cost, efficiency, safety, or significance. The result of an evaluation process is an evaluation as product (i.e., an evaluation report for intended uses by intended users).

Intended Users and Uses of CIPP Model Evaluations

The key users of evaluations for program improvement purposes are supervisors and program staffs. For accountability and public policy purposes, key users include policy boards, an organization's top officials, the program's funder, similar organizations, researchers, beneficiaries, taxpayers, government officials, news media, the public, and other special interest groups.

The main uses of evaluations are to:

- Guide and strengthen enterprises.
- Issue accountability reports.
- Help disseminate effective practices.
- Increase understanding of the involved phenomena.
- As appropriate, make decision makers, stakeholders, and consumers aware of programs or other **evaluands** that proved unworthy of further use.

Standards for Evaluations

Professional standards for evaluations are the principles commonly agreed to by specialists in the conduct and use of evaluations for measuring an evaluation's utility, feasibility, propriety, accuracy, and evaluation accountability. Basically, the CIPP Model is an organized approach to meeting the evaluation profession's standards as defined by the Joint Committee on Standards for Educational Evaluation (1981, 1994, 2011). It is adaptable for application by a wide range of users, including evaluators, program specialists, researchers, developers, policy groups, administrators, committees or task groups, and laypersons as well.

Overview of the CIPP Categories

The CIPP Model's core concepts are denoted by the acronym CIPP, which, as noted earlier, stands for an entity's context, inputs, processes, and products.

Context evaluations assess needs, problems, assets, and opportunities, as well as relevant contextual conditions and dynamics. According to the CIPP Model, those conducting programs should acquire (or conduct) and use context evaluations to define program goals and priorities, and to make sure the goals are targeted to address significant, assessed needs and problems. The evaluator provides program decision makers with context evaluation reports during program planning to inform the process of goal setting and to help program staff to take into account relevant environmental dynamics. Throughout the evaluation, the evaluator updates the context evaluation information as appropriate. At the evaluation's end, the evaluator presents clients with up-to-date context evaluation information to help them and their constituents judge the previously set goals and priorities and especially to interpret the significance of program outcomes in consideration of both the targeted beneficiaries' assessed needs and circumstances in the program's environment.

Input evaluations assess a program's strategy, action plan, staffing arrangements, and budget for feasibility and potential cost-effectiveness to meet targeted needs and achieve goals. An input evaluation may be comparative, as in identifying and assessing optional ways to achieve goals, or noncomparative, as in assessing a single plan and its components. According to the CIPP Model, those who plan programs can beneficially obtain and employ input evaluation findings to help plan their programs, write winning funding proposals, allocate resources, assign staff, schedule work, and ultimately help others judge a program's plans and budget.

Input evaluations assist program planning by identifying and assessing alternative program strategies, the management plan and budget, possible program performance measures, and alternative service providers. In conducting and reporting input evaluations, the evaluator provides information to support the client's planning process. The bottom-line concern of input evaluations is to help decision makers plan and budget on how to best meet the assessed and targeted needs of the intended beneficiaries. Decision makers often use input evaluation reports to identify and compare the relative merits of relevant, existing program approaches that have been applied elsewhere and/or to stimulate the staff to create better, innovative solutions, especially when existing approaches are judged inadequate to meet the assessed needs of the program's targeted beneficiaries and to achieve the program's goals. Near

the end of the client's initial planning process, the evaluator completes the input evaluation work by closely examining and assessing the client's specific activity plans, schedule, staffing plan, and budget.

Often, clients find the succession of context and input evaluation reports to be useful in writing program funding proposals. Moreover, the client likely finds a record of obtained context and input evaluation findings to be useful for accountability purposes if and when critics raise questions about why the program was initiated, targeted, planned, and budgeted as it was.

Process evaluations monitor, document, assess, and report on the implementation of plans. Such evaluations provide feedback throughout a program's implementation and later report on the extent to which the program was carried out as intended and needed. Process evaluations help staff keep activities moving efficiently and effectively, take stock of their progress, identify implementation issues, adjust their plans and performance to assure program quality and on-time delivery of services, and document that actual process. Later, the client can find the record of process evaluation findings and how they were addressed to be useful in helping the broad group of users to understand and judge program implementation and expenditures and also determine why outcomes turned out as they did. In particular, program staff, overseers, and constituents may examine the implementation's documentation to judge whether a program's possibly deficient outcomes were due to a weak strategy or to inadequate implementation of the strategy.

Product evaluations identify and assess costs and outcomes—intended and unintended, short term and long term. These evaluations provide feedback during a program's implementation on the extent that program goals are being addressed and achieved. Ongoing product evaluation helps those responsible for program implementation to keep the program focused on achieving important outcomes at a reasonable cost and to maintain a record of important achievements as well as shortfalls. At the program's end, product evaluations identify and assess the program's full range of outcomes, anticipated as well as unanticipated, positive as well as negative. Ultimately, a retrospective product evaluation helps the client and the broader group of users to gauge the effort's cost-effectiveness in achieving goals, meeting beneficiaries' targeted needs, and, in many cases, producing unexpected benefits and sometimes producing bad outcomes. The key questions addressed are:

Did the program achieve its goals?

Did it successfully address the targeted needs and problems?

What were the unexpected outcomes, both positive and negative?

Were the program's outcomes worth their costs?

In summing up long-term evaluations, the product evaluation (Did it succeed?) component may be further divided into four subparts of assessments: reach to the targeted communities or groups of beneficiaries; effectiveness; sustainability; and **transportability.** These product evaluation subparts ask, Were the right beneficiaries reached? Were the targeted needs and problems addressed effectively? Were the program's accomplishments and mechanisms to produce them sustained and affordable over the long term? Did the strategies and procedures that produced the accomplishments prove or at least show promise to be transportable, adaptable, and affordable for effective use elsewhere?

A product evaluation's most important purpose is to help program staffs use interim product evaluation findings to maintain **focus** on achieving important outcomes and to identify and address deficiencies in the program's progress toward achieving successful outcomes. Ultimately, those responsible for programs are advised to use evaluations to identify, assess, and report summatively on the program's outcomes: positive and negative, anticipated and unanticipated. According to the CIPP Model, the other main purpose of product evaluations is to help program managers, overseers, funders, and constituents obtain and use sufficient, appropriate evidence to judge whether a program's accomplishments were significant and worth the cost.

Formative and Summative Roles of Context, Input, Process, and Product Evaluations

Evaluations based on the CIPP Model focus on two main roles: formative and summative. Table 2.1 summarizes key features of formative and summative evaluation roles.

A formative evaluation proactively assesses a program from start to finish. It regularly issues feedback to assist the formulation of goals and priorities, provide direction for planning by assessing alternative courses of action and draft plans, guide program management by assessing and reporting on implementation of plans

and interim results, and supply a record of collected formative information and how it was used.

Typically, program sponsors expect program staffs to obtain or conduct formative evaluations before and throughout a program to guide planning and implementation, to help assure success, and to document activities and costs. In accordance with the CIPP Model, those who plan and carry out programs should obtain and apply formative evaluation to help set program goals; develop program plans and budgets; systematically identify and address emerging problems and issues as they arise; help assure program quality; where needed, take corrective actions; and track and provide direction for improving interim results. Program staff should document formative evaluation findings for use in completing the program's final summative evaluation.

A summative evaluation is a comprehensive evaluation of a program after it has been completed. It draws together and supplements previous evaluative information to provide an overall judgment of the program's value. Such evaluations help interested audiences decide whether a program—refined through development and formative evaluation—achieved its goals, met targeted needs, made a significant contribution, is devoid of bad outcomes, and is worth what it cost.

According to the CIPP Model, those who conduct programs are expected to obtain and report summative evaluations that assess a program's quality, accomplishments, weaknesses, impact, side effects, fiscal accountability, and cost-effectiveness. These summative evaluations should provide the program's constituency and, as applicable, society at large with a comprehensive, credible assessment of a program's value.

Consistent with its improvement orientation, the CIPP Model places priority on proactive delivery of evaluation reports to guide the planning and implementation of developmental efforts. In this formative role, context, input, process, and product evaluations respectively provide information of use in setting goals and priorities, developing plans for achieving the goals, guiding the implementation of plans, and providing feedback on accomplishments. Prior to and during the course of an improvement program, the evaluator submits reports to the evaluation client that identify needs to be met, identify and assess alternative approaches to meeting the needs, monitor and appraise progress in carrying out program plans, and document, assess, and report on the program's succession of outcomes. The evaluator issues these formatively oriented reports in

TABLE 2.1. Formative and Summative Roles of Evaluations

Aspects	Formative Roles	Summative Roles
Audiences	Program directors and staffs	Sponsors, consumers, other interested stakeholders, interested outside parties
When conducted	Prior to and during implementation	After completion of implementation or a cycle of implementation
Use	Guiding decision making	Addressing accountability requirements and summing up and assessing outcomes
Purpose	Program improvement and quality assurance	Rendering an overall judgment of the program
Functions	Provides timely feedback for improvement	Informs consumers about the program's value (e.g., its quality, cost, utility, practicality, competitive advantage, resilience, and safety)
Orientation	Prospective and proactive	Retrospective and retroactive
Foci	Needs, problems, assets, opportunities, goals, alternative strategies, plans, implementation, and interim outcomes	Program history, final outcomes, costs, and side effects
Particular types of services	Supports goal setting, planning, and management	Supports funders and consumers in deciding what if any use of the finished program is warranted and whether it should be continued
Nature of evaluation plans	Emergent, flexible, interactive, responsive	Relatively fixed, not emergent, interactive, or responsive
Variables/criteria	All aspects of an evolving, developing program	A comprehensive set of dimensions, including quality, worth, cost, probity, equity, significance, safety, and practicality
Methods	Interviews, document analysis, observation, checklists, rating scales, photography, case studies, hearings, surveys, etc.	Checklists, case studies, focus groups, surveys, rating scales, photography, hearings, compilation of formative findings, and synthesis of available evidence
Reports	Periodic, often informal, responsive to client and staff requests	Culminating report of what was attempted, done, and accomplished; identification of the full range of outcomes; comparison with critical competitors; and assessment of the program's cost-effectiveness
Relationship between formative and summative evaluations	Often provides the bulk of information for summative evaluations	Mainly compiles, assesses, and adds to previously collected formative evaluation information

a timely manner to help program staffs work through the various program stages toward achieving successful outcomes. In general, the CIPP Model employs formative evaluation to supply evaluation users—such as policy boards, administrators, and program staffs—with timely, valid information that can be used in identifying an appropriate area for development; formulating sound goals, activity plans, schedules, and budgets; successfully carrying out and, as needed, improving work plans; strengthening existing programs or ser-

vices; periodically deciding whether and, if so, how to repeat or expand an effort; publicizing effective practices; contributing to knowledge in the area of service; and meeting a financial sponsor's requirements for interim reports.

Beyond its primary orientation of improvement-oriented formative evaluation, the CIPP Model advocates and provides direction for conducting retrospective, summative evaluations to serve a broad range of stakeholders. They include funding organizations, persons receiving or considering use of the sponsored services, policy groups and program specialists outside the program being evaluated, and researchers. In the summative report, the evaluator refers to the store of formative context, input, process, and product information and obtains other information needed to enhance comprehensiveness, objectivity, and credibility. The evaluator uses this information to address the following retrospective questions: Was the program (or other evaluand) keyed to clear goals based on assessed beneficiary needs? Was the effort guided by a relevant strategy, defensible operational design, functional staffing plan, effective and appropriate process of stakeholder involvement, and a sufficient, appropriate budget? Were the plans executed competently and efficiently and modified as needed? Did the effort succeed, in what ways and to what extent, and why or why not? Potential consumers need answers to such summative questions to help assess the quality, cost, utility, and competitiveness of products and services they might acquire and use. Other stakeholders might want evidence on the extent to which their tax dollars or other types of support yielded responsible actions and worthwhile outcomes.

> ## BOX 2.1. Formative and Summative Evaluations
>
> Michael Scriven coined the terms *formative* and *summative evaluation* in 1967, and emphasized their differences both in terms of the goals of the information they seek and how the information is used. When applied in education, formative evaluation is often characterized as assessment for learning, which is contrasted with summative evaluation, which is assessment of learning.
>
> The Council of Chief State School Officers (CCSSO) defines *formative assessment* as "a process used by teachers and students during instruction that provide feedback to adjust ongoing teaching and learning to improve students' achievement of intended instructional outcomes."
>
> Robert Stake is often quoted as having stated at a meeting, "when the cook tastes the soup, that's formative and when the guest tastes the soup, that's summative."

If evaluators effectively conduct, document, and report formative evaluations, they will have much of the information needed to produce a defensible summative evaluation report. Such information will prove invaluable to insiders and outsiders engaged to summatively evaluate a project, program, service, or other entity. Upon the improvement program's completion, the evaluator synthesizes the formative evaluation reports, supplements them as needed with additional information, and then provides the right-to-know audiences with a summative accountability report.

An Illustration of Formative and Summative Uses of Evaluation

To illustrate how the theory of formative and summative evaluations can be translated into practice, consider how a school district's central administration might secure and use formative and summative evaluation services to help the district carry out a credible, data-based approach to reform its teacher evaluation system. Assume that the district contracted with a local university's evaluation center to conduct and report the needed formative and summative evaluations. In contracting with the center, the district's superintendent made clear that initially timely, formative evaluation reports would be needed to help the school district's personnel department successfully plan and carry out the needed teacher evaluation reform program. The district's superintendent also emphasized that at the end of the developmental process it would be critically important for the evaluation center to provide the board of education, the district's administration and staff, the local teachers union, and the local community with a credible summative evaluation report assessing the teacher evaluation reform effort in terms of quality, accomplishments, fairness, and cost-effectiveness.

Table 2.2 is a summary of the succession of formative and summative evaluation reports that the evaluation center might appropriately issue and the associated uses that school district groups would appropriately make of the reports. The column at the left denotes whether the reports listed in the middle column are formative or summative. The middle column lists the succession of formative and summative evaluation reports, whereas the column at the right lists school district uses of the reports. In the main, this chart shows how systematic, formative evaluation can be instrumental in helping an evaluation client group employ data-based

TABLE 2.2. Illustrations of Formative and Summative Evaluation Reports and How a School District Might Use the Reports to Reform Its Teacher Evaluation System

Evaluation Roles	Evaluation Reports	District Uses of Reports
Formative evaluation	*Context evaluation*: Evaluate and report on the present teacher evaluation system's technical strengths, weaknesses, costs, and credibility.	*Goal setting*: Confirm the need to reform the teacher evaluation system, identify problems to be solved, set goals for needed improvements, and delineate criteria for assessing the replacement system.
Formative evaluation	*Input evaluation* (*general*): (1) Identify and assess teacher evaluation systems that arguably are working well in other districts, (2) organize teacher evaluation system design teams and engage them to create competing, innovative teacher evaluation system plans, (3) assess and report on the strengths and weaknesses of the identified alternative teacher evaluation systems.	*Planning*: Choose a teacher evaluation approach to serve as the framework for developing the district's new evaluation system. Subsequently, develop an action plan, schedule, and budget.
Formative evaluation	*Input evaluation* (*specific*): Assess and report on the district's plan for executing and managing the teacher evaluation system reform program.	*Design and start-up*: Debug and finalize the specific teacher evaluation reform management plan; then put the plan into action.
Formative evaluation	*Process evaluation*: Monitor the reform program's implementation; issue a succession of interim, process improvement-oriented reports; and maintain documentation on the reform program's actual implementation.	*Implementation*: Use periodic feedback to keep the reform program on track, to address and correct identified deficiencies or problems, and, as needed, to improve the reform program's design.
Formative evaluation	*Product evaluation*: Keep track of and issue periodic reports on reform program outcomes, for example, clarity, appropriateness, and functionality of formats for job descriptions; assessed validity and reliability of teacher performance ratings based on newly constructed evaluation instruments; and assessed efficiency and security of a new system for storing and retrieving teacher evaluation records.	*Recycling and problem solving*: Decide to sustain the present developmental course, or recycle it to strengthen development plans to better assure achievement of the desired outcomes.
Summative evaluation	*Summative accountability report*: Maintain throughout the evaluation's formative stages a complete record of formative context, input, process, and product evaluation reports and how the client group used the reports. Synthesize the reports into a summative accountability report that documents and assesses the reform program's background, design and execution, and outcomes and that culminates with conclusions concerning the merit and worth of the new teacher evaluation system. Deliver and explain the final report in separate sessions to the school district's administration, teaching faculty (with administrators present), and board of education.	*Program accountability and next steps*: Decide whether the new program is worth sustaining and whether it should be adopted as is, should be recycled and strengthened in significant ways, or abandoned. Also, as needed, use the evaluation center's summative accountability report to defend the reform effort—to school district governors, staff, teachers' union, and constituents—and to justify the decision to adopt, recycle, or reject the new system.
Formative evaluation	*Mainstreaming systematic evaluation*: If the new program is to be adopted or recycled for improvement, advise the school district's leaders on how to usefully build systematic formative evaluation into the operation of the new teacher evaluation system.	*Mainstreaming system evaluation*: If the new teacher evaluation system is adopted, arrange for ongoing monitoring and evaluation of the system to assure and, over time, improve its correct functioning.

feedback to assure the quality and success of a developmental effort. The chart also shows how a synthesis of formative evaluation reports—supplemented as needed with additional information—can provide the client with a firm foundation for meeting the requirements for institutional and public accountability.

Table 2.3 presents an overall conceptual summary of the uses of the CIPP Model for both formative and summative evaluations. The matrix's eight cells encompass much of the evaluative information required to guide enterprises and produce credible, and therefore defensible, summative evaluation reports.

Key Evaluation Questions

As a further application of the format in Table 2.3, Table 2.4 summarizes the types of formative and summative questions to be addressed by context, input, process, and product evaluation.

The Philosophy and Code of Ethics Underlying the CIPP Model

The CIPP Model is strongly oriented to service and the principles of a free society. It calls for evaluators and clients to identify and involve rightful beneficiaries, clarify their needs for assistance, obtain information of use in designing responsive programs and other areas of assistance, assess and help guide effective implementation of the intervention, and ultimately assess the intervention's value (e.g., its quality, worth, probity, equity, feasibility, cost, efficiency, safety, or significance). The thrust of CIPP evaluations is to provide sound information and judgments that will help service providers regularly assess and improve services and make effective and efficient use of resources, time, and technology to serve the well-being and targeted needs of rightful beneficiaries appropriately, equitably, and frugally.

TABLE 2.3. The Relevance of Four Evaluation Types to Formative and Summative Evaluation Roles

Evaluation Roles	Context	Input	Process	Product
Formative evaluation: Proactive application of CIPP information and judgments to assist decision making, program implementation, quality assurance, and recordkeeping for accountability	Guidance for identifying needed interventions, determining goals, and setting priorities *by assessing and reporting on needs, problems, risks, assets, and opportunities*	Guidance for choosing a program strategy (and possibly an outside contractor) and settling on a sound implementation plan and budget *by identifying, assessing, and reporting on alternative strategies and resource allocation plans and subsequently closely examining and judging the operational plan and budget*	Guidance for executing the operational plan *by monitoring, documenting, judging, and repeatedly reporting on program activities and expenditures*	Guidance for continuing, modifying, adopting, or terminating the program *by identifying, documenting, assessing, and reporting on intermediate and longer-term outcomes, including side effects*
Summative evaluation: Retrospective use of CIPP information to sum up the program's value (e.g., its quality, efficiency, cost, feasibility, probity, equity, safety, impacts, worth, or significance)	Judging goals and priorities *by comparing them to assessed needs, problems, risks, assets, and opportunities*	Judging the implementation plan and budget *by comparing them to the targeted needs, problems, and risks; contrasting the plan and budget with critical competitors; and assessing their compatibility with the implementation environment and compliance with relevant codes, regulations, and laws*	Judging program implementation *by fully describing and assessing the actual process and costs, comparing the planned and actual processes and costs, and assessing compliance with relevant codes, regulations, and laws*	Judging the program's success *by comparing its outcomes and side effects with targeted needs and stated goals, examining its cost-effectiveness, and, as feasible, contrasting its costs and outcomes with competitive programs; also interpreting results against the effort's outlay of resources and the extent to which the operational plan was both sound and effectively executed*

TABLE 2.4. Types of Formative and Summative Questions to Be Addressed by Context, Input, Process, and Product Evaluations

Context	Input	Process	Product
		Formative evaluation	
• What are the highest-priority needs in the program area of interest? • What beneficiary group should be served? • What is an appropriate breakout of the target group's needs? • What are an apt definition and prioritization of goals for addressing the assessed needs? • What assets are potentially available to assist in achieving the goals?	• What are the most promising potential approaches to meeting the targeted needs and achieving the stated goals? • How do these alternatives compare on past uses, potential for success, costs, political viability, feasibility, etc.? • How can the needed intervention be most effectively designed, staffed, funded, and implemented? • Is the produced action plan sound and workable? • What are predictable barriers to effective implementation?	• To what extent is the program proceeding on time, within budget, and effectively? • What, if any, impediments to successful implementation need to be addressed? • If necessary, how can the design be improved? • How can the implementation be strengthened (e.g., special training for staff, reallocation of resources, updating of the schedule)?	• To what extent is the program effectively addressing the targeted needs? • To what extent is the program achieving its goals? • What, if any, unexpected accomplishments are emerging? • What, if any, negative effects are emerging? • What side effects (positive or negative) are emerging? • How can the implementation be modified to maintain or increase success or eliminate bad outcomes?
		Summative evaluation	
• To what extent did this intervention address high-priority needs? • To what extent did the program's goals reflect the targeted needs? • To what extent did the goals take account of barriers to success? • To what extent did the goals incorporate use of available assets to enhance prospects for success? • To what extent were the stated goals taken seriously and addressed?	• What strategies were considered? • What strategy was chosen and, compared with other viable strategies (re prospects for success, feasibility, costs), why? • How well was the chosen strategy converted to a sound, feasible work plan?	• To what extent was the program carried out as planned or modified with an improved plan? • How effectively did staff identify and overcome problems of implementation? • How well was program implementation documented? • How well was the program executed?	• To what extent did this program successfully address the originally assessed needs and stated goals? • What, if any, were the unanticipated positive outcomes? • What, if any, were the unexpected negative effects? • What conclusions can be reached in terms of the program's quality, impacts, integrity, cost-effectiveness, sustainability, and broad applicability?

Involving and Serving Stakeholders

CIPP evaluations must be grounded in the democratic principles of equity and fairness. A key concept used in the model is that of evaluation stakeholders: those who are intended to use the findings, those who may otherwise be affected by the evaluation, and those expected to contribute to the evaluation. Consistent with the Joint Committee's *Program Evaluation Standards* (1981, 1994, 2011), evaluators should reach out to all relevant stakeholder groups and engage at least their representatives in hermeneutic and consensus-building processes. The evaluator should engage them to help affirm and clarify foundational values, identify pertinent issues and threats to the evaluation's success, define evaluation questions, clarify evaluative criteria, identify and obtain needed information, assess draft reports, interpret findings, and secure appropriate uses of finalized evaluation reports. To succeed, program evaluations must validly address the questions and concerns of interested stakeholders.

Since information empowers those who hold the information, the CIPP Model emphasizes the importance of even-handedness in involving and informing, as feasible, all of a program's stakeholders. Moreover, evaluators should strive to reach and involve those most in need and those with little access to and influence over services. While evaluators should control the evaluation process to ensure its integrity, CIPP evaluations accord beneficiaries and other stakeholders more than a passive recipient's role. Evaluators are charged to keep stakeholders informed and provide them appropriate opportunities to contribute and use findings. Involving all levels of stakeholders is considered ethically responsible because it equitably empowers the disadvantaged as well as the advantaged to help define the appropriate evaluation questions and criteria, provide evaluative input, critique draft reports, and receive, review, and use evaluation findings. Involving all stakeholder groups is also wise because sustained, consequential involvement positions stakeholders to contribute information and valuable insights and inclines them to study, understand, accept, value, and act on evaluation reports.

We understand that substantial, sustained involvement of the full range of a program's stakeholders is an elusive goal. Many stakeholders lack the time, interest, or motivation to engage, over time, in understanding, making input to, and using findings from a program evaluation. Some stakeholders won't respond

---

BOX 2.2. Stakeholder Experiment

The World Heart Federation stresses that "the success of an evaluation depends largely on the participation of program stakeholders. The best way to ensure active participation of the different groups involved is to include them in those stages of evaluation planning that either matter to them or that depend on them."

A six-step framework for conducting evaluation of public health programs, published by the Centers for Disease Control and Prevention (CDC), emphasizes the importance of stakeholder engagement. The framework is as follows:

1. Engage stakeholders.
2. Describe the program.
3. Focus the evaluation.
4. Gather credible evidence.
5. Justify conclusions.
6. Ensure use and share lessons learned.

To evaluate the impact of an Integrative Graduate Education and Research Traineeship program (IGERT) involving the collaborative training of doctoral students across biology, statistics, and mathematics, an evaluator involved doctoral students (IGERT trainees), IGERT faculty mentors in three departments (Biology, Mathematics, and Statistics), the industry partners, university administrators, and the funder. The follow-up evaluation after the IGERT trainees' graduation required her to reach even more stakeholders—their employers and supervisors.

---

to invitations to become involved. Others may accept a role in the evaluation process, such as membership on an evaluation review panel, but fail to attend meetings or otherwise carry through on their commitments. Despite these difficulties, evaluators can employ many procedures to enhance stakeholder participation. These procedures include setting up and meeting periodically with a broadly representative review panel that is chaired by one of the stakeholders—preferably the evaluation client—holding town meetings, interviewing members of a representative group of stakeholders, conducting focus groups, holding feedback workshops with the key decision makers, issuing periodic **newslet-**

ters, operating a website that maintains up-to-date information on the evaluation's progress and results, and issuing progress reports in local newspapers or over TV or radio. The key point is that it is ethically appropriate and in the interest of securing effective impact of an evaluation for evaluators to plan and carry out pertinent measures to keep interested stakeholders informed about and involved in the evaluation process.

Those who design and conduct program evaluations need to plan, budget, and employ effective means to engage stakeholders in program evaluations, such as the following:

- Specifically budget for stakeholder engagement activities.
- Systematically identify parties with legitimate interests in the evaluation.
- Announce and provide opportunities for stakeholders to provide inputs for evaluations.
- Issue periodic information about the evaluation's progress and make it accessible to interested stakeholders.
- Create mechanisms by which stakeholders keep themselves informed about the evaluation and contribute their inputs.

Table 2.5 is a list of selected approaches that evaluators may employ to meaningfully engage stakeholders. Evaluators should exercise foresight and make effective use of such stakeholder engagement approaches. In particular, they should collaborate with the evaluation's client to select approaches that both parties deem most useful and feasible. The evaluator should then schedule and budget for use of the selected approaches. Throughout the evaluation, the evaluator and client should collaborate systematically and effectively to employ the selected approaches and use the generated stakeholder feedback to help ensure the evaluation's quality and impacts and responsiveness to stakeholders.

Table 2.6 provides a further look into the importance of stakeholder engagement by summarizing the key advantages of the **stakeholder engagement procedures** defined in Table 2.5 to both the evaluator and the evaluation stakeholders. As the table clearly indicates, the advantages of applying the stakeholder engagement procedures to both the evaluator and the involved stakeholders argue strongly for evaluators to carefully plan and budget for using these stakeholder engagement procedures in their evaluations. Evaluators should carefully select applicable stakeholder engagement procedures and employ them to help guarantee the evaluation's success and impacts and to assure that the involved stakeholders receive benefits from being involved in the evaluation and are strongly inclined to study and use the findings.

The Evaluation Client as Evaluation-Oriented Leader

A key aim of evaluation work based on the CIPP Model is to support and assist **evaluation clients** to effectively carry out the role of evaluation-oriented leaders. Evaluation-oriented leadership is one of society's most important roles. The role is embodied in evaluation clients who acquire a sound concept of evaluation; gain a commitment to secure useful, valid evaluations; develop skills for carrying out client responsibilities in evaluation; exercise leadership in helping stakeholders understand and value sound evaluation findings; take the initiative in obtaining needed evaluation services; and help assure that contracted evaluations are accurate, ethical, useful, and applied. The most important outcomes of exercising evaluation-oriented leadership are program improvement, accountability, credibility, and, overall, assuring that targeted beneficiaries receive effective, reasonably priced, accountable services. Evaluation-oriented leadership is needed in a wide range of public, commercial, and professional fields, notably school and university administration, public administration, legislative leadership, military leadership, health care, philanthropy, business, social services, financial services, agriculture, food services, transportation, construction, tourism, hotel and restaurant management, public media, community and economic development, technology, research, manufacturing, and more. Evaluators should regularly encourage and assist leaders in the wide array of public, commercial, and professional service areas to evaluate programs and services, communicate and cooperate effectively with evaluators and program stakeholders, and educate and assist constituents to make sound uses of evaluation. An underlying principle of the CIPP Model is that securing, focusing, facilitating, and using systematic evaluation are among a leader's most important responsibilities because valid evaluation is essential to help assure a program's quality, integrity, safety, cost-effectiveness, accountability, and credibility.

TABLE 2.5. Evaluation Stakeholder Engagement Approaches

Evaluation stakeholder review panel

Panel that is representative of key evaluation audiences and that meets regularly through the course of the evaluation to critique the clarity and accuracy of evaluation plans and reports. Preferably, the evaluation's client chairs the panel.

Town hall meetings

Publicly announced meetings that are open to all interested parties for the purposes of sharing information on evaluation plans and reports and soliciting stakeholder inputs. Typically, the evaluator chairs such meetings.

Interviewing stakeholders

Interviews to obtain stakeholder inputs in response to the evaluation's questions. Interviewees should be representative of the program's stakeholders. Typically, the evaluator or members of the evaluation team conduct interviews and report results of the interviews.

Focus group

A group of approximately seven to ten stakeholders who are representative of the subject program's key stakeholder perspectives and which typically is engaged at an evaluation's end to deliberate and issue advice on the most defensible and potentially productive uses of the evaluation's findings. Typically, the evaluator or a member of the evaluation team coordinates and documents the focus group deliberations.

Feedback workshops

Periodic workshops in which the client and a group of stakeholders selected by the client present their judgments to the evaluator concerning the accuracy and clarity of previously reviewed draft evaluation plans and reports. Preferably, the evaluation's client chairs the feedback workshop.

Evaluation newsletters

Periodic newsletters to keep interested stakeholders apprised of the evaluation's progress and of opportunities to make inputs to the evaluation. Typically, the evaluator or a member of the evaluation team edits and assures appropriate, effective dissemination of the newsletters.

Evaluation website

Website open to all interested parties to keep interested stakeholders informed of the evaluation's plans and progress. The evaluator or a member of the evaluation team develops, regularly updates, and manages the website.

Dedicated program evaluation listserv

A computerized listserv open to all interested stakeholders and oriented to keeping the members informed about the evaluation's progress. The evaluator or a member of the evaluation team develops, regularly updates, and manages the listserv.

Periodic webinars focused on the evaluation's progress and needs for stakeholder inputs

Webinars that invite interested stakeholders to sign up and join a computerized session dedicated to updating stakeholders on the evaluation's progress and inviting their inputs. The evaluator or a member of the evaluation team develops, regularly updates, and manages the webinar.

Releases to the media

Periodic releases to the media to obtain their assistance in keeping the public informed about the evaluation's purpose, progress, and findings. The evaluator, pursuant to advance contractual agreements with the client, prepares the releases, shares prerelease versions with the client, uses the client's feedback (on accuracy and clarity) as appropriate, finalizes the releases, and delivers them to selected media outlets.

TABLE 2.6. Benefits to Evaluators and Stakeholders Deriving from the Evaluator's Employment of Stakeholder Engagement Procedures

Stakeholder Engagement Procedures	Main Advantages to the Evaluation	Main Advantages to the Engaged Stakeholders
Evaluation stakeholder review panel	• Engenders stakeholder interest in the evaluation. • Helps identify issues of clarity and accuracy in evaluation materials. • Inclines involved stakeholders to value and use the evaluation's findings. • Secures stakeholders' assistance in data collection. • Involved stakeholders are informed about the evaluation and can provide other stakeholders with accurate information about the evaluation's focus, progress, and potential utility.	• Positions them to help assure that the evaluation will address questions of importance to stakeholders. • Positions them to help assure that evaluation reports are clear, accurate, and of practical use. • Positions them to inform the evaluator about other stakeholders' concerns about the evaluation. • Gives them early access to the evaluation's findings. • Provides them with the information they need to help others understand, assess, and use the evaluation.
Town hall meetings	• Insulates the evaluator against possible charges that the evaluation is being conducted behind closed doors and being monitored by only a select group of stakeholders. • Provides evaluator an opportunity to hear concerns about the evaluation, learn what evaluation questions are most important to those attending the meeting, hear judgments about the subject program, and obtain cooperation in collecting information and disseminating findings.	• Affords an opportunity to stakeholders not on the Stakeholder Review Panel to be apprised of the evaluation's focus and progress, to offer inputs for consideration in the evaluation, to learn how they can keep informed about the evaluation, and to find out they may become involved in the process.
Interviewing stakeholders	• Provides stakeholders' responses to the evaluation's questions. • Provides a source of in-depth qualitative information for use in adding meaning to the evaluation's quantitative findings. • Ensures engagement of selected stakeholders.	• Provides the interviewed stakeholders an opportunity to present both factual responses to the evaluation's questions and their judgments of the subject program. • Increases their knowledge of the evaluation's purpose and key questions and likely inclines them to be interested in reading, making use of the evaluation's reports, and positions them to help others understand the evaluation's purpose and potential utility.
Focus group	• An invaluable means of getting stakeholders' perceptions of the meaning and potential utility of the evauation's findings. • Produces stakeholders who, as well-informed opinion leaders about the evaluation, are in a position to help other stakeholders understand and make use of the evaluation's findings. • Ensures engagement of selected stakeholders.	• Places selected stakeholders in a position to delve into the evaluation's findings and present individual and shared perspectives on the evaluation's quality and potential utility and to offer advice on how the evaluator can best and appropriately promote and support the use of evaluation findings. • Is an excellent means for the involved stakeholders to increase their understanding of the concept and procedures of systematic evaluation.

(continued)

TABLE 2.6. *(continued)*

Stakeholder Engagement Procedures	Main Advantages to the Evaluation	Main Advantages to the Engaged Stakeholders
Feedback workshops	• Provides a mechanism for regularly receiving critiques of the accuracy and clarity of draft evaluation plans and reports from the client and other key stakeholders. • Provides a forum for obtaining stakeholders' assistance in collecting data. • Helps ensure that the key clients will keep apprised of the evaluation's progress and maintain a strong interest in making use of the evaluation's findings.	• Affords the client a means of keeping touch with the evaluation and assuring that it is effectively addressing questions that are important to the program's staff. • Provides the program's staff early information about the evaluation's emerging findings and opportunities to use these early findings in program improvement processes. • Provides a forum to air any concerns about the evaluation's operations and, with the evaluator, to solve any problems, especially in the evaluation's field operations.
Evaluation newsletters	• Provides a convenient outlet for keeping interested stakeholders informed about the evaluation. • Provides a growing directory of stakeholders who are likely targets for getting the evaluation findings used. • Provides a means of documenting the evaluation's focus and progress. • Provides an outlet, as appropriate, for capsulizing and releasing interim and final evaluation findings. • Helps keep the evaluation on the minds of stakeholders.	• Regularly updates stakeholders through carefully prepared releases on the evaluation's focus, progress, and, as appropriate, interim findings. • Helps stakeholders increase their understanding of and appreciation for systematic program evaluation. • Provides a convenient means of storing evaluation progress reports for later reference.
Evaluation website	• Provides a convenient, inexpensive means of keeping interested stakeholders informed about the evaluation. • Provides a growing directory of persons who are interested in the evaluation. • Demonstrates the evaluator's professional approach to keeping interested persons informed about the evaluation.	• Regularly updates interested persons through carefully prepared releases on the evaluation's focus, progress, and, as appropriate, interim findings. • Gives access to information about the evaluation at any times that are convenient to different interested parties.
Dedicated program evaluation listserv	• Provides an efficient means of developing a list of interested stakeholders. • Provides an efficient mechanism for continuously updating information on the evaluation's progress and making the information readily accessible to interested stakeholders.	• Affords interested stakeholders an opportunity to sign up to an efficient service for keeping informed about the evaluation. • Provides continuous access to information about the evaluation that is being stored at the listserv site.
Periodic webinars focused on the evaluation's progress and needs for stakeholder inputs	• Provides a mechanism for identifying stakeholders who are sufficiently interested in being informed about the evaluation and obtaining their inputs. • Provides scheduled opportunities to update interested stakeholders on the evaluation's progress, to hear their inputs, and to listen to their exchanges with each other.	• Provides scheduled opportunities for receiving updates on the evaluation. • Provides opportunities to engage with the evaluator and other stakeholders in in-depth discussions of the evaluation.
Releases to the media	• Helps publicize and, as warranted, legitimize the evaluation. • May acquire for the evaluator influential allies in the press for seeing to it that the evaluation's findings are effectively disseminated.	• Provides a convenient, credible source of information on the media's representation and commentary on the evaluation.

Improvement Orientation

A fundamental tenet of the CIPP Model is that *the evaluation's purpose is not only to prove, but also—and more importantly—to improve*. Evaluation is thus conceived first and foremost as a functional activity oriented in the long run toward stimulating, aiding, and abetting efforts to strengthen and improve enterprises. The model also posits that some programs or other services will prove unworthy of attempts to improve them or will be found overly expensive and thus should be discredited or terminated. By helping stop unneeded, unsustainable, corrupt, or hopelessly flawed efforts, evaluations can serve an improvement function through assisting organizations to free resources and time for worthy efforts. Also, the model charges evaluators to identify and report valuable lessons from both failed and successful efforts.

Objectivist Orientation

The CIPP Model's epistemological orientation is objectivist, not relativist. Objectivist evaluations are based on the theory that moral good is objective and independent of personal or merely human feelings. Such evaluations are firmly grounded in ethical principles, such as the United Nations' Universal Declaration of Human Rights and the U.S. Bill of Rights; strive to control bias, prejudice, and conflicts of interest in conducting assessments and reaching conclusions; invoke and justify appropriate and (where they exist) established technical standards of quality; obtain and validate findings from multiple sources; search for best, unambiguous answers, although these may be difficult to find; set forth and justify the best available conclusions about the program or other evaluand; report findings honestly, fairly, and as circumspectly as necessary to all right-to-know audiences; subject the evaluation process and findings to independent assessments against pertinent professional standards; and identify needs for further investigation. Fundamentally, objectivist evaluations are intended over time to lead to conclusions that are correct—not correct or incorrect relative to an evaluator's or other party's predilections, position, preferences, or point of view. The model contends that when different objectivist evaluations are focused on the same object in a given setting, when they are keyed to fundamental principles of a free society and to agreed-on criteria of merit, when they meaningfully engage all stakeholder groups in the quest for answers, and when they conform to the evaluation field's standards, different, competent evaluators will arrive at fundamentally equivalent, defensible conclusions.

Standards and Metaevaluation

The model calls for evaluators to meet the professional standards for evaluations and subject their evaluations to both formative and summative metaevaluations. The main standards invoked in the model require evaluations to meet professionally defined requirements for utility, feasibility, propriety, accuracy, and evaluation accountability. The five groups of standards are summarized in Table 2.7.

At a minimum, evaluators should conduct their own formative and summative metaevaluations. They should use the formative metaevaluation to guide the evaluation work and correct deficiencies along the way. In the final evaluation report, the evaluators should state and explain their judgments of the extent to which the evaluation met each of the relevant Joint Committee (2011) standards. As feasible, the evaluation should be subjected to an external, independent metaevaluation. Preferably, a party other than the evaluators, such as the client or a private foundation, should choose and fund the external metaevaluator. This helps avoid any appearance or fact of the evaluator's possible **conflict of interest** having influenced the selection of the metaevaluator and the content of the external metaevaluation report. The external metaevaluator's report should be made available to all members of the right-to-know audience. A checklist designed to facilitate systematic application of the Joint Committee (2011) *Program Evaluation Standards* in metaevaluations is available online (see the box at the end of the table of contents).

The Importance of Negotiating Advance Agreements

In the process of deciding to conduct an evaluation, the evaluator and client should negotiate and document a contract or **memorandum of agreement** on how the evaluation will be conducted, what it will produce, what funds it will receive, and who will see its results. Such an agreement must assure that the evaluation will be conducted ethically and legally and will comply with professional standards for evaluations, that is, utility, feasibility, propriety, accuracy, and evaluation accountability (Stufflebeam, 2000b).

Negotiating and documenting an evaluation agreement are important for ensuring the evaluation's suc-

TABLE 2.7. Summary Statements of the 30 Metaevaluation Standards of the Joint Committee on Standards for Educational Evaluation, Grouped into the Five Main Requirements of Utility, Feasibility, Propriety, Accuracy, and Evaluation Accountability

The **Utility Standards** are intended to ensure that an evaluation is aligned with stakeholders' needs such that process uses, findings uses, and other appropriate influences are possible.

U1 Evaluator Credibility. Evaluations should be conducted by qualified people who establish and maintain credibility in the evaluation context.

U2 Attention to Stakeholders. Evaluations should devote attention to the full range of individuals and groups invested in the program or affected by the evaluation.

U3 Negotiated Purposes. Evaluation purposes should be identified and revisited based on the needs of stakeholders.

U4 Explicit Values. Evaluations should clarify and specify the individual and cultural values underpinning the evaluation purposes, processes, and judgments.

U5 Relevant Information. Evaluation information should serve the identified and emergent needs of intended users.

U6 Meaningful Processes and Products. Evaluation activities, descriptions, findings, and judgments should encourage use.

U7 Timeliness and Appropriate Communication and Reporting. Evaluations should attend in a timely and ongoing way to the reporting and dissemination needs of stakeholders.

U8 Concern for Consequences and Influence. Evaluations should promote responsible and adaptive use while guarding against unintended negative consequences and misuse.

Feasibility Standards are intended to ensure that an evaluation is viable, realistic, contextually sensitive, responsive, prudent, diplomatic, politically viable, efficient, and cost-effective.

F1 Project Management. Evaluations should use effective project management strategies.

F2 Practical Procedures. The procedures should be practical and responsive to the way the program operates.

F3 Contextual Viability. Evaluations should recognize, monitor, and balance the cultural and political interests and needs of individuals and groups.

F4 Resource Use. Evaluations should use resources effectively and efficiently.

Propriety Standards are intended to ensure that an evaluation will be conducted properly, fairly, legally, ethically, and justly with respect to (1) evaluators' and stakeholders' ethical rights, responsibilities, and duties; (2) systems of relevant laws, regulations, and rules; and (3) roles and duties of professional evaluators.

P1 Responsive and Inclusive Orientation. Evaluations should be responsive to stakeholders and their communities.

P2 Formal Agreements. Evaluation agreements should be negotiated to make obligations explicit and take into account the needs, expectations, and cultural contexts of clients and other stakeholders.

P3 Human Rights and Respect. Evaluations should be designed and conducted to protect human and legal rights and maintain the dignity of participants and other stakeholders.

P4 Clarity and Fairness. Evaluations should be understandable and fair in addressing stakeholder needs and purposes.

P5 Transparency and Disclosure. Evaluations should provide complete descriptions of findings, limitations, and conclusions to all stakeholders unless doing so would violate legal or propriety obligations.

P6 Conflicts of Interests. Evaluators should openly and honestly identify and address real or perceived conflicts of interests that may compromise the evaluation.

P7 Fiscal Responsibility. Evaluations should account for all expended resources and comply with sound fiscal procedures and processes.

(continued)

TABLE 2.7. *(continued)*

Accuracy Standards are intended to ensure that an evaluation employs sound theory, designs, methods, and reasoning in order to minimize inconsistencies, distortions, and misconceptions and produce and report truthful evaluation findings and conclusions.

A1 Justified Conclusions and Decisions. Evaluation conclusions and decisions should be explicitly justified in the cultures and contexts where they have consequences.

A2 Valid Information. Evaluation information should serve the intended purposes and support valid interpretations.

A3 Reliable Information. Evaluation procedures should yield sufficiently dependable and consistent information for the intended uses.

A4 Explicit Program and Context Descriptions. Evaluations should document programs and their contexts with appropriate detail and scope for the evaluation purposes.

A5 Information Management. Evaluations should employ systematic information collection, review, verification, and storage methods.

A6 Sound Designs and Analyses. Evaluations should employ technically adequate designs and analyses that are appropriate for the evaluation purposes.

A7 Explicit Evaluation Reasoning. Evaluation reasoning leading from information and analyses to findings, interpretations, conclusions, and judgments should be clearly and completely documented.

A8 Communicating and Reporting. Evaluation communications should have adequate scope and guard against misconceptions, biases, distortions, and errors.

Evaluation Accountability Standards are intended to ensure that an evaluation is systematically, thoroughly, and transparently documented and then assessed, both internally and externally, for its utility, feasibility, propriety, and accuracy.

E1 Evaluation Documentation. Evaluations should fully document their negotiated purposes and implemented designs, procedures, data, and outcomes.

E2 Internal Metaevaluation. Evaluations should use these and other applicable standards to examine the accountability of the evaluation design, procedures employed, information collected, and outcomes.

E3 External Metaevaluation. Program evaluation sponsors, clients, evaluators, and other stakeholders should encourage the conduct of external metaevaluations using these and other applicable standards.

Note. From Joint Committee on Standards for Educational Evaluation (2011). Copyright © 2011 Joint Committee on Standards for Educational Evaluation. Reprinted by permission.

cess. This process establishes a trusting relationship between an evaluator and a client and documents their agreements. Such agreements are important for holding each party accountable for discharging their agreed-upon responsibilities and resolving disputes over disagreements that may emerge regarding a host of managerial, funding, implementation, reporting, and other matters. Moreover, written advance agreements are useful for assuring those who will be affected by the evaluation findings that the evaluation was a fairly conducted, professional study, with allegiance to the prin-

ciples of sound evaluation and grounding in advance, printed agreements.

In applying the CIPP Model, the importance of negotiating advanced evaluation agreements has been confirmed repeatedly. Daniel Stufflebeam, the model's creator, instinctively included advance evaluation contracting in one of his early applications of the model and, ever since, has almost always insisted on negotiating advance written evaluation agreements.

The benefits of advance evaluation contracting were demonstrated in a politically charged evaluation done at the request of the National Education Association (NEA) (House, Rivers, & Stufflebeam, 1974). NEA had asked the three evaluators to evaluate Michigan's first-in-the-nation state educational accountability system. Although his colleagues thought a verbal agreement with NEA would suffice, Stufflebeam insisted on first contacting and discussing the projected evaluation with all parties that might be positively or negatively affected by the evaluation. He agreed to proceed with developing a contractual agreement with NEA only after hearing the concerns of all the stakeholders. Following exchanges with school district personnel, the state officials who were engaged in administering the educational accountability system, NEA officials, and others, Stufflebeam and his colleagues negotiated a contract with NEA for conducting the evaluation. This contract was designed to assure that the evaluation would be technically sound, transparent, independent, and fair to all of the evaluation's right-to-know audiences. At the end of the detailed evaluation process, the evaluation team issued a report that was highly critical of the accountability system. Key findings were that the accountability system had been hastily designed, that evaluation instruments were being used before being sufficiently validated, and that unfortunately an arguably inferior accountability system was being imposed, quite unfairly and with harmful effects, on all of Michigan's public school districts. Some leading members of the evaluation profession, upon seeing press accounts of the negative evaluation report, originally asked the three evaluators if they had served as NEA's biased, hired guns. When presented with the actual report, they disabused themselves of that notion, especially after reading the appended evaluation contract. That early application of evaluation contracting was influential in convincing many leading professional evaluators of the time that it was important to negotiate with their clients advanced contracts that would help guarantee an evaluation's soundness, integrity, independence, credibility, and viability.

There was one notable time when Stufflebeam didn't negotiate an advance agreement with a client, and his team and his university got burned. Western Michigan University had contracted with the National Assessment Governing Board (NAGB) for Stufflebeam and his team members Richard Jaeger and Michael Scriven to complete two rounds of formative evaluations of NAGB's project to set achievement levels on the National Assessment of Educational Progress (NAEP). Both formative evaluations were completed with simi-

lar findings showing that NAGB's achievement levels, which were based on a modified Angoff procedure, were unreliable, otherwise flawed, and in need of substantial improvement. NAGB's oversight group, the U.S. Congress, was dissatisfied with NAGB's progress report because the achievement levels project had been subjected only to formative evaluations and was found wanting. Congress demanded that NAGB obtain a summative evaluation of the project. NAGB then asked Stufflebeam and his team to conduct the needed summative evaluation. Because federal funding of NAGB was at stake and Congress wanted to receive the summative evaluation report post haste, NAGB asked Stufflebeam and his team to proceed directly with the summative evaluation and without a contract. The NAGB representative said that taking time to negotiate a contract for the summative evaluation would delay the needed summative evaluation so much that it would fail to meet the demands from Congress. Stufflebeam and his team agreed to proceed without a written contract. They promptly conducted the needed summative evaluation work, found that the achievement levels procedures were fatally flawed, and submitted a prerelease version of their report to NAGB. Upon receiving the draft report, NAGB immediately "fired" the evaluators, which technically it couldn't do because there was no contract. Stufflebeam and Jaeger finalized the summative evaluation report and sent it to NAGB. Eventually, NAGB shared the report with Congress. The U.S. House of Representatives voted to defund NAGB, but the Senate rejected the House decision and asked the U.S. Government Accountability Office (GAO) to evaluate the NAGB achievement levels project. GAO's report corroborated the Stufflebeam, Jaeger, Scriven findings. NAGB continued with application of its achievement levels project. Stufflebeam's university was never reimbursed for the summative evaluation work. This account is a sad illustration of what can go wrong when an evaluator fails to ground the evaluation in a sound advance set of written agreements.

The CIPP Model's Values Component

Figure 2.1 summarizes the basic elements of the CIPP Model in three concentric circles and portrays the central importance of defined values. The inner circle denotes the core values that should be defined and used to undergird a given evaluation. The wheel surrounding the values is divided into four evaluative foci associ-

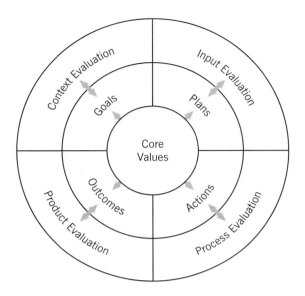

FIGURE 2.1. Key components of the CIPP Evaluation Model and associated relations with programs.

ated with any program or other endeavor: goals, plans, actions, and outcomes. The outer wheel indicates the type of evaluation that serves each of the four evaluative foci: context, input, process, and product evaluation. Each two-directional arrow represents a reciprocal relationship between a particular evaluative focus and a type of evaluation.

The goal-setting task raises questions for a context evaluation, which in turn provides information for validating or improving goals. Planning improvement efforts generates questions for an input evaluation, which correspondingly provides judgments of plans and direction for strengthening plans. Program actions bring up questions for a process evaluation, which provides judgments of activities plus feedback for strengthening staff performance. Outcomes, including accomplishments, lack of accomplishments, and side effects, command the attention of product evaluations, which ultimately issue judgments of outcomes and identify needs for achieving better results.

These relationships are made functional by grounding evaluations in core values, referenced in the scheme's inner circle.

Evaluation's root term is *value*. This term refers to any of a range of ideals held by a society, group, or individual. The CIPP Model calls for the evaluator and client, using appropriate inputs from stakeholders, to identify and clarify the values that will undergird particular evaluations. Examples of educational values—applied in evaluations of U.S. public school programs—are success in helping students meet a state's mandated academic standards; helping children develop basic academic skills; helping each child to fulfill her or his potential for educational development; assisting and reinforcing the development of students' special gifts and talents; upholding human rights; meeting the needs of disabled and underprivileged children; developing students as good citizens; instilling in students an understanding and respect for the principles of a free, democratic society; ensuring equality of opportunity; effectively engaging parents in the healthy development of their children; nurturing and developing the school's primary resource, its teachers; attaining excellence in all aspects of schooling; conserving and using resources efficiently; ensuring the safety of employed facilities, products, and procedures; maintaining separation of church and state; employing research and innovation to strengthen teaching and learning; and maintaining accountability. Essentially, evaluators should take into account a set of pertinent societal, institutional, program, and professional and technical values when assessing programs or other entities.

The values provide the foundation for deriving or validating particular evaluative criteria. Selected criteria, along with stakeholders' questions and the characteristics and needs of particular programs, help clarify an evaluation's information needs. These in turn provide the basis for selecting and constructing the evaluation instruments and procedures, accessing existing information, collecting new information, and defining interpretive standards.

A values framework also provides a well-knit point of reference for detecting unexpected defects and strengths. For example, through broad values-oriented surveillance, an evaluator might discover that a program excels in meeting students' targeted academic needs but has serious deficiencies, such as racist practices, unsafe equipment, teacher burnouts, wasting of resources, or graft. On the positive side, examination of a program against a backdrop of appropriate values might uncover unexpected positive outcomes, such as strengthened community support of schools, invention of better teaching practices, or more engaged and supportive parents.

The CIPP Model in the Form of a Logic Model

The CIPP Model not only provides a format for evaluating individual programs and projects, but is also geared to a systems view of evaluation. In this latter orientation, the model is concentrated on providing ongoing evaluation services to an organization's decision makers, especially top-level administrators. The model's systems orientation is illustrated in the flow model that appears in Figure 2.2.

Beginning in the upper left-hand corner, Figure 2.2 denotes the general operations of a school district, federal agency, hospital, private business, and some other organization (or a component of such an organization). The indicated context evaluation component denotes that, periodically, the organization needs to subject its operations to an assessment of system needs, problems, assets, opportunities, and existing goals. The need for such a context evaluation is especially present when the organization needs to conduct strategic planning or respond to accreditation requirements.

The Context Evaluation

Such a context evaluation would assess the needs of the organization's clients/beneficiaries, such as a school district's students, a hospital's patients, or a department store's customers; collect and examine information about problems in the organization that need to be solved (such as communication with customers, staff morale, safety, financial stability, poor outcomes, or community support); and assess the soundness and sufficiency of the organization's goals and priorities. The context evaluation would also seek to identify opportunities for helping to meet assessed needs and solve underlying problems. Relevant opportunities might be in the form of government funding programs, advanced technologies, or a charitable foundation with a program to support improvement efforts such as those being contemplated in the subject organization.

An organization's context evaluation may be motivated from inside the organization as a regular "state of the organization" assessment, as an early step in a strategic planning effort, or as a response to criticisms from staff, beneficiaries, funders, or constituents about the organization's **mission** and/or performance. The organization might also need a context evaluation to respond to forces outside the organization, as when an accrediting organization requires a self-study or a funding agency requires a "needs assessment" as a basis for justifying a funding request. Context evaluations that respond to such requests may be targeted on specified areas of concern, such as a university's engineering college, or focused more generally on a wide range of organizational functions, including policy, administration, staffing, facilities, services, products, and public relations. Context evaluations are especially useful for identifying needs to be met and diagnosing problems that must be solved in an organization's improvement effort. In general, such context evaluations aid in system renewal; promote services that are of improved quality, responsiveness to beneficiaries, and efficiency; help improve outcomes; and communicate the organization's involvement in systematically using evaluation to set goals for continually improving the organization's services.

Ideally, the context evaluation results would lead to a decision about whether to initiate a program improvement project. If decided in the negative, the organization would continue with program operations as usual. However, if a decision was made to mount an improvement effort, then pertinent organizational decision makers would clarify and stipulate the needs that must be met, the associated problems that have to be solved, and the improvement goals to be achieved. Next, they would consider whether some acceptable, "ready-made" solution already exists. If so, they could adapt the solution, install it, and tailor a specific evaluation to monitor and help guide its application.

The Input Evaluation

If no satisfactory solution were found, then, according to the flowchart, the organization's decision makers would conduct an input evaluation. Such an evaluation would search the relevant literature; query personnel in other organizations that may have dealt successfully with similar program improvement needs; draw on the ingenuity and creativity of the organization's staff, beneficiaries, and constituents; and possibly consult outside experts. Subsequently, as in use of the Advocate Teams Technique (to be explained later in this chapter), the organization could engage one or more teams to compete in creating, detailing, and proposing unique program improvement plans. The organization would then evaluate the alternative plans against preset criteria, including their projected feasibility and efficacy for meeting the targeted beneficiary needs, solving the underlying problems, and achieving the program improvement goals.

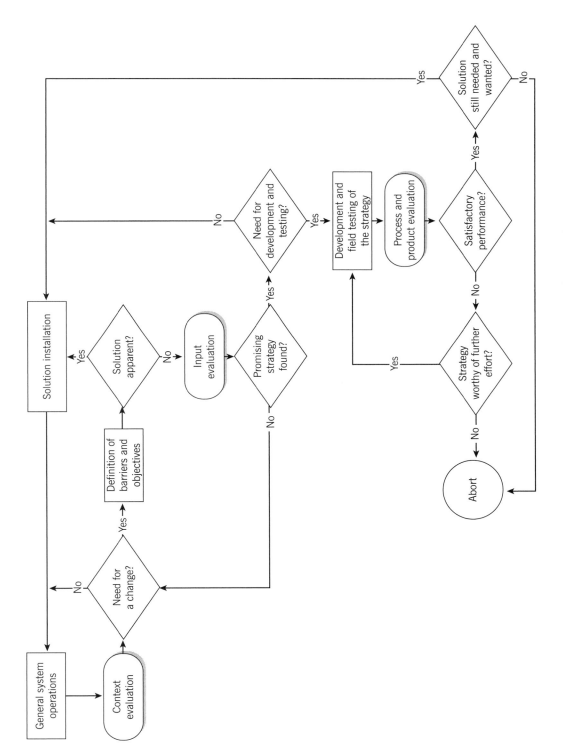

FIGURE 2.2. Flowchart of a CIPP evaluation in fostering and assessing system improvement.

The organization's decision makers would use the input evaluation results to determine whether a sufficiently promising program improvement strategy had been found to warrant proceeding with its further development. If not, according to the flowchart, the organization's decision makers would reconsider whether the contemplated program improvement effort was sufficiently important to warrant a further search. If so, the organization's decision makers would recycle their search for an acceptable program improvement strategy.

If, however, a promising program improvement strategy had been found, then the organization's decision makers would decide whether or not the strategy could justifiably be installed without further testing. If much were known about the strategy and the staff were confident in being able to install and operate it, then the organization's leaders likely would turn their attention to incorporating the program improvement strategy into regular organizational operations.

Overlapping Process and Product Evaluations

If the decision makers decided to test the strategy further, they would plan and conduct a field test of the strategy. In accordance with the flowchart, they would activate the strategy and subject it to process and product evaluations over whatever period of time would be required to debug and routinize stable implementation of the strategy. The process evaluation would entail engaging a **resident observer** to closely monitor and document the intervention's operations. Key process evaluation questions include the following: Are the intervention's operations consistent with the intervention's specifications? Is the intervention working equally well in all areas where it is being applied? Is the intervention being conducted on schedule and within its budget? Are those charged with managing and operating the intervention appropriately skilled, and are they supportive of the effort? To address these and related process evaluation questions, the on-site process and product evaluator would collect and analyze stakeholder interview data and relevant project documents. As appropriate, he or she would maintain a photographic record of observable project events. He or she would also observe project operations. Periodically, the on-site evaluator would compile interim process evaluation reports, submit them to predefined recipients, and sit down with key decision makers to go over the results. The on-site evaluator would maintain documentation of the project's execution for later reference and use in preparing the final summative evaluation report.

While conducting the process evaluation, the on-site evaluator would also collect data related to the effort's accomplishments. In particular, he or she would seek evidence about the extent to which the intervention was meeting the beneficiaries' targeted needs and overcoming the previously identified problems and barriers. The on-site evaluators likely would use the same procedures as were applied in conducting the process evaluation. Ultimately, he or she would compile and provide the predetermined audience with a product evaluation report containing both quantitative and qualitative information as well as judgments about the effort's success in goal achievement and its possible unanticipated outcomes. Ultimately, the evaluator would compile and synthesize the accumulated store of context, input, process, and product evaluation into the final summative report. Further steps would include face-to-face presentation of the findings to the right-to-know audiences.

If the program improvement effort has not performed satisfactorily or is viewed as too costly, the organization's leaders might conclude that no further effort is warranted. In accordance with this conclusion, they would abort the effort. Organizations have often reached such conclusions at the end of federally supported projects, when the grantee had insufficient local funds to support the effort's continuation. As shown in the bottom right-hand corner of Figure 2. 2, even if the program improvement effort had succeeded, the organization's leaders might decide that the previously required effort was no longer needed, and, accordingly, they would terminate the program improvement effort. Under the assumption that the effort was successful and the solution it afforded was still needed and wanted, the organization's staff would activate the proven improvement strategy as a regular part of organizational operations and subject it to ongoing monitoring, evaluation, and improvement, as appropriate.

The preceding depiction of evaluation in the context of an organization's ongoing needs for periodic reflection and problem solving points up a number of important features of a systems approach to evaluation.

1. Evaluation should be an integral part of an organization's regular operations and not just a specialized activity involved in innovative projects.

2. An organization's implementation of the CIPP Model (or any other evaluation approach) is only part of the total mosaic of informal and **formal evaluation** that goes on in the organization.

3. Evaluations have a vital role in stimulating, focusing, and planning program improvement.

4. The employment of context, input, process, or product evaluation is indicated only if information beyond what already exists is needed, not by the inherent value in doing each kind of evaluation. Each of these kinds of evaluation should be conducted only if it is essential to provide the client group with credible evaluative input.

5. The installation of new or improved programs should provide for systematically evaluating, over time, their operation and contributions to the success of the overall organization.

6. Systematic evaluation of new or improved programs provides not only guidance for making them work, but also documentation of their execution and accomplishments for use in issuing accountability reports and in storing lessons learned.

7. Although the CIPP Model includes no special, consistently applied provisions for formulating and testing hypotheses, when fully implemented it accumulates a comprehensive set of information on an intervention's context, input, process, and products for use in interpreting why an effort did or did not succeed.

Delineation of the CIPP Categories and Relevant Procedures

This section presents a more specific discussion of each type of evaluation. Table 2.8 provides a convenient overview of the essential meanings of context, input, process, and product evaluation. It defines these four types of studies according to their objectives, procedures, and uses. This section describes procedures that evaluators have found useful for conducting each type of evaluation. No one evaluation would likely use all of the procedures referred to here. They are presented to give an idea of the range of qualitative and quantitative procedures that are potentially applicable in CIPP evaluations.

Context Evaluation

Context evaluation assesses needs, problems, assets, and opportunities within a defined environment. Needs are those things that are necessary or useful for fulfilling a **defensible purpose.** Problems are impediments to overcome in meeting and continuing to meet targeted needs. Assets include accessible expertise and services, usually in the local area, that could be used to help fulfill the targeted purpose. Opportunities especially include funding programs that might be tapped to support efforts to meet needs and solve associated problems. Defensible purposes define what is to be achieved related to the institution's mission while adhering to **ethical standards** and legal standards.

While context evaluation is often referred to as needs assessment, the latter term is too narrow since it focuses on needs and omits concerns about problems, assets, and opportunities. All four elements are critically important in designing sound programs, projects, and services and should be considered in context evaluations. A context evaluation's main objectives are to:

- Set boundaries on and describe the setting for the intended service.
- Identify intended beneficiaries and assess their needs.
- Identify problems or barriers to meeting the assessed needs.
- Identify relevant, accessible assets and funding opportunities that could be used to address the targeted needs.
- Provide a basis for setting improvement-oriented goals.
- Assess the clarity and appropriateness of improvement-oriented goals.
- Identify basic criteria against which to judge outcomes of a targeted program or other improvement effort.

Context evaluations may be initiated before, during, or even after a project, program, or other intervention. In the before case, organizations may carry out context evaluations as narrowly bounded studies to help set goals and priorities in a particular area. When an evaluation is started during or after a project or other intervention, institutions often conduct and report a context evaluation in combination with input, process,

TABLE 2.8 Four Types of Evaluation

Context Evaluation	Input Evaluation	Process Evaluation	Product Evaluation
Objectives			
To define the relevant context, identify the targeted beneficiaries and assess their needs, identify assets and opportunities for addressing the needs, diagnose problems underlying the needs, and judge whether program goals and priorities are sufficiently and appropriately responsive to the assessed needs	To identify and assess system capabilities, alternative program strategies, and (as appropriate) alternative external contractors; assess the chosen strategy's procedural design, budget, schedule, staffing, and stakeholder involvement plans; and help assure that the selected inputs are responsive to targeted program goals and beneficiary needs	To identify or predict defects in the procedural design or its implementation, provide information for preprogrammed implementation decisions, affirm activities that are working well, and record and judge procedural events and activities	To identify intended and unintended outcomes; relate them to goals and assessed needs and to context, input, and process information; and judge accomplishments in such terms as quality, worth, probity, equity, cost, safety, and significance
Procedures			
Uses such procedures as system analysis, survey, document review, records analysis, demographic analysis, secondary data analysis, hearings, interviews, focus groups, diagnostic tests, case studies, site visits, epidemiological studies, historical analysis, literature reviews, and the Delphi technique	Uses such procedures as document analysis, interviews, background checks, literature search, visits to exemplary programs, advocate teams studies, pilot trials, and content analysis	Employs resident observers or visiting investigators to monitor the program's implementation, identify potential procedural barriers and unanticipated ones, obtain information for implementation decisions, document the actual process and costs, photograph progress, obtain staff-kept diaries, and regularly interact with and provide feedback to staff and other stakeholders	Uses such procedures as objective measurement, rating scales, checklists of expected outcomes, documentation of participation, interviews, photographic records, cost-effectiveness analysis, goal-free evaluation, experimental design, trend studies, surveys, and qualitative and quantitative analyses
Relation to decision making in the improvement process and to accountability			
For planning needed changes, that is, deciding on the setting to be served; the goals associated with meeting needs or using opportunities; the priorities for budgeting time and resources; and objectives associated with solving problems. Also, for providing a basis for judging goals, priorities, and outcomes.	For determining sources of support, solution strategies, and procedural designs, that is, for structuring, staffing, scheduling, and budgeting improvement activities. Also for determining and applying criteria for judging implementation.	For implementing and refining the program design and procedure, that is, for effecting process and quality control. Also, providing a log of the actual process and program costs for later use in judging implementation and interpreting outcomes.	For deciding to continue, modify, or refocus a program. Also for documenting and preserving a clear record of effects (intended and unintended, positive and negative), for comparison with assessed needs, targeted goals, and costs.

and product evaluations. Here, context evaluations are useful for judging established goals, identifying new needs that emerge during the course of the intervention, and helping the audience assess the effort's worth in meeting beneficiaries' needs.

A context evaluation's methodology may involve collecting a variety of information about members of the target population and their surrounding environment and conducting various types of analysis. A usual starting point is to ask the clients and other stakeholders to help define the **evaluation boundaries.** Such boundaries might pertain to a geographic location, program or administrative sectors within the organization, a targeted group of the organization's beneficiaries, and a time frame. Subsequently evaluators may employ a variety of techniques to generate and test hypotheses about needed services or changes in existing services. These techniques might include reviewing documents, analyzing demographic and performance data, conducting hearings and community forums, conducting focus group sessions, interviewing beneficiaries and other stakeholders, and, in the case of education, administering a pretest.

The evaluators might construct a survey instrument to investigate identified hypotheses concerning the existence of beneficiaries' needs. Then they could administer it to a carefully defined sample of stakeholders. The evaluators could also make the survey instrument available more generally to anyone who wishes to provide input. They would analyze the two sets of responses separately.

Evaluators should examine existing records to identify performance patterns and background information on the target population. In education, these might include immunization records; enrollment in different levels of courses; attendance; school grades; test scores; honors; graduation rates; participation in extracurricular activities; participation in special education; participation in free and reduced-fee meal programs; participation in further education; housing situations; employment and health histories; disciplinary records; or feedback from teachers, parents, former students, counselors, coaches, health personnel, librarians, custodians, law enforcement officers, administrators, or employers.

The evaluators might administer special **diagnostic tests** to members of the target population. They might engage an **expert review panel** to visit, closely observe, and identify needs, problems, assets, and opportunities in the targeted environment. The evaluators might conduct focus group meetings to review the gathered information. They might use a consensus-building technique such as Delphi to solidify agreements about priority needs and goals. They might conduct case studies of selected targeted beneficiaries or beneficiary groups. These procedures contribute to an in-depth perspective on the system's functioning and highest-priority needs.

Often audiences need to view an effort within both its present setting and its historical context. Considering the relevant history helps decision makers avoid past mistakes. Thus, the methodology of context evaluation includes **historical analysis** and literature review as well as methods aimed at characterizing and understanding current environmental conditions. After the initial context evaluation, organizations often need to continue collecting, organizing, filing, and reporting context evaluation data, since needs, problems, assets, and opportunities are subject to change.

In some situations, the evaluator should look beyond the local context to ascertain whether a program has widespread relevance. For example, a successful early childhood program might produce a ripple effect that eventually improves early childhood programming far beyond the program's setting. In such cases, the evaluator would judge the program not only on its worth in addressing the needs of targeted beneficiaries, but also its significance in serving beneficiaries outside the program's area of operation. To the extent a context evaluation shows that a proposed program has widespread significance, the program developer can make an especially strong case for external financial support.

Context evaluations have a wide range of possible constructive uses. A context evaluation might provide a means by which an administrator communicates with constituents to gain a shared conception of the organization's strengths and weaknesses, needs, assets, opportunities, and priority problems. A program developer could use context evaluation information to support a request for external grants or contracts. A university might use a context evaluation to convince a funding agency that it directed a proposed project at an urgent need or to convince a state legislature to increase the institution's funding. A social service organization might use context evaluation information to formulate objectives for staff development or to identify target populations for priority assistance. A school would use a context evaluation to help students and their parents or advisors focus their attention on developmental areas requiring more progress. An institution also could use context evaluation information to help decide how to make the institution stronger by cutting marginally important or ineffective programs. Similarly, such an organization could profitably employ a context evaluation to set the foundation for strategic planning. And, as observed at the beginning of this chapter, a home owner might use a context evaluation to set priorities for a home renovation project.

Context evaluation information is particularly useful when an organization needs to assess the worth and significance of what an intervention accomplished. Here the organization assesses whether the investment in improvement effectively addressed the targeted needs of intended beneficiaries. The evaluator also refers to context evaluation findings to assess the appropriateness of goals and relevance of project plans. Similarly, the evaluator uses context evaluation findings to examine how the intervention's process is affecting improvements outside the local setting. Considering such uses, an organization can benefit greatly by establishing, keeping up-to-date, and using information from a regularly updated **evaluation database.**

The concept of context evaluation has wide applicability and can be of critical importance. Consider its applicability in military operations. To plan and mount an invasion, military planners must have accurate information about the terrain to be invaded. Otherwise they may create and mount an invasion plan that due to previously undetected obstacles won't succeed, but instead will result in the avoidable death and wounding of many invading soldiers. As a case in point, amphibious assault vehicles bogged down in too shallow water far from the shores of Tarawa in the U.S. Marine Corps' World War II invasion of this Pacific atoll. Consequently, the amphibious vehicles were like sitting ducks in the waters far from the shores of Tarawa and, sadly, many Marines were needlessly killed or wounded. Unfortunately, the military planners had failed to adequately assess the depth of water lying off the selected invasion beach by taking into account variations in water depth due to high and low tides. Analogously, many soldiers avoidably drowned in the Allies 1944 invasion of the Normandy Coast's Omaha Beach, because they were disembarked from their landing crafts in water that was much deeper than predicted. Sound context evaluations in advance of these invasions, including a valid assessment of water depths and tides off Tarawa and Omaha Beach could have helped prevent these disasters.

Before leaving this discussion of context evaluation a caveat is in order. Evaluators should be selective in their use of available procedures for context evaluations. They should not unnecessarily try to apply all or a large number of the procedures identified above. In choosing procedures they should be guided by an assessment of what information is needed to meet the Joint Committee Standards requirements, especially for utility and accuracy, but they should also keep the investigation within reasonable bounds of feasibility. Of course, they should also take care to meet requirements for propriety and evaluation accountability. This caveat regarding the employment of multiple procedures applies to input, process, and product evaluation, as well as context evaluation.

Input Evaluation

An input evaluation primarily helps prescribe and arrange for conducting a program by which to meet targeted needs and goals. Also, if an external contractor is to be chosen, an input evaluation helps decision makers identify and assess the relevant qualifications of alternative potential contractors. Input evaluations search out and critically examine potentially relevant approaches, including the one already being used. Input evaluation is a precursor of the success or failure and efficiency of a change effort. Initial decisions to allocate resources constrain change projects. A potentially effective solution to a problem will have no possibility of impact if a planning group does not at least identify it and assess its merits. If one is needed, the most qualified external contractor is unlikely to be found if there is no search for and assessment of potentially qualified alternative contractors. Beyond assisting in the selection of a program strategy and contractor, an input evaluation informs interested parties about what programmatic approach was chosen and why, as well as the qualifications and reasons for choosing a particular, external contractor (if one was engaged). In this sense, input evaluation information is an important source of a developer's accountability for designing, staffing, and budgeting an improvement effort.

An input evaluation should identify and rate relevant approaches (including associated equipment and materials) and assist decision makers in preparing the chosen approach for execution. When applicable, it should identify, assess, and rate the qualifications of potentially qualified, interested external contractors. It should also search the client's environment for political barriers, financial or legal constraints, and available resources. The input evaluation's overall intent is to help decision makers examine alternative strategies for addressing the assessed needs of targeted beneficiaries, choose (as applicable) a qualified external contractor, evolve a workable plan and appropriate budget, and develop an accountability record for defending its procedural and resource plans and, as applicable, selection of an external contractor. Another important function of an input evaluation is to help program leaders avoid the wasteful practice of pursuing proposed innovations that predictably would fail or at least waste resources.

Evaluators conduct input evaluations in several stages that occur in no set sequence. An evaluator might first review the state of practice in meeting the specified needs and objectives. This could include a number of possible components:

- Reviewing relevant literature.
- Visiting exemplary programs.
- Consulting experts and representatives of government.
- Querying pertinent information services (especially, those on the World Wide Web).
- Reviewing a pertinent article in *Consumer Reports* or similar publications that critically review relevant available products and services.
- Inviting and supporting the development of creative proposals from involved staff.
- Contacting pertinent professional organizations to identify qualified contractors who might be interested and available to conduct the needed project.

Evaluators might organize this information in a special planning room. They might engage a special study group to investigate it or conduct a special planning seminar to analyze the material. The evaluators would use the information to assess whether potentially acceptable solution strategies (and external contractors) exist. They would rate promising approaches on relevant criteria. Examples are:

- Responsiveness to assessed needs of targeted beneficiaries
- Amelioration of targeted organizational problems
- Responsiveness to stated goals
- Utilization of special funding programs or other relevant opportunities

- Potential effectiveness
- Cost
- Political viability
- Administrative feasibility
- Staffing
- Potential for important impacts outside the local area

Next, the evaluation planning team could advise the decision makers about whether they should seek a novel solution and possibly, also, an external contractor to proceed with the program. In seeking an innovation, the client and evaluators might determine criteria that the innovation should meet, structure a request for proposal, obtain competing proposals, and rate them on the chosen criteria. Subsequently, the evaluators might rank the potentially acceptable proposals and suggest how the institution could combine their best features. They might conduct a hearing to obtain additional information. They could ask staff and administrators to express concerns or make recommendations. They would appraise resources and barriers that the institution should consider when installing the intervention. The planning group could then use the accumulated information to design and budget for what they see as the best combination strategy and action plan.

Criteria for evaluating detailed funding proposals could include:

- Grasp of what type of intervention is needed
- Quality of the technical plan
- Qualifications of the proposed project director
- Qualifications of supporting staff
- Positive attitudes of staff toward the project
- Adequate provision for stakeholder engagement
- Reasonableness of the projected cost
- Sufficiency of funds for the project
- Adequacy and appropriateness of the budget
- **Track record** of the proposing group
- **Political sensitivity** and **viability**
- Innovativeness
- Administrative feasibility of the work plan
- Appropriateness of the schedule
- Sufficiency of organizational support

- Adequate arrangements for fiscal accountability
- Provisions for process and product evaluations

Input evaluations have several applications, the chief one being the preparation of a proposal for submission to a funding organization or policy board. Another application is to assess one's existing practice, whether or not it seems satisfactory, against what is being done elsewhere and proposed in the literature. Input evaluation has been used in the Dallas Independent School District; the Des Moines, Iowa, public schools; and the Shaker Heights, Ohio, School District. These institutions used it to decide whether locally generated proposals for innovation would likely be cost-effective. The public school district for Detroit also used input evaluation to generate and assess alternative architectural designs for new school buildings. The United States Marine Corps used input evaluation to replace the Corps' system for evaluating officers and enlisted personnel; they did so by identifying and evaluating a wide range of personnel evaluation systems used by other military branches and by industry; engaging planning teams to invent new creative approaches; evaluating the capacity of all identified approaches to address the Corps' need for the new system; judging the alternatives against professional standards for sound personnel evaluations; and, ultimately, selecting and installing the preferred new approach. In addition to informing and facilitating planning decisions, input evaluation records help authorities defend their choice of one course of action above another or one contractor over another. Administrators and policy boards can find input evaluation records useful when they must publicly defend sizable expenditures for new programs.

The **Advocate Teams Technique** is a procedure designed specifically for conducting input evaluations. This technique is especially applicable when institutions lack the effective means to meet targeted needs and stakeholders hold opposing views on what strategy the institution should adopt. The evaluators convene two or more teams of experts and stakeholders. They give the teams the objectives, background data on needs, specifications for a solution strategy, and criteria for evaluating the teams' proposed strategies. They may staff these teams to match members' preferences and expertise to proposed alternative strategies; evaluators should do so, especially if stakeholders severely disagree about what type of approach to accept. The advocate teams then compete, preferably in isolation from one another, to develop a winning solution strategy. A

panel of experts and stakeholders rates the advocate team reports against the predetermined criteria. The institution might also field-test the teams' proposed strategies. Subsequently, the institution would choose and operationalize the winning strategy. Alternatively, it might combine and operationalize the best features of the two or more competing strategies.

The Advocate Teams Technique provides a systematic approach for:

- Designing interventions to meet assessed needs
- Generating and assessing competing strategies
- Promoting innovation and creativity
- Exploiting bias and competition in a constructive search for effective alternatives
- Addressing controversy and breaking down stalemates that stand in the way of progress
- Involving personnel from the adopting system in devising, assessing, and operationalizing improvement programs
- Documenting why a particular solution strategy was selected

Additional information, including a technical manual and the results of five field tests of the technique, is available in Reinhard (1972).

Process Evaluation

A process evaluation includes an ongoing check on a plan's implementation and documentation of the process. One objective is to provide staff and managers feedback about the extent to which they are carrying out planned activities on schedule, as planned and budgeted, and efficiently. Another is to detect flaws in the guiding plans and to guide staff in improving the procedural and budgetary plans appropriately. Typically, staff cannot determine all aspects of such plans when a project starts. Also, they must alter the plans if some initial decisions are unsound or not feasible. Still another objective is to periodically assess the extent to which participants accept and can carry out their roles. A process evaluation should contrast activities and expenditures with the plan and budget, describe implementation problems, and assess how well the staff addressed them. It should document and analyze the effort's costs. Finally, it should report how observers and participants judged the process's quality.

The linchpin of a sound process evaluation is the process evaluator. More often than not, staff failure to obtain guidance for implementation and to document their activities and expenditures is due to failure to assign an appropriate person to do this work. Sponsors and institutions too often assume erroneously that the managers and staff will adequately evaluate process as a normal part of their assignments. They can routinely do some review and documentation through activities such as staff meetings, minutes of the meetings, and periodic accounting reports. However, these do not fulfill the requirements of a sound, systematic process evaluation reflecting an independent perspective. Experience has shown that usually project staffs can effectively meet the requirements of a sound process evaluation only by assigning an evaluator to provide ongoing review, feedback, and documentation.

A process evaluator has much work to do in monitoring and documenting an intervention's activities and expenditures. Initially, the process evaluator may review the relevant strategy, work plans, budget, and any prior background evaluation to identify what planned activities they should monitor. Possible examples are delivering services to beneficiaries, hiring and training staff, supervising staff, conducting staff meetings, monitoring and inspecting work flow, securing and maintaining equipment, ordering and distributing materials, developing other needed materials, controlling finances, documenting expenditures, managing program information, and keeping constituents informed.

With process evaluation issues such as those mentioned above in mind, the process evaluator could develop a general schedule of data collection activities and begin carrying them out. Initially, these activities probably should be as unobtrusive as possible so as not to threaten staff, get in their way, or constrain or interfere with the process. As rapport develops, the process evaluator can use a more structured approach. At the outset, the process evaluator should obtain from the program's director an overview of how the work is going. He or she could visit and observe centers of activity, review pertinent documents (especially the work plans, budgets, accounting reports, and minutes of meetings), attend staff meetings, and interview key participants. The evaluator then could prepare a brief report summarizing the process evaluation's data collection plan, initial findings, and observed issues. He or she should highlight existing or impending process problems that the staff should address. The evaluator could then deliver this report at a staff meeting.

The evaluator might invite the staff's director to lead a discussion of the report. The project team could then use the report for decision making as it sees fit. Also, the process evaluator could apprise project staff of plans for further data collection and the subsequent report and ask them to react to the plans. Staff could then identify what information they would find most useful at the next meeting. They could also suggest how the evaluator could best collect certain items of information, and they might agree to facilitate the collection of needed information. Subsequent methods to collect process information might include observations, **staff-kept diaries,** interviews, or questionnaires. The evaluator should ask the staff when they could best use the next evaluation report.

Using this feedback, the evaluator would schedule future feedback sessions. He or she would modify the data collection plan as appropriate and proceed accordingly. The evaluator should continually show that process evaluation helps staff carry out its work through a kind of quality assurance and ongoing problem-solving process. He or she should also sustain the effort to document the process and lessons learned.

The evaluator should periodically report on how well the staff carried out the work plan and integrated it into the surrounding organizational environment. He or she should describe main deviations from the plan and should note variations concerning how different persons, groups, or sites are carrying out the plan. He or she should also characterize and assess the ongoing planning activity and record of expenditures.

Staff members use process evaluation to guide activities, correct faulty plans, and maintain accountability records. Some managers use regularly scheduled process evaluation feedback sessions to keep staff on their toes and abreast of their responsibilities. Process evaluation records are useful for accountability, since funding agencies, policy boards, and constituents typically want objective and substantive confirmation of whether grantees did what they had proposed and expended allocated funds appropriately. Process evaluations can also help external audiences learn what was done in an enterprise and at what cost in case they want to conduct a similar effort. Such information is useful to new staff as part of their orientation to what has gone before. Moreover, process evaluation information is vital for interpreting product evaluation results. One needs to learn what was done in a project before judging why program outcomes turned out as they did.

Product Evaluation

The purpose of a product evaluation is to measure, interpret, and judge an enterprise's outcomes. Its main objectives are to ascertain the extent to which the evaluand met the needs of all the rightful beneficiaries and to assess the extent to which project goals were achieved. Feedback about outcomes is important both during an activity cycle and at its conclusion. A product evaluation should assess intended and unintended outcomes and positive and negative outcomes. Moreover, evaluators often should extend product evaluation, beyond the completion of a project work plan, to assess long-term outcomes.

A product evaluation should gather and analyze stakeholders' judgments of the enterprise. Sometimes it should compare the effort's outcomes with those of similar enterprises. Frequently, the client wants to know whether the enterprise achieved its goals and was worth the investment. If appropriate, evaluators should interpret whether poor implementation of the work plan caused poor outcomes. Finally, a product evaluation should usually view outcomes from several vantage points: in the aggregate, for subgroups, and sometimes for individuals.

Product evaluations follow no set algorithm, but many procedures are applicable. Evaluators should use a combination of procedures. This helps them make a comprehensive search for outcomes and cross-check the findings from use of different procedures.

To assess performance beyond goals, evaluators need to search for unanticipated outcomes, both positive and negative. They might conduct **hearings** or group interviews to generate hypotheses about the full range of outcomes and follow these up with **clinical investigations** intended to confirm or disconfirm the hypotheses. They might conduct case studies of the experiences of a carefully selected sample of participants to obtain an in-depth view of the program's effects. They might survey, by telephone or mail, a sample of participants to obtain their judgments of the service and their views of both positive and negative outcomes. They might ask participants to submit concrete examples of how the program or other service influenced their work or well-being. These could be written pieces, other work products, or new job status. The evaluator might engage observers to identify program and comparison groups' achievements. They might also compare identified program achievements with a comprehensive checklist of outcomes of similar programs or services. Also, they

might compare recently assessed outcomes with outcomes identified at one or more prior points in time. Trend analysis can be invaluable when outcome variables have been measured repeatedly (e.g., prior to, during, and after a period of intervention).

Evaluators might conduct a goal-free evaluation (Scriven, 1973). Accordingly, the evaluator would engage an investigator to determine the effects of an intervention. The evaluator purposely would not inform the goal-free investigator about the intervention's goals. The point is to prevent the investigator from developing tunnel vision focused on stated goals. The evaluator then contrasts identified effects with the program beneficiaries' assessed needs. This provides a unique approach to assessing the intervention's value, whatever its goals.

Program evaluation findings may be reported at different stages. Evaluators may submit interim reports during each program cycle. These reports should show the extent to which the intervention is addressing and meeting targeted needs and achieving project goals. End-of-cycle reports may sum up the results achieved. Such reports should interpret the results in light of assessed needs, costs incurred, and the extent to which the plan was successfully carried out. Evaluators may also submit follow-up reports to assess long-term outcomes. In such reports, evaluators might analyze the results in the aggregate, for subgroups, and for selected individuals.

People use product evaluations to decide whether a given program, project, service, or other enterprise is worth continuing, repeating, or extending to other settings. A product evaluation report also should provide direction for modifying the enterprise or replacing it so that the institution will more cost-effectively serve the needs of all members of the targeted beneficiaries. It should also help potential adopters decide whether the approach merits their serious consideration. Product evaluations have psychological implications. By showing signs of growth or superiority to competing approaches, they reinforce the efforts of both staff and program recipients; or they may dampen enthusiasm and reduce motivation when the results are poor.

Regarding the latter point, evaluators should not publicly release product evaluation findings too soon. A program requires time to achieve results for which it should be held accountable. Premature release of a product evaluation report might unjustly discourage continuation of the program because no results were found. If public reports of product evaluation are delayed for a reasonable amount of time, the evaluator might discover late-blooming, important outcomes that would support the program's continuation. In addition, an evaluator can stifle program staff members' creativity by being overzealous in conducting and reporting product evaluations during a program's exploratory stage. Of course, the evaluator can respond appropriately to staff requests for ongoing formative product evaluation findings; usually, such early interim results should be shared only with the program's staff members as an aid to their quest for success. Rules of thumb are that evaluators should be low key in conducting product evaluations early in a program and should not report product evaluation findings beyond the program staff until they have had ample time to install and stabilize procedural plans. The evaluator should distribute product evaluation findings to right-to-know audiences after the program has had a fair chance to mature and produce its outcomes. Clearly, evaluators need to exercise professional judgment and discretion in deciding matters of conducting and reporting product evaluation findings.

Figure 2.3 illustrates the appropriate relationship between the relative prevalence of process and product evaluations across an enterprise's time line. As shown, process evaluation appropriately dominates in the early

> **BOX 2.3. The CIPP Model as an Evaluation Guide**
>
> The CIPP Model is unique as an evaluation guide as it allows evaluators to evaluate the program at different stages, namely: before the program commences by helping evaluators to assess needs and at the end of the program to assess whether or not the program had an effect, especially in meeting assessed needs.
>
> The CIPP Model allows you to ask formative questions at the beginning of the program, then later gives you a guide of how to evaluate the program's impact by allowing you to ask summative questions on all aspects of the program.
>
> - *Context:* What needs to be done? Vs. Were important needs addressed?
> - *Input:* How should it be done? Vs. Was a defensible design employed?
> - *Process:* Is it being done? Vs. Was the design well executed?
> - *Product:* Is it succeeding? Vs. Did the effort succeed?

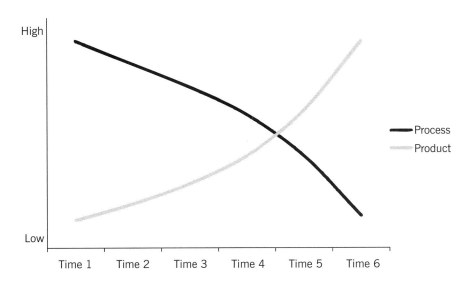

FIGURE 2.3. Hypothetical relationships of relative prevalence of process and product evaluation across an enterprise's time line.

stages of an evaluation, with product evaluation playing a much lesser role. As the evaluation matures, the relative prevalence of process and product evaluations reverses, with product evaluation increasing and process evaluation playing a less important role.

Product evaluation information is an essential component of an accountability report. When authorities document significant achievements, they can better convince community and funding organizations to provide additional financial and political support. If authorities learn that the intervention made no important gains, they can cancel the investment. This frees funds for worthy interventions. Moreover, other developers can use the product evaluation report to help decide whether it would be wise to pursue a similar course of action.

The CIPP Evaluation Model Checklist

The CIPP Evaluation Model Checklist, a comprehensive checklist for use in planning and assessing CIPP Model–based program evaluations, is available online (see the box at the end of the table of contents). The full-length checklist provides separate but correlated practical checkpoints for evaluators and clients to follow in carrying out their individual and joint evaluation activities.

Checklist 2.1 (at the end of this chapter) provides a summarized version of the CIPP Evaluation Model Checklist's checkpoints related to the evaluator's responsibilities. Although it provides a useful starting point for planning an evaluation based on the CIPP Model, evaluators are advised to consult and use the full-length checklist as they delve into detailed planning of an evaluation.

Advice on Applying the Full-Length CIPP Evaluation Model Checklist

The full-length CIPP Evaluation Model Checklist is a tool used by both evaluators and evaluation clients. This checklist is designed to facilitate collaboration by both parties in their individual and joint efforts to plan, carry through, and apply sound effective evaluations. In the early stages of planning an evaluation, both parties can walk through the checklist together as a guide for reviewing and fleshing out the evaluation's initial

evaluation design and, subsequently, for finalizing its budget and contract. Throughout the evaluation process, the checklist can help both parties uncover and address problems that may arise. We advise both evaluators and evaluation clients to study and make regular use of this checklist before, during, and following the evaluation process. They will find the checklist to be a useful, detailed guide for assuring the evaluation's integrity, soundness, utility, and impact. As needed, the evaluator and client should supplement their understanding of the checklist by consulting the related resources referenced in the body of the checklist and especially its appendix. In individual evaluation cases, either the evaluator or the client may initiate use of the checklist.

At a general level, the evaluator and client should review and discuss the relevant sets of checkpoints to develop a mutual understanding of their individual and joint evaluation responsibilities. As they proceed to address particular parts of the evaluation process, they should consult and apply the pertinent checklist components as needed. In this respect, each of the checklist's 12 main components is a distinct, subchecklist that provides guidance for the particular part of an evaluation (e.g., the budget, contractual agreements, context evaluation, input evaluation, process evaluation, impact evaluation, effectiveness evaluation, transportability evaluation, or metaevaluation). It cannot be overemphasized that, in almost all evaluations, the evaluator and client need to communicate throughout the entire evaluation process. The full-length CIPP Evaluation Model Checklist is an invaluable guide to facilitate such exchange and collaborative planning, as well as problem solving. In general, we advise evaluators and their clients to study, embrace, and use the checklist to plan and conduct sound evaluations that contribute effectively to program improvement and accountability and other intended beneficial uses of findings.

Summary

The CIPP Evaluation Model treats evaluation as an essential concomitant of improvement and accountability within a framework of appropriate values and a quest for clear, unambiguous answers. It responds to the reality that evaluations of innovative, evolving efforts typically cannot employ controlled, randomized experiments or work from published evaluation instruments, both of which yield far too little pertinent information; experiments focus narrowly on outcome variables, and published data collection instruments almost inevitably lack validity for an evaluation's specific questions. The CIPP Model is configured specially to enable and guide comprehensive, systematic examination of social and education programs that occur in the dynamic, septic conditions of the real world, not the controlled conditions of experimental psychology, double-blind experiments in medicine, and split-plot crop studies in agriculture. The model also allows **information collection** plans and devices to be tailored to the evaluation's particular questions and the evaluation needs of the client and other stakeholders. CIPP Model–based evaluations may use experimental designs and standardized tests in the context of a broader, more comprehensive approach to evaluation but only when the circumstances of the assessed project permit their appropriate use. Fundamentally, the model is keyed to professional standards for sound evaluation and requires that evaluations be evaluated against such standards.

The model sees evaluation as essential to societal progress and the well-being of individuals and groups. It contends that societal groups cannot make their programs, services, and products better unless they learn where they are weak and strong. Developers and service providers cannot be sure their goals are worthy unless they validate the goals' consistency with sound values and responsiveness to beneficiaries' assessed needs. Developers and service providers cannot make effective plans and wise investment of their time and resources if they do not identify and assess options. They cannot earn continued respect and support if they cannot show that they have responsibly carried out their plans and produced beneficial results. They cannot build on past experiences if they do not preserve, study, and act on lessons from failed and successful efforts. Nor can they convince consumers to buy or support their services and products unless their claims for the value of these services are valid and honestly reported. Institutional personnel cannot meet all of their evaluation needs if they do not both contract for external evaluations and build and apply capacity to conduct internal evaluations. Evaluators cannot defend their evaluative conclusions unless they key them to both sound information and clear, defensible values. Moreover, internal and external evaluators cannot maintain credibility for their evaluations if they do not subject them to metaevaluations against appropriate standards. The CIPP Model

employs multiple methods, is based on a wide range of applications, is supported by an extensive theoretical and pragmatic literature, and is operationalized in the referenced CIPP Evaluation Model Checklist. Above all, the CIPP Evaluation Model is keyed to the proposition that the evaluation's purpose is not only to prove but, more importantly, to improve.

REVIEW QUESTIONS • • • • • • • • • •

1. What are the similarities and differences between the concepts of needs assessment and context evaluation?

2. What is the essential meaning of input evaluation, and what are at least two illustrations of its use?

3. What is the Advocate Teams Technique, and what is its use in evaluations based on the CIPP Model?

4. What is the relationship between the concepts of context, input, process, and product evaluations and the concepts of formative and summative evaluations?

5. What are examples of the uses of process evaluations for formative and summative purposes?

6. What is meant by the CIPP Model's objectivist orientation?

7. What is the role of values in the CIPP Model, and how are these identified and applied?

8. What is meant by the claim that the CIPP Model is a social systems approach to evaluation, and what is the practical significance of this orientation?

9. List and define at least five procedures for engaging stakeholders in a program evaluation.

10. Suppose you were asked to conduct a product evaluation of a state's long-standing policy to prohibit smoking in public buildings. What might you look at within the product evaluation's subparts of impact/reach, effectiveness, sustainability, and transportability?

11. What is goal-free evaluation, and what is its potential and unique use in conducting an evaluation based on the CIPP Model?

12. What is the CIPP Model's concept of and rationale for supporting the role of the evaluation-oriented leader?

13. What is the CIPP Model's stance on the relative importance of proving versus improving a program's effectiveness?

14. As a capstone exercise, find a client who wants a particular program evaluated and is willing to engage with you in planning an evaluation of the program. Use the checklist in Table 2.8 to interview the client and develop a general plan for the evaluation. If the client is then serious about supporting and cooperating with an actual evaluation of the program, download the full-length CIPP Evaluation Model Checklist and apply it with the client to develop a specific plan for the evaluation.

SUGGESTIONS FOR FURTHER READING

Alkin, M. C. (2004). *Evaluation roots: Tracing theorists' views and influences.* Thousand Oaks, CA: Sage.

Alkin, M. C. (2013). *Evaluation roots: Tracing theorists' views and influences* (2nd ed.). Thousand Oaks, CA: Sage.

Candoli, I. C., Cullen, K., & Stufflebeam, D. L. (1997). *Superintendent performance evaluation: Current practice and directions for improvement.* Norwell, MA: Kluwer.

Evers, J. (1980). *A field study of goal-based and goal-free evaluation techniques.* Unpublished doctoral dissertation, Western Michigan University.

Guba, E. G., & Stufflebeam, D. L. (1968). Evaluation: The process of stimulating, aiding, and abetting insightful action. In R. Ingle & W. Gephart (Eds.), *Problems in the training of educational researchers.* Bloomington, IN: Phi Delta Kappa.

House, E. R., Rivers, W., & Stufflebeam, D. L. (1974). A counter-response to Kearney, Donovan, and Fisher. *Phi Delta Kappan, 56,* 19.

Joint Committee on Standards for Educational Evaluation. (2011). *The program evaluation standards: A guide for evaluators and evaluation users* (3rd ed.). Thousand Oaks, CA: Sage.

Nevo, D. (1974). *Evaluation priorities of students, teachers, and principals.* Unpublished doctoral dissertation, The Ohio State University, Columbus, OH.

Nicholson, T. (1989). Using the CIPP Model to evaluate reading instruction. *Journal of Reading, 32*(40), 312–318.

Reinhard, D. (1972). *Methodology development for input evaluation using advocate and design teams.* Unpublished doctoral dissertation, The Ohio State University, Columbus, OH.

Stufflebeam, D. L. (1966b, January). *Evaluation under Title I of the Elementary and Secondary Education Act of 1967.* Address delivered at the Title I Evaluation Conference sponsored by the Michigan State Department of Education, Lansing, MI.

Stufflebeam, D. L. (1967a). The use and abuse of evaluation in Title III. *Theory into Practice, 6,* 126–133.

Stufflebeam, D. L. (1969). Evaluation as enlightenment for decision making. In A. Walcott (Ed.), *Improving educational assessment and an inventory of measures of affective behavior.* Washington, DC: Association for Supervision and Curriculum Development.

Stufflebeam, D. L. (1971a). The use of experimental design in educational evaluation. *Journal of Educational Measurement, 8*(4), 267–274.

Stufflebeam, D. L. (1985). Stufflebeam's improvement-oriented evaluation. In D. L. Stufflebeam & A. J. Shinkfield, *Systematic evaluation* (pp. 151–207). Norwell, MA: Kluwer.

Stufflebeam, D. L. (1997). *Strategies for institutionalizing evaluation: Revisited.* Kalamazoo: Western Michigan University, The Evaluation Center.

Stufflebeam, D. L. (2000). Lessons in contracting for evaluations. *American Journal of Evaluation, 22*(1), 71–79.

Stufflebeam, D. L. (2002). CIPP evaluation model checklist. Available at *www.wmich.edu/evalctr/checklists.*

Stufflebeam, D. L. (2003a). The CIPP Model for evaluation. In T. Kellaghan & D. L. Stufflebeam (Eds.), *The international handbook of educational evaluation* (pp. 31–62). Norwell, MA: Kluwer.

Stufflebeam, D. L. (2003b). Institutionalizing evaluation in schools. In T. Kellaghan & D. L. Stufflebeam (Eds.), *The international handbook of educational evaluation* (pp. 775–806). Norwell, MA: Kluwer.

Stufflebeam, D. L. (2004). The 21st-century CIPP Model: Origins, development, and use. In M. C. Alkin (Ed.), *Evaluation roots* (pp. 245–266). Thousand Oaks, CA: Sage.

Stufflebeam, D. L. (2005). CIPP Model (context, input, process, product). In S. Mathison (Ed.), *Encyclopedia of evaluation* (pp. 60–65). Thousand Oaks, CA: Sage.

Stufflebeam, D. L. (2013). The 21st-century CIPP Model: Origins, development, and use. In M. C. Alkin (Ed.), *Evaluation roots* (2nd ed., pp. 243–260). Thousand Oaks, CA: Sage.

Stufflebeam, D. L., & Coryn, L. S. (2014). *Evaluation theory, models, and applications* (2nd ed.). San Francisco: Jossey-Bass.

Stufflebeam, D. L., Foley, W. J., Gephart, W. J., Guba, E. G., Hammond, R. L., Merriman, H. O., et al. (1971). *Educational evaluation and decision making.* Itasca, IL: Peacock.

Stufflebeam, D. L., Jaeger, R. M., & Scriven, M. S. (1992, April). *A retrospective analysis of a summative evaluation of NAGB's pilot project to set achievement levels on the National Assessment of Educational Progress.* Paper presented at the annual conference of the American Educational Research Association, San Francisco, CA.

Stufflebeam, D. L., & Webster, W. J. (1988). Evaluation as an administrative function. In N. Boyan (Ed.), *Handbook of research on educational administration* (pp. 569–601). White Plains, NY: Longman.

Webster, W. J. (1975, March). *The organization and functions of research and evaluation in large urban school districts.* Paper presented at the annual conference of the American Educational Research Association, Washington, DC.

Zhang, G., Zeller, N., Griffith, R., Metcalf, D., Shea, C., Williams, J., et al. (2010, October). *Using the CIPP Model as a comprehensive framework to guide the planning, implementation, and assessment of service-learning programs.* Paper presented at the annual conference of the National Evaluation Institute, Williamsburg, VA.

CHECKLIST 2.1. A Summary Version of the CIPP Evaluation Model Checklist

Directions: Review the following checkpoints with your client and check (✓) the ones that are applicable to the evaluation you are planning. Then proceed to work out your evaluation plan. For additional, specific guidance download and use the full-length CIPP Evaluation Model Checklist, available online (see the box at the end of the table of contents). Note that the CIPP Model's product evaluation component is divided into its subparts of impact, effectiveness, sustainability, and transportability evaluations.

___	**1. Designing Evaluations**	Develop an initial, general evaluation design to provide direction for budgeting and contracting the evaluation. As the evaluation proceeds add specificity to the design to assure its utility, feasibility, propriety, accuracy, and accountability.
___	**2. Budgeting Evaluations**	Determine as completely as possible the funds needed to complete the evaluation at high levels of quality, professionalism, and fiscal accountability.
___	**3. Contracting Evaluations**	Ground CIPP Model evaluations in explicit, printed advance agreements with the client, and, as needed, upgrade the agreements throughout the evaluation.
___	**4. Context Evaluation**	As needed, design, conduct, and report a context evaluation to assess needs, problems, assets, opportunities, area dynamics, and program goals.
___	**5. Input Evaluation**	Identify and assess alternative goal-achievement strategies and subsequently assess and provide feedback on the client's management plan and budget.
___	**6. Process Evaluation**	Monitor, document, assess, and provide feedback on the program staff's implementation of the adopted program plan.
___	**7. Impact Evaluation**	Assess the program's reach to the targeted beneficiaries and its impacts on the program's environment.
___	**8. Effectiveness Evaluation**	Document, assess, and report on the quality, cost-effectiveness, and significance of program outcomes.
___	**9. Sustainability Evaluation**	Assess and report the extent to which the program's contributions are or will be institutionalized and sustained over time.
___	**10. Transportability Evaluation**	Assess and report on the extent to which the program's approach has been or could be successfully applied elsewhere.
___	**11. Feedback Workshops**	Plan and conduct periodic, face-to-face or teleconference feedback sessions to engage the client group in reviewing draft evaluation plans and reports for their accuracy and clarity. Use the obtained feedback to improve the assessed evaluation materials.
___	**12. The Final Synthesis Evaluation Report**	Compile and disseminate to right-to-know audiences a summative evaluation report that reports what was attempted, done, and accomplished; what lessons were learned; the bottom-line assessment of the program; and the extent to which the evaluation adhered to the metaevaluation standards.
___	**13. Metaevaluation**	Assess and attest to the extent to which the evaluation has met, partially met, or not met each of the 30 Joint Committee (2011) program evaluation standards. Also, advise the client to obtain an independent metaevaluation of the evaluation.

CHAPTER 3

A Case Illustrating Application of the CIPP Model to Evaluate a Self-Help Housing Project

"The Spirit of Consuelo: I want to spend my heaven doing good on Earth."
—CONSUELO ZOBEL ALGER

This chapter illustrates and explains the CIPP Model's correct, effective application based on an 8-year evaluation of the Consuelo Foundation's self-help housing project for 75 low-income families in Hawaii. Ultimately, the foundation used the evaluation both to assure the project's success and to strengthen the foundation's approach to evaluating other projects in Hawaii and the Philippines. The chapter identifies 11 key ingredients that contributed to the subject evaluation's effectiveness.

Overview

Evaluation is an essential part of the Consuelo Foundation's history of developing and delivering effective, values-based services to many poor people and abused and neglected women and children in Hawaii and the Philippines. This chapter describes the Foundation's use of the CIPP Model to evaluate its flagship project, titled **Ke Aka Ho'ona** (The Spirit of Consuelo).[1]

That evaluation, spanning 8 years from 1994 through 2002, assessed the Foundation's first, major project. It was a self-help housing and **community development** project for low-income families in Hawaii. The 2002 report on that evaluation—by Stufflebeam, Gullickson, and Wingate—is titled *The Spirit of Consuelo:*

An Evaluation of Ke Aka Ho'ona. That report is the exemplar referenced throughout this chapter. Interested persons may obtain and study a copy of the report, which is available from The Evaluation Center, Western Michigan University, Kalamazoo, Michigan [269-345-3266; *http://wmich.edu/evaluation*].

The remainder of this chapter summarizes the **Ke Aka Ho'ona** project and references the evaluation of Ke Aka Ho'ona to highlight 11 important ingredients of the Foundation's approach to and use of systematic evaluation. These include evaluation-oriented leadership; grounding project planning and evaluations in explicit values; using professional standards to guide and judge evaluations; employing a planning grant to focus, design, and budget an evaluation; adopting and applying an explicit, proven approach to evaluation; employing multiple qualitative and quantitative information collection methods; reporting formative and summative findings; budgeting adequately and frugally for evaluation; employing a range of **evaluation expertise**; and using evaluation findings for improvement, **accountability,** and recording and applying lessons learned.

The Ke Aka Ho'ona Project

The Ke Aka Ho'ona project had a number of remarkable features. The project required the husband and wife of each involved family (or sometimes another pair of builders, such as two brothers) to devote 10 hours each Saturday and Sunday over a period of 10 months to building their house. Children were not allowed at the building site, and each family had to arrange for the care of the children during the weekends when parents were away constructing the houses. Accordingly, the families sacrificed time away from their children and worked long hours each week—typically in the hot sun—to obtain the long-range benefits of home ownership. Many of the builders had no prior construction experience, and some were quite out of shape considering the hard physical labor they would experience over the 10-month period. The work they performed in building their own houses was credited in the amount of about $7,500 of sweat equity against their home mortgage (of about $50,000); also, their involvement in constructing most parts of their house was deemed important for learning how to keep their homes in good repair. From its outset, the project required all participants to subscribe to covenants and rules for producing and maintaining high-quality houses; keeping properties in good repair; and keeping the community safe and free of violence, drug and alcohol abuse, crime, and domestic abuse. Moreover, the project focused heavily and effectively on the positive growth and development of the community's children and stressed the importance of giving back to help needy people in the larger community outside Ke Aka Ho'ona.

Evaluation Ingredient 1: Evaluation-Oriented Leadership

In 1993, Patti Lyons, president of the **Consuelo Foundation,** invited the Western Michigan University Eval-

uation Center to evaluate the Ke Aka Ho'ona project. Because the Center was conducting, a 7-year study of housing rehabilitation for the John D. and Catherine T. MacArthur Foundation (a rehabilitation being carried out by Chicago's Local Initiatives Support Corporation and grass-roots community development corporations throughout Chicago) the Center's staff members were immediately interested to learn about similar work in Hawaii.

Though funded at a level of more than $10 million, the housing work in Chicago had been an uphill struggle. It was one thing to rehab rundown houses in a slum area, but it was quite another matter to place poor families in the houses and see them succeed in maintaining the houses and also bringing order, safety, and stability to their crime-ridden neighborhoods. Unfortunately, many of Chicago's previously rehabbed houses in disadvantaged neighborhoods had deteriorated and taken on their former blighted status. As expressed by an official of Chicago's South Shore Bank, most inner-city rehab projects were prone to fail, not only because of the crime in the streets, but because the persons placed in the houses lacked employment and employable skills. He observed that without resources for maintaining the properties, families could enjoy the houses for a while, but inevitably they would fail to keep them up. Also, fixing up old houses had little to do with combating the deeper problems of crime, drugs, and poverty. This was especially so when isolated rehabbed houses were interspersed among rundown properties in slum neighborhoods. (It is noteworthy that the Consuelo Foundation's Ke Aka Ho'ona project produced 75 houses on a single 12-acre plot. Like the Chicago project, Ke Aka Ho'ona occurred in an area with high levels of poverty and crime. However, because the houses were concentrated in a single area, the Ke Aka Ho'ona houses became a fenced community that acquired a measure of insularity from the negative influences of the surrounding, problem-filled Waianae Coast environment.)

As The Evaluation Center's leaders considered President Lyons's invitation, they wondered if she and her colleagues had found or would find ways to provide housing for poor people so that over time they would maintain their homes, pay for them, and build a safe, healthy community environment for their families. The Center's staff members were glad to learn that President Lyons wanted answers to the same questions. Moreover, she wanted the evaluation to be built into her foundation's project from its beginning. And, possibly most important, she wanted the project's staff to make systematic use of evaluation throughout the project to identify and address problems as they arose, assure the project's eventual success, identify particular housing and community development approaches that could succeed for the long term, and record lessons learned that could be used to assure soundness of future efforts.

Throughout The Evaluation Center's experience in evaluating the Ke Aka Ho'ona project, Patty Lyons effectively carried out the role of evaluation-oriented leader. She believed in the importance of obtaining candid, critical evaluation feedback throughout project development and implementation. She stressed the importance of systematic evaluation to the foundation's policymakers and staff members. She and her staff used evaluation throughout the project and beyond for decision making, for examining how the implementation of such decisions worked out in practice, for communicating progress to the foundation's board and other interested parties, and basically for problem solving and accountability. Moreover, she ensured that evaluations of foundation efforts would be grounded in explicit values and keyed to assessing the organization's success in pursuing and fulfilling its mission. Nothing is more important for an evaluation's success than having it commissioned, overseen, and used by evaluation-oriented leaders, such as President Patti Lyons.

Fortunately, a strong commitment to obtaining and using evaluation to ensure the success of the foundation's efforts permeated the entire Consuelo Foundation. Like President Lyons, board members and foundation staff were keenly focused on obtaining and applying lessons from targeted needs assessments and systematic assessments of project plans, processes, and outcomes. It was advantageous that this group of evaluation-oriented leaders was averse to using evaluation as window dressing; instead, they wanted honest feedback—both the bad news and the good—that they could use to set projects on a solid foundation, to guide and strengthen project operations, and ultimately to record lessons learned for future reference. Of course, they welcomed the evaluations' good news about the project's success as well as valuable lessons learned that they could share with other community development groups throughout the United States and across the world. One implication of evaluation-oriented leadership is that evaluation educators should deliver evaluation training to administrators as well as evaluators, through both preservice and in-service education programs.

Evaluation Ingredient 2: Values

The core term in evaluation is *values*. Ideally, evaluations assess enterprises in terms of explicit, defensible values. Such values form the basis for institutional missions, project goals, and project approaches. Unfortunately, many evaluation clients do not stipulate clear values for reference in structuring and evaluating their enterprises. This was not the case with the Consuelo Foundation. From the outset of The Evaluation Center's assignment for evaluating Ke Aka Ho'ona, in 1994, it was clear that all Consuelo Foundation efforts were grounded in and were expected to be evaluated against the foundation's core values.

The Consuelo Foundation had been founded in 1988 by its namesake, Mrs. Consuelo Zobel Alger. In defining her vision for the foundation, she stipulated that its mission was "to operate or support projects in Hawaii and the Philippines that improve the life of disadvantaged children, women, and families." She charged the foundation to especially serve the poorest of the poor and, in its Hawaii work, to give priority to native Hawaiians but also to serve persons of other ethnic backgrounds. She stated, "What matters in life is not great deeds, but great love. St. Therese of the Child Jesus did what I want to do in life . . . to let fall from heaven a shower of roses. My mission will begin after my death. I will spend my heaven doing good on Earth."[2]

Consistent with Mrs. Alger's mandate, the Consuelo Foundation's quest has been to help establish "communities in Hawaii and the Philippines in which disadvantaged children, women, and families achieve dignity, self-esteem, and self-sufficiency resulting in renewed hope for those who have lost it and hope to those who never had it." Flowing from this vision, the Consuelo Foundation was focused on three overarching project goals:

1. Reduce the incidence of child abuse and neglect and improve the quality of life of exploited children.
2. Strengthen families and neighborhoods.
3. Enhance the well-being and status of underprivileged women. (Consuelo Zobel Alger Foundation, 1999)

The Consuelo Foundation adopted a set of eight stated values to guide its work in pursuing the foundation's mission, vision, and goals: spirituality, individual worth, caring and nurturing, participation and reciprocity, prevention, creativity and innovation, teamwork and collaboration, and Philippine and Hawaii connectedness (Consuelo Zobel Alger Foundation, 1999).

Consistent with these values, The Evaluation Center evaluators stressed the foundation's holistic approach to serving the underprivileged. It has often been shown that in tackling deep-rooted and systemic social problems, piecemeal and quick-fix approaches have little lasting worth. Terry George, who served as the foundation's chief project officer during the early stages of the Ke Aka Ho'ona project, described the foundation's community development approach as follows:

> Our community development approach is comprehensive rather than piecemeal, preventive rather than palliative, and long-term rather than short-term. We also take an assets approach rather than a deficits approach to community building. In other words, we look for what is right in families and communities and seek to deepen that, rather than looking for what is wrong and seeking to treat that. We also believe that communities everywhere contain the talent and potential to solve their own problems if they adhere to common values and if they receive the kind of support they need to strengthen their capacity to work together. Our work, therefore, is in essence the building of capacities: in individuals, in families, and in communities. (George, 2000, p. 118)

Ke Aka Ho'ona initially served working poor families in the project's early increments. All of these families qualified for low-interest mortgages and thus did not represent the poorest of the poor that Consuelo Zobel Alger stipulated in her statement of the foundation's vision. However, in the final increments, the project included very poor families that could not qualify for mortgages but were accepted into the project on a rent-to-own basis. The Evaluation Center's staff judged this overall succession of first serving families with moderate levels of assets for success and subsequently serving higher-risk families to be appropriate and prudent. In our judgment, this new foundation needed to "learn to crawl before it walked," and that is what it did.

As evidenced earlier, in undertaking the evaluation assignment for the Consuelo Foundation, the Evaluation Center's staff found the organization's plans, overall approach, and efforts to be firmly grounded in a clear mission and set of defensible values that stemmed directly from Mrs. Alger's vision. The foundation's values helped the contracted evaluators to focus their collection, analysis, interpretation, and reporting of evaluative information in an appropriate way.

Evaluation Ingredient 3: Evaluation Standards

Just as projects should be grounded in explicit, defensible values, project evaluations should be guided by and assessed against professionally defined standards for sound evaluations. Accordingly, the contract for evaluating Ke Aka Ho'ona stipulated that the evaluation work would be keyed to the 30 Joint Committee (1994) *Program Evaluation Standards*. These standards are grouped into four categories:

1. *Utility:* The **utility standards** are intended to ensure that an evaluation will serve the information needs of intended users, while also ensuring that the focal project will be thoroughly examined for its quality and impact. The seven utility standards are labeled Stakeholder Identification, Evaluator Credibility, Information Scope and Selection, Values identification, Report Clarity, Report Timeliness and Dissemination, and Evaluation Impact.

2. *Feasibility:* The three feasibility standards are intended to ensure that an evaluation will be realistic, viable, prudent, diplomatic, and frugal. The labels of these standards are Practical Procedures, Political Viability, and Cost-Effectiveness.

3. *Propriety:* The eight propriety standards are intended to ensure that an evaluation will be conducted legally, ethically, and with due regard for the welfare of those involved in the evaluation, as well as those affected by its results. The labels of these standards are Service Orientation, Formal Agreements, **Rights of Human Subjects,** Human Interactions, Complete and Fair Assessment, Disclosure of Findings, Conflict of Interest, and Fiscal Responsibility.

4. *Accuracy:* The 12 accuracy standards are intended to ensure that an evaluation will reveal and convey technically adequate information about the features that determine a project's merit and worth. The Accuracy Standards are labeled Project Documentation, Context Analysis, Described Purposes and Procedures, Defensible Information Sources, Valid Information, Reliable Information, Systematic Information, Analysis of Quantitative Information, Analysis of Qualitative Information, **Justified Conclusions,** Impartial Reporting, and Metaevaluation.

(The 1994 Joint Committee *Program Evaluation Standards* did not break out the Accuracy category's Metaevaluation standard into the separate category of Evaluation Accountability that is found in the 2011 edition of the Joint Committee Project Evaluation Standards. Essentially, the 2011 Standards break out the 1994 edition's Metaevaluation standard into the three **Evaluation Accountability standards** of Evaluation Documentation, **Internal Metaevaluation,** and **External Metaevaluation.**)

The evaluation of Ke Aka Ho'ona was keyed to meeting the full range of the 1994 Joint Committee *Program Evaluation Standards.* The final evaluation report included the evaluators' documented judgments of whether the completed evaluation met, partially met, or did not meet each of the 30 Joint Committee standards. The evaluators also recommended to President Lyons that the foundation contract with an independent metaevaluator to evaluate the Evaluation Center's final report. Ideally, the foundation would have secured an independent metaevaluation of the evaluation in order to obtain assurance that the Center's conclusions and recommendations were fully justified and worthy of use for decision making and issuing public communications. However, the foundation's president and board deemed such corroborative assessment as unnecessary, based on their confidence in the evaluation's compliance with accepted standards of the evaluation profession.

Evaluation Ingredient 4: Metaevaluation

Unfortunately, in our experience, client groups are reluctant to fund independent metaevaluations. A basic recommendation of this chapter is that in the initial negotiation process the evaluator should strongly advise the client to arrange for and independently fund an external evaluator to conduct an independent metaevaluation of the project evaluation. The most important role for such an external metaevaluator is to deliver a summative metaevaluation report to help the client and other stakeholders judge the relevance and validity of the final evaluation findings. In some projects, it can also be useful to engage the independent metaevaluator to conduct formative metaevaluations throughout the project to help guide the project evaluation and assure its soundness.

Whether or not the client funds an independent metaevaluation, the project evaluator should conduct for-mative metaevaluation, keyed to professional standards for evaluations, to guide and continually strengthen the evaluation work, as needed. Ultimately, at the evaluation's end, the project evaluators should append to the final report their attestation of the extent to which the evaluation met each of the standards that guided the evaluation. The evaluator should back up each of these metaevaluation judgments with a statement of the factual basis for the judgment. An appendix to the report titled *The Spirit of Consuelo: An Evaluation of Ke Aka Ho'ona* referenced throughout this chapter includes a completed Attestation Form that presents The Evaluation Center teams' attestation of the extent to which their evaluation of Ke Aka Ho'ona ultimately met each of the 30 Joint Committee (1994) program evaluation standards.

As noted earlier, the project evaluator bears clear responsibility for metaevaluation. He or she should:

- Conduct ongoing formative metaevaluation to help assure that all relevant evaluation standards are being met.
- Fully and transparently document the evaluation process and results.
- Cooperate with the external metaevaluator, if one has been appointed, to help meet her or his information needs.
- Append to the final evaluation report an attestation—with justifications—of whether the evaluation met, partially met, or failed to meet each of the relevant metaevaluation standards.

The main points in this section are that the client and evaluator should agree at the outset that the contracted evaluation work will be grounded in professional standards for evaluation. The project evaluator should consistently adhere to the requirements of the standards; fully document the actual evaluation process; and assess her or his evaluation both formatively to guide the evaluation and summatively to assess and report how well the evaluation adhered to the standards. Finally, the client should contract with an external evaluator to conduct at least an independent, summative metaevaluation of the project evaluation and release the summative metaevaluation findings of both the project evaluator and the independent metaevaluator, if one was appointed, to all right-to-know audiences for their review and use.

Evaluation Ingredient 5: Evaluation Planning Grant

Upon being invited to conduct a comprehensive, long-term evaluation of Ke Aka Ho'ona, The Evaluation Center's director requested and obtained an initial short-term planning grant. This grant enabled him to become acquainted with the project, its beneficiaries and staff, as well as the project's environment before designing, budgeting, and contracting for the long-term evaluation. Such initial planning grants support evaluators, clients, and other stakeholders to develop sound understanding, rapport, and agreements on which to plan and budget the ensuing, often multiyear evaluation work. Nevertheless, having worked out a sound plan and budget to guide the subsequent evaluation work, it remains important to revisit the evaluation plan and budget regularly and revise them as appropriate.

Providing a selected external evaluator with a planning grant is a more prudent way to plan for an evaluation than is the typical **Request for Proposal (RFP)** approach. Whereas the grant approach allows the evaluator, as he or she plans the evaluation, to learn firsthand of stakeholder needs and interests and of a project's context, the relatively sterile RFP approach typically causes the prospective evaluators to guess about important focusing matters and often leads to key assumptions that later prove wrong. What is more, the RFP approach prevents evaluators, at the outset of their planning, from developing a rapport with the project's stakeholders and consulting them in the course of identifying priority questions and intended uses of findings and formulating key evaluation planning decisions. The RFP approach allegedly affords a sponsor the opportunity to consider the relative merits of alternative evaluators and different evaluation plans. But this is not a strong advantage when the competing evaluation contractors draw up their plans in the absence of any meaningful exchange with the project's stakeholders. Of course, in the case of providing a single, selected evaluator with a planning grant, the client should carefully select an evaluator with relevant experience and excellent credentials. Nevertheless, the sponsoring organization can hedge its bet in choosing an evaluator by first only agreeing to an initial, short-term, small planning grant.

A decided advantage of a small **evaluation planning grant** is that both the client and evaluator can terminate their relationship if the evaluation planning project does not culminate in a mutually satisfactory evaluation plan and set of supporting financial agreements. In such an unfortunate circumstance, the "wastes" of client resources and evaluator time are minimal, compared to what could be the case in implementing a defective evaluation plan. Also, the client can use lessons learned from an aborted evaluation planning effort to search out and negotiate better evaluation agreements with a different evaluator.

In securing a preliminary grant for planning the evaluation of the Ke Aka Ho'ona self-help housing project, The Evaluation Center requested and obtained a cost-reimbursable grant of $12,000. Such grants should be both small and cost-reimbursable, so that only those funds needed to conduct the planning are expended. In the case of the Ke Aka Ho'ona planning effort, The Evaluation Center used only about half of the authorized $12,000 amount.

Clearly, the recommendation that client groups provide evaluation planning grants has its limits. It reflects the unique circumstance in which the client chooses the evaluator before seeing any proposal. Sometimes, laws or codes require a sponsor to seek and assess multiple evaluation proposals, so that a fair level of competition is offered and possible charges of selecting cronies or friendly critics are dispelled. In addition, the sponsor is thereby able to choose the most cost-effective proposal from an array of proposals. Even in the face of first seeking and assessing multiple proposals, however, the client group should consider the likely merits of subsequently providing the tentatively chosen evaluator with an evaluation planning grant. In such cases, the first round of evaluation proposals should be examined to assess the proposer's track record and qualifications for conducting an evaluation of the type being sought. The subsequent evaluation planning grant should focus on producing a responsive, sound evaluation design, work plan, and budget. However, often the client should retain the option of funding or not funding the follow-up evaluation, depending on the evaluation plan's quality, responsiveness to client needs, and feasibility.

Evaluation Ingredient 6: A Systematic Evaluation Approach

Foundations, school districts, government agencies, and other organizations can benefit substantially by adopting a systematic approach to evaluation. Typically, project evaluations are team efforts. Usually, they also engage a wide range of stakeholders in various aspects of the evaluation process. Effective involvement of interested and involved parties in obtaining and using evaluation findings requires that they share a common concept of evaluation, including its key terms and guiding standards. Such a shared evaluation approach facilitates efficient communication and cooperation in an evaluation. In adopting a particular evaluation approach, an organization has the enduring advantage of being able to use it repeatedly, which helps the organization's board and staff to learn and embrace a common evaluation language and to cooperate efficiently and effectively in the conduct and use of the organization's evaluations.

Foundations and other organizations may choose from a number of viable, published approaches to evaluation (Stufflebeam & Coryn, 2014; Stufflebeam & Shinkfield, 2007).[3] The evaluation of Ke Aka Ho'ona employed the CIPP Evaluation Model (see Chapter 2 and Stufflebeam, 2000a). This model presents a comprehensive approach to assessing *context,* including the nature, extent, and criticality of beneficiaries' needs, relevant assets, and pertinent environmental forces; *inputs,* including the responsiveness and strength of project strategies, work plans, and resources; *process,* including documentation and assessment of project operations; and *product,* including the extent, desirability, and significance of intended and unintended outcomes. To gain additional insights into project outcomes, as seen in Chapter 2 of this book, the product evaluation component may be divided into four parts: (1) impact, regarding the project's reach to the intended beneficiaries; (2) effectiveness, regarding the quality, desirability, and significance of outcomes; (3) sustainability, concerning the project's institutionalization and long-term viability; and (4) transportability, concern-

ing the utility of the project's meritorious features in other settings.

The framework for evaluating Ke Aka Ho'ona included proactive and retrospective applications of context, input, process, and product evaluations. Thus, the evaluation would provide ongoing formative evaluation to guide ongoing project operations and an end-of-project summative evaluation to meet project accountability requirements and inform interested parties of the project's assessed value.

Evaluation Ingredient 7: Multiple Data Collection Methods

Multiple methods were used to gather information for each component of the evaluation of the Ke Aka Ho'ona project. Table 3.1 lists the primary methods used. The X's in the matrix's cells indicate which parts of the evaluation model were addressed by which methods. The aim was to address each type of evaluation with at least two data collection methods.

Table 3.2 shows the data collection methods in relationship to project years, with the X's indicating which methods were applied during each project year. Not every method was applied every year. However, at least three methods were employed during each project year. It is noteworthy that the evaluation's collection of pertinent information was reduced by discontinuation of the environmental analysis and project profile procedures about midway into the evaluation, due to the foundation's need to reduce the evaluation's costs.

Each method is characterized and discussed below.

Environmental analysis involved gathering contextual information in the forms of available documents

TABLE 3.1. Data Collection Methods Related to Evaluation Types

Method	Context	Input	Process	Impact	Effectiveness	Sustainability	Transportability
Environmental analysis	X		X				
Project profile		X				X	
Traveling observer			X	X	X	X	
Case studies			X		X	X	
Stakeholder interviews	X	X	X	X	X	X	X
Goal-free evaluation			X		X		X
Photographs	X	X	X	X	X	X	X

TABLE 3.2. Data Collection Methods in Relationship to Project Years

Method	1994	1995	1996	1997	1998	1999	2000	2001	2002
Environmental analysis	X		X						
Project profile	X	X	X	X	X				
Traveling observer	X	X	X	X	X	X	X	X	
Case studies		X		X			X		
Stakeholder interviews	X	X	X	X	X	X	X	X	
Goal-free evaluation			X		X				
Task/reports/feedback workshops	X	X	X	X	X	X	X	X	X
Synthesis/final report							X	X	X

and data concerning such matters as area economics, population characteristics, related projects and services, and the needs and problems of the targeted population. It also involved interviewing persons in various roles in the area and visiting pertinent projects and services. Individuals interviewed for this aspect of the evaluation included area school teachers and administrators, government officials, Catholic Charities' personnel, Department of Hawaiian Home Lands personnel, local social workers, the local police, and others.

The foundation considered the environmental analysis to be important and useful early in the Ke Aka Ho'ona project, when the foundation was still clarifying the target population and examining its needs relating to Hawaii's economy and social/cultural context. The procedure was discontinued when the foundation experienced serious financial problems, especially in its stockholdings in the Philippines, and needed to cut back the evaluation as well as other foundation efforts. Foundation staff decided that a continuing environmental analysis was not among their high priorities and instructed the evaluators to concentrate on observing and analyzing what was happening at the Ke Aka Ho'ona project site. This change in the evaluation somewhat limited the evaluation's ability to assess the relevance of a Ke Aka Ho'ona approach to Hawaii's evolving economic and social environment.

A **project profile** characterized the project, including its mission, goals, plan, constituents, staff, timetable, resources, progress to date, accomplishments, and recognitions. This was the evaluation's qualitative version of a regularly updated (largely qualitative) database. From the evaluation's beginning, the evaluation team wrote and periodically updated a relatively large

and growing document that profiled the project as it was established and as it evolved. Especially included was commentary concerning which project features remained stable, which ones changed, and what new ones were added. Early in the evaluation, the evaluators prepared the Project Profile report, submitted the draft to the foundation's staff, and discussed it with them. In following years, as the report grew in size, the staff found that they were reading a lot of what they had read before. For subsequent editions, they therefore asked for updates that highlighted the information that had changed or was added, so they could verify its accuracy and clarity. Like the environmental analysis, the project profile procedure was also discontinued during the final 3 years of the evaluation because of the need to cut costs. In the future, it would seem wise to set up and maintain a project profile as a computerized database. Clients could then access and use the profiled information on a need-to-know basis, and the evaluators would be able to maintain an up-to-date profile of an evolving project and draw information from it for their various reports, including the final summative evaluation report.

Traveling observers design and carry out a systematic procedure to monitor and assess both project implementation and project outcomes along the way, while also gathering information from groups and enterprises outside the project area. The traveling observer is a method in that, as in naturalistic inquiry and ethnography, the observer is the instrument of data collection. These observers are referred to as traveling observers when their assignment includes traveling across sites to collect information about the project and its surrounding environment. Observers who conduct their work solely at a single project site are called resident researchers. Typically, both types of observers serve as liaisons for evaluation team members who visit the project site periodically. Both traveling observers and resident researchers develop and employ an explicit protocol—called a **Traveling Observer Handbook**—that is tailored to the questions, information needs, and circumstances of the particular evaluation. Over time, three different traveling observers participated in evaluating Ke Aka Ho'ona. These individuals performed the following tasks:

- Conducted interviews with project participants; maintained a newspaper clippings file pertaining to the project or pertinent environmental issues.
- Served as advance persons for preparing the way for the lead investigators to be both efficient and effective during their periodic **site visits.**
- Collected and reviewed documents pertaining to the project.
- Especially helped identify and assess the project's effects on the project's children and youth.
- Kept a photographic record of developments at the project site, including especially progress in construction, but also meetings and other interactions among project participants.
- Conducted interviews pertaining to case studies involving selected families in the community.
- Conducted interviews with representatives of various groups throughout the island of Oahu.

An invaluable aspect of the traveling observers' work was their briefing of the lead evaluators on their arrival in Hawaii to help them become as current as possible with recent issues and events in the project, on the Waianae Coast, and in Hawaii, in general.

The evaluators learned early on that it was not productive to include the traveling observer in the feedback sessions to go over with foundation leaders and staff the findings in the interim, formative evaluation reports. Too often, the presence of the traveling observer in the feedback session resulted in friction, including defensive reactions by both members of the project staff and the traveling observer. Such defensiveness was counterproductive to useful, frank discussions of the findings. The feedback process worked much better in the absence of the traveling observer who had collected and interpreted much of the information being

discussed. In general, evaluators should employ the traveling observer methodology to capture first-hand accounts of project activities and surrounding dynamics and to facilitate the efficient work of the visiting evaluators. However, as a rule of thumb, the evaluators should not engage the traveling observers in helping to brief the project's director and staff on draft reports and in having frank discussions of the reports.

Case studies were conducted as repeated interviews with a panel of participants over time, followed by a synthesis of their perspectives on the project. Case studies were undertaken in project years 2, 4, and 7. Additional families were added to the panel each year. Originally, the case studies were intended to track the experiences of individual families over time. However, it was deemed that anonymity of the families included in the case studies was essential but could not be guaranteed in such a small, intact community. Therefore, instead of jeopardizing the families' privacy, the case study focus shifted from individual families to the collective perceptions of the selected families about the project and its impacts on them. Thus, the total Ke Aka Ho'ona project was the case.

Because case study participants were constantly on site and involved in all phases of their community, the evaluation treated them as **key informants.** The lead evaluators informed these key informants that they, rather than the project evaluators, were the experts as to identifying and reporting life and happenings in Ke Aka Ho'ona. The evaluators worked with these key informants as colleagues in the effort to understand and record valuable lessons from the Ke Aka Ho'ona experience. The lead evaluators periodically interviewed the key informants to gain their perspectives on the project's impacts on the families' quality of life and relationships; needs of children, the Ke Aka Ho'ona, and Waianae communities; and the extent to which beneficiaries were influenced to help other needy parties, including those outside of the Ke Aka Ho'ona community. A special protocol was used to guide the case study interviews. The project evaluators looked for changes over time in the key informants' perceptions of the project's quality and success, particular issues, and how well these issues were being resolved.

Stakeholder interviews were conducted with virtually all the families who built their own houses, the project's staff members, the outside contractors who provided the house builders with on-the-job training and support, board members and administrators of the foundation, area school teachers and administrators, area merchants, community service personnel in Waianae, and community developers in Honolulu. Interview protocols were tailored to each group of interviewees and used to guide the interviews and later to organize and analyze the information obtained.

The majority of interviews were conducted with the co-builders who built houses in each annual increment of houses. These interviews occurred about 3–6 months after the families moved into their new houses. The interviews acquired information about the builders' perceptions of the community; the process they experienced in building the houses; the nature and quality of the construction and community development outcomes; the project's impacts on their lives and especially those of their children; the extent to which the project was fulfilling the foundation's mission and values; the type and quality of services delivered by the foundation; and matters related to sustaining and improving the Ke Aka Ho'ona community. The protocol that guided the interviews changed only slightly from year to year. The families were highly cooperative and forthcoming in helping the investigators understand the developing project, identify key issues related to project improvement, and assess the project's success in relationship to their family's needs and the broader values-based **vision** for the community that had been projected by the Consuelo Foundation.

Interviews of other parties were interspersed throughout 7 years of the evaluation. Most of these interviews followed set protocols, but others were more informal, especially when unplanned-for opportunities arose to obtain insights from certain knowledgeable parties. Overall, the interview procedure yielded a wealth of information for this evaluation.

Typically, the evaluation's two lead evaluators conducted the interviews over a period of about one hour. One evaluator conducted the interview, while the other took notes and sometimes interjected follow-up questions. This two-person conduct of the interviews was deemed needed because the foundation prohibited the tape recording of interviews. Interviews were scheduled with about 90 minutes between them, so that following an interview the evaluators immediately could write up the interview. This was deemed important to assure that key responses were not forgotten and to merge the notes, recollections, and interpretations of both interviewers.

With regard to the use of interviews in evaluating Ke Aka Ho'ona, application of the procedure yielded a great deal of valuable information. However, most of this information was qualitative, in-depth information. In future evaluations of Ke Aka Ho'ona or similar projects, it would be beneficial for the interview protocols to include both open-ended questions to yield the needed qualitative information and a rating scale to obtain supplementary quantitative information.

Goal-free evaluations were conducted in years 3 and 4. A goal-free evaluation is one that is conducted by a highly competent evaluator who is not knowledgeable of the project being studied. This technique is especially useful for identifying and assessing unexpected project outcomes. The **goal-free evaluators** are told that their study of background information pertaining to the project will not include any information concerning the project's goals. The goal-free evaluator's assignment is to enter the project's site and the surrounding community and find out what the project actually did and achieved. Questions addressed included:

- What positive and negative effects flowed from the project?
- How were these effects judged regarding criteria of merit, such as quality of construction, quality of communication and collaboration within the community, quality of organization and administration, integration into the larger community, giving back to the larger community, and so on?
- How significant were the project's outcomes compared with the assessed needs of the families involved and the needs of the surrounding environment?

Thus, this technique seeks not to determine whether the project achieved what it set out to achieve, but to determine and judge what it actually accomplished. Observed achievements are credited regardless of project goals, and then they are assessed for their significance. Significance is gauged against the participants' assessed needs and those of the surrounding, broader community. A goal-free evaluator gives a project credit for what it did and achieved and how important that was, not necessarily for whether it achieved what it was intended to achieve.

Obtaining a defensible, valuable goal-free evaluation requires several key components. First, the lead evaluator must select a field researcher who is experienced and proficient in constructing a wide range of evaluation tools and in conducting intensive field-based research. The field researcher should also be schooled and experienced in designing, conducting, and reporting goal-free studies. Sociologists, anthropologists, ethnographers, project evaluators, and investigative journalists are examples of the kind of specialist who might be qualified and chosen to do a goal-free evaluation. Second, an up-to-date needs assessment in the area of the project is required because goal-free findings must be interpreted in terms of their relevance to the assessed needs of targeted beneficiaries. The third essential component of a successful goal-free evaluation is a dedicated search to determine and document what the subject project actually did. The final required component is a product evaluation in the form of a wide-ranging search for project outcomes—both positive and negative (i.e., a comprehensive product evaluation).

In this evaluation, the lead evaluator selected two sociologists with track records of conducting excellent ethnographic studies in the project's geographic area. The contract for their goal-free evaluation services included a requirement that they develop a **goal-free evaluation manual** tailored to guide the explorative inquiry they would conduct; project the kinds of information they would seek and the expected sources of such information; project the type of final report they would produce; and ensure that their evaluation would adhere to the Joint Committee (1994) *Program Evaluation Standards*. These evaluators proved to be highly resourceful in pursuing their assignment and producing unique, highly interesting sets of findings. Especially interesting in their reports were the perspectives of different area groups on what the Ke Aka Ho'ona project was achieving and how it was impacting the larger community. The project's staff and the foundation's leaders found the goal-free evaluation reports to be highly informative and useful and to add unique value to the overall evaluation.

Experience has shown that clients and other project stakeholders are keenly interested in the results of competently conducted and reported goal-free evaluations. They welcome findings that confirm that the project is achieving its goals, and they are receptive to learning about positive outcomes that are outside the project's goals. The last named are often referred to as side effects. Of course, side effects may be either positive or negative. Accordingly, clients and other stakeholders often want to know whether the project produced deleterious side effects, as well as unanticipated positive side effects. The full range of goal-free evaluation findings takes on added meaning when their importance is gauged in terms of the assessed needs of targeted beneficiaries. A sound, goal-free evaluation report is especially useful to evaluation clients in delivering information on area groups' perceptions of a project's operations, accomplishments, and value. Overall, the goal-free evaluation technique is highly applicable to the evaluation of projects conducted by foundations and other types of organizations.

Photographs were taken throughout the evaluation of Ke Aka Ho'ona. The photos were of planning activities at foundation headquarters; planning, construction, and events at the project site; houses, yards, and the Community Center at the project site; various locations of interest in the Waianae area; project beneficiaries; project staff, project contractors; and officials of the foundation. The photographs were invaluable in revealing and documenting poverty-related conditions in the Waianae area; the start-up, progression, and conclusion of construction at the project site; the participation of beneficiaries, project staff, foundation officials, and contractors; the apparent quality of completed project grounds, houses, and the Community Center; evidence over time of residents' good maintenance of their properties; the involvement of beneficiaries in social services provided by the foundation; and the great joy of the beneficiary adults and their children upon realizing their dream of home ownership. The photographs provided a clear record over time of the project's implementation and accomplishments and were useful in conveying interim feedback to the project's staff and officials of the foundation. The pictures proved invaluable in reprising and reinforcing the verbal messages in the final evaluation report. Significantly, photographs are useful in obtaining, documenting, and reporting findings for each type of evaluation, as seen in Table 3.1.

Clearly, evaluations of a foundation's projects can be greatly enhanced by employing multiple data collection methods. Fortunately, the evaluation discipline provides a rich cornucopia of such methods. Here we have illustrated the use of seven methods that proved especially useful in the evaluation of Ke Aka Ho'ona. Subsequent chapters in this book present and discuss 15 data collection procedures for use in project evaluations: literature review, interviews, traveling observer, resident researcher, site visits, surveys, rating scales, focus groups, hearings, **public forums,** observations, case studies, goal-free evaluations, knowledge tests, and **self-assessment devices.** Foundations and their evaluators should consider these data collection procedures when planning project evaluations.

Evaluation Ingredient 8:
Formative and Summative Reports

The CIPP Model, as implemented in the evaluation of Ke Aka Ho'ona, produced and delivered both formative and summative reports. Formative reports were presented periodically during each project year both in face-to-face meetings and more informally via correspondence and telephone calls. Preliminary and final versions of the summative evaluation were provided during the last 3 years in both printed reports and meetings of project staff, board members, and a broader group of stakeholders.

Formative reports presented foundation leaders and staff with periodic feedback keyed to helping them review and strengthen project plans and operations. Each formative report was sent first as a draft to a panel of foundation personnel, including foundation administrators and project staff. Members of the evaluation team subsequently conducted a **feedback workshop** for the panel. Each such workshop was aimed at and organized to achieve two-way feedback. The evaluators briefed the panel on the recent formative findings and oriented them to the evaluation's planned next steps. The panel's role included reacting to the evaluation's report and planned next steps and expressing how they could facilitate future data collection activities. Based on the exchange, the evaluators subsequently finalized and submitted the formative report, updated their data collection plans, and availed themselves of the panel's relevant offers of assistance in collecting additional information. This ongoing process of communication and cooperation between evaluators and project stakeholders greatly supported the evaluation's effectiveness. The process provided a continuing basis for the evaluators to assist project decision making and accountability; it assisted in keeping findings and reports relevant to stakeholder interests and needs; and, in general, it served to keep the evaluation on the foundation's "front burner." Often, during the feedback sessions, focused on draft reports, the client group would use the reported information to formulate decisions relating to project implementation. A 2001 *Feedback Workshop Checklist,* by Gullickson and Stufflebeam, for use in planning and conducting feedback workshops, is available at *http://wmich.edu/evaluation/checklists.*

The evaluation's final summative report was largely retrospective. It summarized and appraised what was done and accomplished during the project's first 7 years. To serve the differential needs of different audiences, the final summative report included three main sections.

Section One, titled *Antecedents,* addressed a broad audience of potentially interested organizations and professionals who might have had no previous knowledge of the Consuelo Foundation, the Ke Aka Ho'ona project, or the Waianae Coast of Oahu, and who might have been interested in the details of Ke Aka Ho'ona. This section conveyed factual information about the Consuelo Foundation, the genesis of the Ke Aka Ho'ona project, and the project's political, economic, and geographic context.

Section Two, titled *Project Implementation,* was intended for use by charitable foundations; local, state, and national government agencies; and social workers and community development specialists. This section was directed especially to groups that might be planning to launch housing and community development projects similar to Ke Aka Ho'ona and might be seeking information on how to organize, schedule, staff, fund, and carry out the various required activities. It was assumed that such an audience would be interested in receiving a factual account of the "nuts and bolts" of Ke Aka Ho'ona. This report on project implementation reflected annual observations and data collection and documentation. It described how the Ke Aka Ho 'ona project was originated, designed, and operated. The evaluators endeavored to keep the account of project implementation factual and descriptive, while reserving their judgments for Section Three. Section Two conveyed information on the project's implementation, with an overview of the whole project plus detailed, factual descriptions of the recruitment and selection of project participants, home financing and financial support, the construction process, and social services and community development activities.

Section Three, *Project Results,* was intended for use by the evaluation's entire audience. This report focused on the evaluation approach and results. It opened with a description of the employed evaluation approach, including the CIPP Evaluation Model, the main data collection methods, and the schedule of data collection activities and reports. This section was followed with a presentation of findings, including assessments of the project's context, inputs, process, impacts, effectiveness, sustainability, and transportability. Basically, this section compared the reached group of beneficiaries with the originally targeted group; assessed the responsiveness, soundness, and feasibility of the project's design and planning process; judged the efficiency and quality of project implementation; assessed the project's effectiveness in meeting beneficiaries' assessed and targeted needs; assessed the project's achievement of its stated goals; identified the project's unintended but beneficial side effects; assessed prospects for the project's long-term viability; and reported on indications of the project's transportability. Section Three also summarized the project's main strengths and weaknesses in regard to addressing the participant families' assessed needs when they entered the project; the pertinent community and individual human needs that the evaluation uncovered during the course of the project; and the Consuelo Foundation's stated values. The report next listed what the evaluators saw as 24 valuable lessons from this evaluation. Finally, the section concluded with a bottom-line assessment, which judged Ke Aka Ho'ona to be highly successful and pointed to areas for improvement.

Each of the three main sections of the final, summative report was followed by a photographic reprise. Included at the end of Section One were pictures of foundation leaders and staff, foundation offices, a map locating the project on the Waianae Coast of Oahu, blighted housing and neighborhoods surrounding the project site, area resource organizations, and close-by pristine beaches and mountains. Notably, these photographs contrasted the area's beauty and its blight.

Images at the end of Section Two included architectural plans, project infrastructure, project staff members, on-site planning activities, project beneficiaries, beneficiaries in the process of constructing their own houses, landscaping taking shape, happy families in front of their new houses, children enjoying their new environment, and a communitywide celebration of what the project had produced.

The pictures at the end of Section Three portrayed a community with attractive houses, impressive yards and stone walls, beautiful flower gardens, well-maintained lawns, exceedingly happy parents and children, an area teacher helping students with their homework in Ke Aka Ho'ona's magnificent community center, and a concluding photograph of Mrs. Consuelo Zobel Alger, under her statement of legacy: "*I want to spend my heaven doing good on Earth.*"[4]

Readers of the final report said the photographic reprises made the evaluation findings clear, believable, and memorable. In fact, the lead evaluator's colleague, Egon Guba—one of the evaluation field's most productive scholars—observed that he would not have believed the evaluation's claims about the project's suc-

cess had he not seen pictures of the participating families, their performing construction tasks in a very hot setting, the impressive three- and four-bedroom houses they constructed, and the overall, well-cared-for community of 75 houses and an impressive community center. When appropriate, evaluators and their clients can find it very beneficial to supplement their narrative and quantitative accounts with photographs of a project's environment, processes, and observed results.

Evaluation Ingredient 9: Budgeting for Evaluation

Sound evaluation requires adequate funding. Such funding should allow an evaluation to meet the information needs of intended users and adhere to the professional standards of sound evaluation. Moreover, **evaluation budgets** should be commensurate with the expected value of the projected evaluative feedback. An evaluation should be frugal in its requests for and use of resources but should be funded at a level to ensure that the evaluation can fully succeed and ultimately be worth what it cost.

A hallmark of the evaluation of Ke Aka Ho'ona was its frugality. From the beginning, the evaluators and the sponsor agreed that full-cost budgets would be approved, that these would be cost-reimbursable, and that the evaluators would constantly seek ways to cut costs. During one period when the foundation encountered fiscal difficulties following a downturn in the Asian stock markets, the evaluation's director charged for only half of the time he spent directing the project. Also, The Evaluation Center discontinued two of the planned evaluation tasks that the foundation found less important than the others. Additionally, the evaluation team was able to save the foundation substantial money for the evaluation by such means as sharing travel costs with other Center projects being conducted in Hawaii.

The cost-cutting limited the amount of evaluation feedback that could be provided, especially relating to relevant developments and needs in the project's surrounding environment. But, on the whole, the evaluation team believed that the evaluation of the project adequately fulfilled the requirements of utility, feasibility, propriety, and accuracy as defined in the Joint Committee (1994) *Program Evaluation Standards*; the foundation's leaders concurred in this judgment.

While the full-cost budgets negotiated for the seven-year evaluation totaled $731,027, due to budget cuts and cost-saving measures, The Evaluation Center actually billed about $200,000 less than this amount. The important points learned from this evaluation's costs are that (1) initially it is wise to budget for the full cost of the projected evaluation, (2) sometimes an evaluation's scope must be reduced in the face of unanticipated problems (such as the sponsor's unexpected funding difficulties) in order to carry through the evaluation's core aspects without canceling it entirely, (3) evaluators should constantly seek ways to make the evaluation as efficient as possible, and (4) in cutting an evaluation's costs, the evaluator and client should ensure that the evaluation meets the most important needs of intended users and adheres to the requirements of professional standards for evaluations.

These four points are so important that both parties to an evaluation should consider making them part of the basic working agreements, if not the formal contract. At the outset of the evaluation of Ke Aka Ho'ona, The Evaluation Center's team informed the foundation that the evaluation would be designed and conducted to comply with these points so as to assure the project's cost-effectiveness. The foundation's president welcomed this orientation to fiscal responsibility. Both parties followed through in implementing a fiscally responsible and frugal approach to funding the evaluation. At the start of each budget period, the evaluation team was able to proceed with confidence that sufficient funds would be available to complete the agreed-upon tasks. The foundation saved substantial funds from what it had expected to spend. Some of the evaluation tasks and budgets were cut, so that the evaluation could survive some of the foundation's financial difficulties. These cuts limited the scope of evaluation findings. However, most of the intended evaluation work got carried out, and the evaluators and client group ultimately judged the overall evaluation to be useful, richly informative, and, overall, cost-effective.

Evaluation Ingredient 10: Evaluation Expertise

Woody Hayes, the famous Ohio State University football coach, titled one of his books, *You Win with People,* to emphasize that his coaching success was largely due to the talents, dedication, and performance of numerous student athletes, assistant coaches, and others. Similarly, from 1994 to 2002, many persons contributed to the Consuelo Foundation's effective use of evaluation. The foundation's board, staff members, and collabora-

tors applied a wide range of specialized knowledge and skills to the foundation's various evaluation processes in such areas as legal, fiscal, and policy analysis; social work; evaluation of project applicants; and quality assurance in house construction. Participants in the project's various forms of evaluation helped assess a wide range of matters related to starting, planning, budgeting, managing, and assuring the project's success. This point is illustrated below with a few examples.

To acquire guidance for planning their inaugural self-help housing project, President Patti Lyons and selected foundation staff members visited and carefully assessed the experiences and accomplishments of several self-help housing projects in California. Input from the visits sensitized and informed foundation board members and staff members concerning such matters as the influence of a project's environment, the selection of beneficiaries, possible roles of beneficiaries in the construction process, possible house designs, project costs, and many other aspects of a complex, self-help housing and community development project, such as Ke Aka Ho'ona.

In choosing participants for each of the seven annual increments of house construction, foundation staff members and their collaborators systematically assessed applicants' qualifications and prospects for successful participation in the project. The assessment process included a detailed application form, criminal **background checks,** credit checks, and a review of each applicant's employment history. Foundation staff members then made home visits and conducted in-depth interviews with applicants who had passed the initial screening procedure. Next, foundation staff members engaged groups of applicants in focus group exchanges and role playing. Staff identified the most promising candidates, and potential lenders subsequently assessed the remaining applicants for their qualifications to receive a home mortgage. Ultimately, the foundation used all the obtained information to choose families for participation in the subject increment of houses.

In the ongoing construction process, the on-site manager of Ke Aka Ho'ona played a key personnel assessment role. She wrote weekly reports that assessed the performance and emotional state of each participant. These reports provided early identification of participants who were experiencing difficulties in the highly stressful building process. (Such stress was often associated with a mom—who had to work with her husband building the family's house for 20 hours each weekend, over a period of 10 months—being separated from the family's children.) The weekly reports were subsequently useful in tracking and assessing efforts to address participants' project-related and family-related needs and problems.

The foundation's librarian made valuable contributions to assessing and clarifying policies for Ke Aka Ho'ona. As is common in innovative efforts, project policies emerge in the course of project experiences, brainstorming, and staff deliberations. Sometimes emergent project policies are inadequate. As a project matures, project leaders need to clarify, validate, and record appropriate, consistent policies. Ke Aka Ho'ona's librarian highlighted all statements in the minutes of project meetings that contained relevance to project policies. Over time, her highlighted minutes helped the Ke Aka Ho'ona team to identify, assess, refine, and clarify policies that would guide the project for the long term. The eventual solidification of sound self-help housing project policies, based on the Ke Aka Ho'ona experience, was to prove useful to the foundation later when it planned and conducted similar projects in the Philippines.

Beyond the evaluation contributions of foundation board and staff members, external assessors contributed to all phases of Ke Aka Ho'ona's construction activities. Government inspectors assessed electrical, plumbing, construction, infrastructure, and other aspects of the building process to ensure the quality and safety of the houses and grounds. Also, by contracting the Western Michigan University Evaluation Center, the foundation obtained an external, professional evaluation perspective on the total project.

The foundation used a wide range of evaluation expertise in its quest to mount a sound project and assure and demonstrate its success. No doubt, the involvement of a wide range of project participants, with various forms of specialized evaluation expertise, contributed to the foundation's effective use of evaluation for decision making, accountability, and institutional learning, and to the project's success.

The main missing element in the mosaic of evaluation expertise was a foundation staff member with a specific assignment to lead and coordinate the full range of foundation evaluation activities. Clearly, evaluation plays a crucial role in the Consuelo Foundation's work. If not already in place, the foundation might consider adding a position of coordinator of foundation evaluations.

Such an internal evaluation leader could provide a wide range of services to ensure continuation and fur-

ther development of the foundation's effective use of evaluation. Among these services are providing a coherent, documented framework for foundation evaluation efforts; drafting foundation evaluation policies and procedures; developing an evaluation operations manual; designing evaluations; leading in selecting external evaluators; conducting internal evaluations; providing evaluation reports to the foundation's administrators and board; training existing and new organizational personnel in the foundation's approach to evaluation; maintaining a database to assist foundation evaluations; maintaining an archive of past evaluations, including key lessons learned; representing foundation interests at professional evaluation meetings; and keeping foundation board members and staff members appraised of relevant developments in the evaluation discipline. Quite likely, the Consuelo Foundation and similar organizations could benefit from designing, staffing, and using services for the role of coordinator of foundation evaluations.

Evaluation Ingredient 11: Using Findings for Improvement, Accountability, and Institutional Learning

In accordance with this book's position that evaluation's most important purpose is not to prove but to improve, the main point of evaluating Ke Aka Ho'ona or any other social service project is to improve services to beneficiaries. The preferred way to do so is to use evaluative feedback early and continually to assess and strengthen project aims, plans, operations, and outcomes. Another evaluative avenue to improvement, though counterintuitive, is to provide a basis for terminating a hopelessly flawed enterprise so that its resources can be retrieved and applied beneficially.

Fortunately, the leaders and staff of the Consuelo Foundation were predisposed to obtain early evaluative feedback on Ke Aka Ho'ona and other foundation ventures, to use the feedback to uncover and address deficiencies as well as identify project strengths that should be nurtured, and to keep project activities firmly addressed to the foundation's mission and keyed to its values. It was important that the foundation's president and board members kept in contact and were involved with the evaluation of Ke Aka Ho'ona throughout the course of the evaluation. They played a critically important role in helping the evaluators identify the most important evaluation questions, especially during the process evaluation phase. They critically appraised draft reports. And they used evaluation findings both to make decisions and to keep interested parties informed about the progress of Ke Aka Ho'ona. The foundation's leaders also considered evaluative feedback on Ke Aka Ho'ona, as they planned other projects in Hawaii and in the Philippines.

A critically important aspect of the foundation's use of evaluation for improvement was the employment of *feedback workshops,* as described above in Evaluation Ingredient 7. By meeting regularly with a cross-section of foundation leaders and project staff, the ongoing evaluation was a regular and effective part of the foundation's process of project oversight and decision making. Through these regular exchanges, the evaluators were able to assist project decision making, and the foundation and project personnel were able to help assure that the evaluation addressed their most important questions and needs for evaluative information.

An Example of Evaluative Impact

A poignant example of the impact of interim evaluation reports on project improvement occurred during the project's first increment of house construction. Eight pairs of co-builders were engaged to do the main construction of the eight houses in the increment. At the outset of this process, the project staff conducted a lottery to assign the house to each of the pairs that would be theirs. Subsequently, the project staff instructed the co-builders to work together in building all eight houses. For example, if one pair had special skills in a task such as roofing, that pair would do much of the roofing work on all eight houses. Similarly, the other seven pairs would be assigned certain tasks—such as framing, painting, or digging holes for post-on-pier foundations—associated with constructing all of the houses.

As the collaborative house construction process unfolded, the evaluation revealed some growing problems: uneven quality in the construction of the different houses and growing dissension among the co-builders. In general, some of the co-builders were working hard and carefully on the house that would be theirs but they were not making the same effort on the other houses. Consequently, discord among the co-builders was growing and threatening the project's success.

The evaluators reported the dysfunctional relationship between early assignment of houses to the co-builder pairs, the subsequent uneven effort by pairs in building all the houses, and the consequent dissension among co-builders. The evaluators noted that, if uncorrected, this flaw in the approach to collaborative house construction could jeopardize the overall success of the Ke Aka Ho'ona project.

Subsequently, the project staff revised the collaborative house construction plan, so that in subsequent house construction increments, houses would not be assigned to pairs of co-builders until all houses in the increment had been completed. As a result, throughout the remainder of the project, the evaluators reported that the collaborative approach to house construction was functioning as intended and that co-builders were getting along quite well as they worked on the different houses. Thus, the benefits of interim evaluative feedback were twofold. First, the evaluation helped the project staff make an early correction in the house construction approach. Second, the lesson learned in the final evaluation report would help the foundation plan similar projects and also assist other groups seeking to replicate the Ke Aka Ho'ona approach.

Use of Evaluative Feedback for Accountability

President Lyons made the external evaluation of Ke Aka Ho'ona part of the foundation's accountability to the foundation's board and to external groups, such as accreditation organizations. The foundation's board commissioned Lyons to write a book on the foundation's early history, especially as reflected in the Ke Aka Ho'ona project. The board stipulated that this book would not be published but would be preserved in the foundation's private archives. The book would inform future foundation leaders of the strengths and weaknesses of past projects, warts and all. In writing the book, Lyons made extensive use of the lessons learned from the evaluation of the Ke Aka Ho'ona project. Her book, which would be of such great use by future foundation leaders, is an apt example of how organizations should preserve and make future uses of lessons learned.

A Few Afterthoughts

It has been many years since The Evaluation Center completed its work in evaluating the Ke Aka Ho'ona project. On a recent trip through Hawaii, the evaluation's director (Daniel Stufflebeam) drove to the Waianae Coast to see how things may have developed or stayed the same in the Ke Aka Ho'ona community and the surrounding environment. He was very pleased to talk with some of the original project beneficiaries. If anything, he observed that the area surrounding Ke Aka Ho'ona had gotten even more depressed than he remembered from visits there in 2002. Numerous area beaches were covered with the shacks and tents of squatters, many of whom likely were homeless.

However, Ke Aka Ho'ona continued to be a beautiful, suburban-like community: an island of plenty in the midst of poverty. Almost all of the houses and lots were in good repair and well maintained. There was a quiet air of tranquility in this community. On the surface, it appeared that the Consuelo Foundation had made many sound decisions in its original selection of families, planning of the community, establishment of covenants, arrangement of mortgages for the participating families, design of houses, management of the construction process, and continuing oversight of the project. Following Stufflebeam's impromptu visit to the project site, he was convinced that evaluation and wise use of findings by foundation and project officials played an important part in what appeared to him to be a continuing success story.

Summary

This chapter illustrates and explains the CIPP Model's correct, effective application. Contracted by Hawaii's Consuelo Foundation, the Western Michigan University Evaluation Center in 1994 launched and conducted an 8-year, formative and summative evaluation of the innovative Ke Aka Ho'ona (Spirit of Consuelo) project. This inaugural project of the foundation helped 75 low-income families, including 155 adults and 235 children, build their own houses, while simultaneously creating a nurturing neighborhood free from violence and substance abuse. The project was located on a 12-acre plot within Oahu's Waianae Coast area, an area plagued by poverty and crime. In each of eight successive increments lasting approximately one year, the foundation assisted between 7 and 17 families to obtain low-interest mortgages and construct their own, high-quality houses, or, for a few families, to participate on a rent-to-own basis. Subsequently, over about 40 years each family, with a mortgage, was expected to pay off the mortgage and an associated land lease. The project's secondary purpose was to afford the new foundation a hands-on learning experience from

which it could build its capacity to plan, conduct, and evaluate effective projects. The evaluation focused on the foundation's mission of serving poor families and abused and neglected women and children in Hawaii and the Philippines; adhered to professional evaluation standards of utility, feasibility, propriety, and accuracy; systematically engaged the full range of project stakeholders in the evaluation process; referenced the foundation's stated positive values in defining evaluative criteria; collected and reported a wide range of relevant qualitative and quantitative information; addressed questions related to the project's context, plans, implementation, and outcomes; continuously informed the project's decision-making process; delivered periodic project accountability reports to the foundation's board; and, in particular, assisted foundation leaders and the project's beneficiaries in pursuing and achieving enduring, positive project outcomes. Through this extensive programming and attendant evaluation experience, the foundation's board, president, and staff conducted an innovative, successful project. The project's success was patently apparent to visitors to the project site, who came from throughout the United States and several other countries to see what had been accomplished. The project's impacts were evident in the excellent living and learning conditions of 390 adults and children; in their pride in what they had accomplished; in the secure, beautiful, well-maintained neighborhood and the well-kept individual properties; in the spirit of community that was beginning to emerge among the 75 families; and in the neighborhood's freedom from violence, substance abuse, crime, and overcrowding. Ultimately, the foundation used lessons learned from this project to strengthen its policies and procedures for planning, conducting, and evaluating other projects in Hawaii and the Philippines.

This chapter was prepared by the director of the evaluation of the Consuelo project and gives an account of an 8-year effort to apply the CIPP Model in conducting formative and summative evaluations of a self-help housing project for a selected group of Hawaii's **working poor** as well as a few families who fit the definition of Hawaii's poorest of the poor. Basically, the chapter discusses 11 important ingredients of the evaluation of the project labeled Ke Aka Ho'ona. These key ingredients are as follows:

- Providing evaluation-oriented leadership.
- Referencing the client organization's values in defining evaluative criteria and interpreting findings.

- Keying the evaluation to professional standards for evaluations.
- Conducting formative metaevaluation to help plan and guide a sound evaluation and conducting and reporting a summative metaevaluation of how well the completed evaluation adhered to the standards of the evaluation profession.
- Employing a cost-reimbursable evaluation planning grant.
- Using the CIPP Model to guide the evaluation.
- Employing multiple qualitative and quantitative data collection methods.
- Reporting formative and summative findings.
- Budgeting adequately and frugally expending the evaluation's funds.
- Engaging a wide range of talented foundation representatives and evaluation team members to carry out the needed evaluation tasks.
- Facilitating the use of findings for project improvement, accountability, and evaluation capacity development.

Overall, the case reported in this chapter represents an exemplary application of the CIPP Model.

REVIEW QUESTIONS • • • • • • • • • •

1. List actions that President Patti Lyons took in the case to deserve the description "evaluation-oriented leader."

2. Reflect on a project with which you are familiar. Then record a concrete example of how you could have used the stated values of the organization that conducted the project to address each of the following: clarifying and validating the project's goals, judging the project's plan of action, judging the project's treatment of project staff, and searching for side effects.

3. In your judgment, what are the pros and cons of clarifying foundational values for use in carrying out a project evaluation?

4. What rationale does this chapter give for starting an evaluation assignment with a separate evaluation planning grant? What are the pros, cons, and applicability of this recommendation?

5. In the Ke Aka Ho'ona case, beyond the Western Michigan University evaluation team, what group conducted the CIPP Model's input evaluation component, and what were the essential features of this input evaluation?

6. In evaluating Ke Aka Ho'ona, what main types of information were collected to carry out the context evaluation, and what was the relevance of the information for carrying out the project?

7. What is the traveling observer technique, what is it for, what is the nature and role of a Traveling Observer's Handbook, and how was the technique employed in evaluating Ke Aka Ho'ona?

8. What is the feedback workshop technique, what was its use in evaluating Ke Aka Ho'ona, where could you find additional information—beyond that provided in this chapter—about the technique, and what do you see as the essential tasks in applying this technique?

9. What are the unique features of the goal-free evaluation technique, how was it applied in evaluating Ke Aka Ho'ona, and what do you see as this technique's pros and cons?

10. Considering this chapter's discussion of budgeting for evaluation, explain and support with examples what is meant by the dual stipulations that an evaluator should budget both adequately and frugally.

11. What does this chapter mean by the role of "evaluation-oriented leader"? Outline a workshop that you might conduct to help administrators learn the responsibilities of an evaluation-oriented leader and how to carry out these responsibilities.

12. Construct an eight-by-two matrix, with the row headings consisting of the Consuelo Foundation's stated values and the column headings being formative reports and summative reports. In each of the matrix's 16 cells, provide a statement of the pertinent value's relevance to providing needed formative or summative feedback.

13. Choose a project that you might propose to evaluate and assume that the client is amenable to awarding an evaluation planning grant in advance of negotiating the larger evaluation agreement. List the objectives and the attendant tasks for conducting this planning grant.

14. For the project you identified in response to Question 13, reference this chapter's discussion of reporting summative evaluation; then outline and explain the main parts of a summative evaluation report that your group might plan to deliver.

15. Given that a main requirement of standards for evaluations is assuring that findings are used, list steps you would take to ensure that all of a project's stakeholders would learn and make appropriate, effective use of the final, summative evaluation findings.

NOTES

1. In the native Hawaiian language, *Ke Aka Ho'ona* roughly means "The Spirit of Consuelo." This project title was chosen in honor of the benefactress who established the Consuelo Foundation: Mrs. Consuelo Zobel Alger.

2. In symbolic commemoration of Mrs. Alger's wishes, the Foundation planted shower trees throughout the Ke Aka Ho'ona community.

3. Sixteen legitimate approaches to program evaluation are reviewed in Stufflebeam and Shinkfield (2007). Chapter 12 summarizes the evaluation of Ke Aka Ho'ona, and Chapters 13 through 18 show how the approaches of experimental design, case study, the CIPP Model, consumer-oriented evaluation, responsive evaluation, and utilization-focused evaluation can be applied to conduct a follow-up evaluation of Ke Aka Ho'ona. Subsequent chapters on the methods of evaluation and on metaevaluation also draw on lessons learned from the evaluation of Ke Aka Ho'ona.

4. Interested readers may view the actual photographs included in the photographic reprises at the end of each subreport in *The Spirit of Consuelo* report by accessing the report at *www.wmich.edu/evalctr*.

....

CHAPTER 4

Evaluation-Oriented Leadership in Launching and Supporting Effective Evaluations

"Without evaluation-oriented leadership, an organization's evaluations will be fewer and less effective than needed; but with strong, sustained evaluation-oriented leadership the organization's decisions and performance will be grounded in values, be guided by timely and relevant information, and be accountable."

This chapter is about the crucial role of evaluation-oriented leadership, especially in launching and supporting effective evaluations. The chapter explains why administrators should acquire and apply evaluation expertise; delineates evaluation tasks that administrators should carry out; provides tools for administrators to employ in fulfilling their evaluation responsibilities; and concludes with a discussion of how evaluators can help administrators develop their evaluation expertise. The chapter's practical contributions are a role definition for evaluation-oriented leaders; a checklist of evaluation-oriented leadership tasks; five key questions to answer—plus general responses—in launching an evaluation; a matrix that identifies and assesses options for choosing a lead evaluator; a matrix for use in staffing an evaluation team; a matrix for use in determining relevant types of evaluation, that is, context, input, process, and/or product; and procedures for engaging stakeholders.

Overview
....

As was illustrated in Chapter 3, organizational administrators can and should play a powerful role in assuring an evaluation's soundness and utility. The president of the Consuelo Foundation, along with her board of directors, determined that the new foundation's inaugural, high-risk flagship project—called Ke Aka Ho'ona— should be evaluated from its beginning and throughout its planning, development, and execution. She decided that the evaluation should be external and independent, and she also chose the contractor who could carry out the needed evaluation work. Throughout the project's course, the president interacted regularly with the evaluator and contributed significantly to focusing the evaluation; engaging the project's full range of stakeholders; ensuring that the evaluation would be keyed to the foundation's core values; critiquing draft evaluation tools and reports for accuracy and clarity; facilitating data collection; fostering the project staff's valuing of evaluation feedback and use of findings; helping disseminate reports to the full range of the intended users and other interested parties; and helping the foundation's board use lessons from this evaluation to assist in their decisions regarding other projects and foundation policies.

In this chapter, we distill lessons from actual evaluations, especially evaluation of Ke Aka Ho'ona, to provide concrete guidance to organizational leaders and evaluators concerning the important process of launching an evaluation, then supporting its execution. In particular, we define the role of evaluation-oriented leader. In the context of that role definition, we discuss how an evaluation-oriented leader can determine the need for an evaluation and confirm its potential for meaningful use, select an appropriately qualified evaluator, work with the evaluator to focus and carry out the evaluation, and foster beneficial uses of findings. Related to these tasks, we provide practical tools for use by evaluation-oriented leaders. The chapter concludes by offering advice for evaluators in helping organizational administrators develop their capacity for effective evaluation-oriented leadership.

The Key Role of an Evaluation-Oriented Leader

In our evaluation experiences, no factor was more important to an evaluation's success than the active leadership and support of the evaluation by an administrator in the organization that housed the subject project. The accomplished evaluation-oriented leaders we have worked with include high officials in federal and state government agencies, school district administrators, university administrators, directors of federally funded research centers and educational laboratories, presidents and other officials in charitable foundations, and generals and other officers in the U.S. military.

Stufflebeam was privileged to work with such evaluation-oriented leaders in many evaluations. These leaders' contributions to effective evaluation in their organizations proved highly influential in developing the CIPP Model. It was on the basis of these valuable collaborations that Stufflebeam conceived of and, in this chapter, has defined and elaborated the concept of evaluation-oriented leader. Based on valued experiences with the above listed and other leaders, we offer the definition of the evaluation-oriented leader, as delineated in Table 4.1.

The Rationale for Evaluation-Oriented Leadership

As is clear from Table 4.1, it is in an evaluator's interest to collaborate with evaluation-oriented leaders. Such leaders provide invaluable support to evaluation efforts. In the Consuelo Foundation case, described in Chapter 3, the president's contributions to the evaluation were crucial to the evaluation's success and impacts at both project and organizational levels. Without her firm, proactive leadership and sustained support, the external evaluation undoubtedly would have had many weak spots. It likely would not have been initiated at the project's outset, nor would it have been carried out interactively to assist in project decision making. Project staff may have been slow to lose their apprehension about being monitored by outside evaluators, and they almost certainly would not have actively and regularly engaged in critiquing draft evaluation tools and reports. The evaluation team's task of acquiring needed information likely would have been hampered, especially if the beneficiaries were unsure of the president's support for the evaluation. Without the leader's active participation in evaluation feedback sessions, the evaluation likely would have had a lesser role in stimulating project improvement. Also, it was crucial that the president keep the foundation's board informed about the evaluation and help them apply the findings from this evaluation to deliberations concerning the foundation's other projects, both in Hawaii and the Philippines and concerning foundation policies. Clearly, the role of evaluation-oriented leadership is critical to the success of evaluations.

The Evaluator's Role in Developing Evaluation-Oriented Leaders

Unfortunately, in our experience effective evaluation-oriented leaders are few and far between. Clearly evaluators need to do all they can to help the administrators, who are their clients; understand and embrace the concept of evaluation-oriented leader; and develop the insights and skills required to carry out this crucial role. To help evaluators address this administrator education function, we offer Checklist 4.1 (at the end of this chapter), which is a checklist of tasks for evaluation-oriented leaders. The checklist breaks out the tasks that an evaluation-oriented leader needs to perform in launching and supporting sound evaluations. Evalua-

TABLE 4.1. The Role of Evaluation-Oriented Leader

An evaluation-oriented leader is a top administrator with responsibilities, authority, and an orientation to assure that her or his organization meets its evaluation needs. This leader projects a strong commitment to systematic, improvement-oriented evaluation and to organizational accountability. He or she articulates and documents a common language of evaluation, including the concept of evaluation to be embraced and applied throughout the organization. This concept explains what evaluation is, why the organization needs it, what entities should be evaluated, what organizational values and criteria should be invoked in evaluations, the standards evaluations should meet, the conceptual framework for guiding evaluations, how evaluations should be conducted, who should be involved, how evaluations should be reported, how findings should be used, and how the organization will support staff members to develop their evaluation skills. The leader regularly and systematically engages stakeholders in supporting data collection, reviewing draft reports for accuracy and clarity, using findings for improving projects and programs, meeting accreditation requirements, and fulfilling accountability requirements.

The prudent evaluation-oriented leader commits the organization to undertake an evaluation only if the projected findings are clearly needed and would be meaningfully applied. He or she eschews any projected evaluation that would be only an academic exercise with no practical value or one whose costs would necessarily exceed its value to the organization. The leader secures and allocates adequate funding of evaluations but also strives to make sure funds used for evaluations are expended efficiently and effectively to address the organization's highest priority needs for evaluations.

After establishing the need for an evaluation and its expected uses, the leader invokes demanding standards in choosing an appropriately qualified evaluator. With inputs from the evaluation's intended users, the leader works with the evaluator to select, for given evaluations, the most relevant types of evaluation (e.g., context, input, process, and/or product). Once the evaluator has produced an acceptable evaluation plan, the leader effectively addresses the evaluation's budgeting needs. Subsequently, the leader arranges to collaborate with the evaluator throughout the evaluation process in engaging stakeholders, facilitating data collection, arranging and supporting reporting occasions, and fostering meaningful formative and summative uses of findings. As warranted in particular evaluations, the leader arranges, funds, and supports an independent, standards-based audit of the evaluation, that is, an independent metaevaluation.

tors can use the definition of evaluation-oriented leader that appears in Table 4.1 and in this checklist to help administrators understand the valuable evaluation role they can play and, with evaluators' mentoring, how they can acquire and employ the skills needed to carry out the role.

Every evaluation-oriented leader we have worked with effectively addressed all or almost all of the checkpoints in Checklist 4.1 Thus, our Checklist of Tasks for Evaluation-Oriented Leaders is not an academic set of notions. Rather, we see it as a practical tool of significant utility to administrators, evaluators, and evaluation educators. We recommend that administrators employ this tool to consider and embrace, in specific terms, the actions they can take to assure that their organization's projects are appropriately, thoroughly, and helpfully evaluated. Similarly, we advise evaluators to use the checklist to mentor evaluation clients on how they can best secure, support, and use evaluation services. We believe this checklist also can serve as an advance organizer for planning and delivering university courses and workshops aimed at helping administrators

develop their capacity to lead, support, and apply sound evaluation services. Similarly, the checklist provides a tool for training evaluators in how they can best help their evaluation clients understand and implement the evaluation-oriented leadership role.

Questions to Answer in Launching an Evaluation

In deciding to launch an evaluation, an administrator/ client must answer five main questions:

1. Should a project or program undergo systematic evaluation?
2. If an evaluation is to be conducted, when should it begin?
3. Who should lead the evaluation?
4. What perspectives and competencies should be represented in the evaluation's team?
5. What types of evaluation should be conducted?

Responsibility for addressing the first three questions lies with the administrator who will be the main client of the evaluation, if one is to be conducted. In addressing these questions, typically the administrator will consult as appropriate with potential evaluation stakeholders, including project staff; other administrators and staff in the organization; external funders, if any; the organization's board members; and possibly others. The client should consult with the prospective evaluator to address the fourth question regarding the projected evaluation team's composition and the fifth question concerning what type of evaluation should be conducted—that is, context, input, process, and/or product evaluation. Below we offer our advice about how clients can best address these five bottom-line questions.

Should a project undergo systematic evaluation? Every project—ranging from those that are small and localized in an organization to those that are large and pervasive in the organization—reports to an administrator, such as a project director. The project is also likely to be overseen by a higher-level administrator, such as a school district superintendent, school principal, college dean, foundation president, government agency head, or military organization commanding general. Each of these administrators is positioned to fulfill the role of evaluation-oriented leader. In that role, the administrator can and should carefully determine whether a particular project under her or his purview should be subjected to systematic evaluation.

Table 4.2 is a matrix designed to help administrators assess cases both for and against subjecting a project or program to a systematic evaluation. The matrix lists compelling and other arguments against proceeding with an evaluation or not mounting such an evaluation. The decision to launch or not launch an evaluation is never cut and dried. We advise administrators to work through Table 4.2, as they deliberate whether or not to initiate an evaluation.

As a first step in using Table 4.2, we suggest that the administrator fill out the matrix by placing checkmarks in the spaces in front of the listed arguments deemed relevant for determining whether or not to conduct an evaluation. Subsequently, the administrator might ask potential evaluation stakeholders independently to complete copies of the matrix. Ultimately, the administrator and colleagues should use the one or more completed matrixes to deliberate about and ultimately decide whether or not to proceed with an evaluation.

If an evaluation is to be conducted, when should it begin? Having decided to evaluate a project, the administrator needs to decide when the evaluation should be conducted. Options are to launch the evaluation before the project begins, when it begins, after the staff has shaken it down and stabilized it, or after it has been completed. Under varying circumstances, any of these starting points may be justified. In general, though, it is desirable to begin the evaluation as early as possible in a project's life.

Table 4.3 is provided to help administrators consider why different evaluations may justifiably be initiated at different times in a project's life. As seen in the chart, it is not always desirable or feasible to activate an evaluation before or concurrent with the evaluation's start-up. In the case of the Ke Aka Ho'ona project, the commissioned evaluation was started when the project began. However, the foundation had conducted what we call initial context and input evaluations in advance of starting the project. The foundation had done so by assessing the needs of Hawaii's working poor for affordable housing (context evaluation) and subsequently by visiting self-help housing projects in California to identify and assess alternative ways of addressing the housing needs of Hawaii's working poor (input evaluation). When the contracted evaluation began, it included retrospective context and input evaluation to help the foundation formulate and assess its project goals and its self-help housing project plan for achieving the goals. Mainly, however, the contracted evaluation proceeded through its 8-year course by systematically conducting process and product evaluations. We suggest that administrators use Table 4.3 to gain a perspective on the reasons to consider in deciding when to start an evaluation.

Who should lead the evaluation? One of an evaluation-oriented leader's most important project evaluation decisions involves selecting the evaluator who will lead the evaluation. Basic to making such a determination is a clear understanding of the generic role of a project's lead evaluator. Table 4.4 provides such a role definition. We recommend that administrators familiarize themselves with the particulars of Table 4.4 and use them to firm up their expectations for the evaluators they hire and to clarify with prospective evaluators the project evaluator's expected role. Moreover, the complexity of the lead evaluator's role denotes that many evaluations need to be conducted by a team of evaluators.

TABLE 4.2. Arguments for and against Launching an Evaluation

Arguments for Evaluating the Project	Arguments against Evaluating the Project
Compelling arguments	
— The project has prospects for significant service to intended beneficiaries. — The organization would experience serious negative consequences if the project fails. — The project is addressed to important, so far intractable problems. — The project arguably would fail in the absence of evaluative feedback. — An external funder requires that the project be evaluated. — Other:	— The project was stabilized in prior years based on evaluation of it, and its renewed implementation will be routine. — No one is interested in or would use the evaluation's findings. — Costs of the evaluation likely would exceed its utility. — Evaluation of this project is less important than other projects in the organization which are more justified in using the organization's limited funds for evaluation. — There are no available funds to support evaluation of the project. — Other:
Other relevant arguments	
— Sufficient funds have been allocated to support the evaluation. — Stakeholder support for the evaluation is already present. — The project is highly innovative. — The project is controversial. — A qualified evaluator is available to lead the evaluation. — There is widespread interest in the project and a clear opportunity to disseminate evaluation findings beyond the local organization. — The project affords the organization a significant opportunity for organizational learning. — Other:	— Political resistance to the evaluation likely would impede or preclude its success. — No appropriately qualified evaluator is available to lead the evaluation. — The organization has little to learn from an evaluation of the project. — Other:

In selecting a lead project evaluator, the evaluation's client can entertain a range of options, including:

- Self-evaluation: charging the project's director to engage the project's staff to conduct a self-evaluation of the project.
- Self-evaluation plus metaevaluation: charging the project director to engage project staff in conducting a self-evaluation of the project and to subject the self-evaluation to an independent metaevaluation.
- The organization's evaluation (or institutional research) office: engaging the organization's evaluation office to conduct the evaluation, if such an office exists.
- The organization's evaluation office plus metaevaluation: engaging the organization's evaluation office to conduct the evaluation, if such an office exists, and requiring that the office's evaluation be subjected to an independent metaevaluation.
- External evaluator: contracting with an independent evaluator.
- External evaluator plus metaevaluation: contracting with an independent evaluator and arranging to have their evaluation assessed by an independent metaevaluator.

Table 4.5 is designed to help administrators assess the strengths and weaknesses of each of these options in selecting a lead evaluator. This chart's row headings represent the different hiring options, while the column headings are the main standards for an evaluation's utility, feasibility, propriety, accuracy, and accountability. The stars in the matrix's cells denote our assessment of each option against the five standards for sound evaluations (with one star being weakest and five stars being strongest).

The star ratings in Table 4.5 reflect our experiences and associated general judgments based on having conducted a wide range of evaluations and metaevaluations. We offer these opinions to administrators as rules of thumb for deciding how to choose a lead evaluator. In general, we believe that the administrator should choose an external evaluator, preferably along with an independent metaevaluator, for projects that are of high risk or evaluations that are especially po-

litically sensitive. Moreover, if the organization has a competent office of evaluation, we see that option as equally strong, especially if an external metaevaluation is to be conducted. Granted, internal/self evaluations will sometimes be sufficient. The added benefit of this option is that it can engage project staff to learn and apply the valuable practice of systematic evaluation, especially if they key their evaluation to the evaluation field's standards and subject their evaluation reports to an independent metaevaluation.

What perspectives and competencies should be represented in the evaluation's team? Beyond choosing the lead evaluator, the evaluation's client should consider whether a "lone ranger" evaluator or a team can better meet the needs for the evaluation. For small projects, a single evaluator can be sufficient. In such cases, the evaluation's client should confirm that the single evaluator has sufficient understanding of the

TABLE 4.3. Examples of Relevant Circumstances Underlying Different Start Times for an Evaluation

Before the Project Begins	When the Project Begins	After Staff Have Stabilized the Project	After the Project Has Been Completed
— Initiating a project depends on first establishing why it is needed. — Project planning would benefit by assessing similar efforts in other settings and/or competing creative ideas about what approach should be employed. — Project planning would benefit by engaging staff in an input evaluation or providing them with findings from an independent input evaluation.	— The project is so challenging that staff needs guidance to carry it out from the start. — Management needs ongoing feedback on the project's progress. — An external funding agency requires periodic reports on the project's initiation and its subsequent progress.	— Staff would be significantly intimidated by an evaluator "looking over their shoulders" if the evaluation began before they had exercised their creativity and stabilized project staffing and activities. — The project has experienced significant shortcomings in midstream; it should be investigated for either improving it or assessing its accountability for effective implementation.	— Following a pilot project's completion, a funding organization requires that it be evaluated before deciding whether to fund its expansion and continuation. — Following completion of a successful project, a funding organization proposes to fund an evaluation of it as a basis for possibly replicating it in a wide range of venues. — Following a project's completion, the organization's top administration or board of directors requests an evaluation of what was done and accomplished.

TABLE 4.4. A Generic Role Description for Project Lead Evaluators

Task Areas	Specific Responsibilities
Client/stakeholder engagement	— Meet with the client to gain an in-depth perspective on the project and the need for evaluating it. — Meet with persons who are representative of the project's stakeholders to get their take on the need for and appropriateness of the projected evaluation. — Identify and obtain inputs from any parties who might be harmed by the evaluation. — Based on interactions with the client and stakeholders, decide whether to proceed with the evaluation, unless not proceeding is not an option. — As appropriate, set up a representative stakeholder review panel and involve them in critiquing draft evaluation plans, tools, and reports.
Designing the evaluation	— Ground the evaluation planning process in the evaluation field's standards. — Develop in-depth knowledge of the subject project. — Engage the client and stakeholders in focusing the evaluation, including what is to be evaluated, the key evaluation questions, foundational values, project success criteria, key evaluation audiences, and intended uses of findings. — Using client and stakeholder inputs, clarify the core evaluation questions, as needed. — Analyze the subject project's political environment. — Conceptualize a general framework within which to conduct the evaluation. — Lay out a data collection plan. — Draft the data analysis plan. — Plan the needed reports and reporting process.
Staffing the evaluation	— Define needed staffing roles for the evaluation (e.g., designated project contacts, evaluation management, instrument construction, field data collection, information management, qualitative and quantitative analysis, report writing and editing, and delivery of findings). — Recruit and orient evaluation team members. — As needed, recruit and orient evaluation subcontractors.
Budgeting the evaluation	— Determine the evaluation's resource requirements. — Prepare the evaluation's budget. — Firm up a schedule of payments to coincide with a schedule of completed evaluation deliverables. — Secure agreement with the client on the evaluation budget.
Contracting the evaluation	— Secure human subjects review board approvals, as needed. — Negotiate a written agreement with the client for the funding and conduct of the evaluation. — Inform right-to-know parties of the terms of the evaluation agreement.
Training evaluation participants	— As needed, provide evaluation training to evaluation staff members, the client, evaluation subcontractors, and interested stakeholders. — As appropriate, use the project evaluation as case material for training the client organization's staff in the concepts and procedures of systematic evaluation.

(continued)

TABLE 4.4. *(continued)*

Task Areas	Specific Responsibilities
Collecting the needed information	— Determine with the client and stakeholders the qualitative and quantitative information needed to address the core evaluation questions. — Obtain or construct the needed evaluation instruments. — Describe the subject project. — Collect specified information. — Verify and correct, as needed, the accuracy of the obtained information. — Provide for secure storage and retrieval of information.
Analyzing and synthesizing the obtained information	— Analyze the qualitative information to address the evaluation's questions. — Analyze the quantitative information to address the evaluation's questions. — Synthesize the quantitative and qualitative information in response to the evaluation's questions.
Reporting and facilitating use of the evaluation's findings	— Prepare and deliver needed interim reports and facilitate use of the reports. — Prepare and deliver the final report. — Facilitate use of the final report. — Prepare a detailed technical appendix and append it to the final report or develop a separate technical report. — Append to the final report an attestation of the extent to which the evaluation measured up to standards of utility, feasibility, propriety, accuracy, and accountability.
Cooperating with an external metaevaluation	— Advise the client to contract for an external metaevaluation of the project evaluation. — Cooperate with any external metaevaluation by responding to the metaevaluator's information requests. — As feasible, use metaevaluation feedback to strengthen the project evaluation.
Overall management of the evaluation	— Coordinate and oversee the work of evaluation staff members. — Coordinate and oversee the work of any evaluation subcontractors. — Assure that obtained information and evaluation reports are kept secure. — Manage and maintain accountability for the evaluation's finances. — Provide the client with progress reports and financial reports as needed. — Foster communication and mutual assistance among those engaged in the evaluation.

TABLE 4.5. Assessment of Options for Selecting a Lead Evaluator

Lead Evaluator Options	Utility	Feasibility	Propriety	Accuracy	Accountability
Self-evaluation	★★	★★★★	★	★	★
Self-evaluation + metaevaluation	★★★	★★★	★★★	★★	★★★
The organization's evaluation office	★★★★	★★★★	★★	★★★★	★★★
The organization's evaluation office + metaevaluation	★★★★★	★★★	★★★★	★★★★★	★★★★
External evaluator	★★★	★★★	★★★★	★★★★	★★★★
External evaluator + metaevaluation	★★★★	★★	★★★★★	★★★★★	★★★★★

project's subject matter; is fully qualified and committed to meet the evaluation field's standards; has the full range of needed technical skills; is an excellent communicator of evaluation findings; and would be credible to the full range of the evaluation's stakeholders. We know of evaluation experts who have possessed this range of qualifications and have delivered excellent evaluation services, all by themselves.

For evaluations that are large, complex, and potentially volatile, however, it is wise to consider appointing an evaluation team. The evaluation client and lead evaluator should collaborate in determining the composition of the team. Table 4.6 is a matrix designed to assist clients and their lead evaluators to select appropriately qualified evaluation team members. The column headings are key areas of expertise needed by an evaluation team, and the matrix's row headings are possible job titles for team members, with each title followed by a blank space for naming a potential team member. The cells of the matrix are left blank so that the client and evaluator can place checkmarks in the cells for which the individual named on the left has the needed qualification. After assigning the checkmarks, the client and evaluator can assess the overall set of qualifications of the projected slate of evaluation team members and do further evaluation team development as needed. This table is a planning tool to help clients and lead evaluators ensure that the slate of evaluation team members will together possess the full range of qualifications. Of course, users of the matrix can adapt it to their particular evaluation situations as appropriate, by, for example, adding evaluation team job titles or needed areas of evaluation expertise.

The matrix in Table 4.6 is a general outline of the type of analysis Stufflebeam used, in collaboration with Dr. Paul Lingenfelter, to develop a team to conduct a 7-year evaluation of a $12 million program funded by the John T. and Catherine T. MacArthur Foundation. That program supported Chicago's Local Initiatives Support Corporation (LISC) in conducting housing rehabilitation and economic development projects in poverty-stricken neighborhoods throughout Chicago.

In that evaluation, Dr. Lingenfelter—an administrator in the foundation—exemplified the best characteristics of the evaluation-oriented leader. He assisted Stufflebeam in defining the team members' qualifications and subsequently recruited and engaged highly qualified team members. In reference to Table 4.6, the key characteristics the evaluation team needed included expertise in community and economic development

and housing rehabilitation. The team also required wide-ranging skills, including managing a large-scale evaluation; conducting site visits in poverty-stricken, dangerous neighborhoods; developing observation schedules, interview protocols, and project profiling templates; conducting economic, statistical, and document analyses; managing a large amount of sensitive data, writing and editing both site-specific and overall program evaluation reports; and communicating findings to neighborhood audiences, LISC, and the sponsoring foundation.

It was essential in this evaluation that field evaluators be sent out who could readily develop rapport with the ethnically diverse residents of these neighborhoods. Although the evaluation team had to have a full complement of methodological skills, it was also vital that they have credibility with the neighborhood project staffs and program beneficiaries. Thus, team members had to be respected for their ethnic characteristics and cultural backgrounds, as well as their evaluation expertise and knowledge of community development and housing construction. The team had to have credibility not only with people at the local program sites, but also with the community developers at LISC and the foundation's staff and board members. Dr. Lingenfelter's collaboration with the lead evaluator in setting and keeping the evaluation on a solid footing was essential to the evaluation's success. To build a competent evaluation team, Stufflebeam and Dr. Lingenfelter worked through the type of analysis reflected in Table 4.6. We offer the table as a general tool that evaluation clients and their lead evaluators can apply to guide the staffing process.

What types of evaluation should be conducted? Launching an evaluation also requires determining the type of evaluation one should start with and what types are to be added later. That is, should the evaluation begin with a context evaluation and subsequently conduct input, process, and product evaluations? Or should it start with a type other than context, and should all or only some of the CIPP Model's components be included?

In answering these questions, the client and evaluator must address the **point of entry issue.** In the context of the CIPP Model, this issue concerns whether the evaluation should begin with a context, input, process, or product evaluation. In addition to determining the evaluation's starting point, the client and evaluator need to determine whether one, two, or three types of evaluation or all of them are needed.

TABLE 4.6. Matrix for Use in Staffing an Evaluation Team

Evaluation Team Jobs and Projected Team Members	Areas of Needed Expertise							
	Evaluation Management	Project Content Expertise	Cultural Knowledge	Field Research Skills	Information Management and Clerical Support Skills	Measurement and Statistics Skills	Qualitative Analysis Skills	Reporting Skills
Evaluation-oriented leader								
Lead evaluator								
Project secretary								
Field researcher no. 1								
Field researcher no. 2								
Field researcher no. 3								
Technical expert no. 1								
Technical expert no. 2								
Technical expert no. 3								
Reporting specialist								
Secretary/editor								

The bases for deciding where to start an evaluation assignment and which types of evaluation to conduct include:

- Relevant evaluations that may have been previously conducted.
- The subject project's history and current state.
- The store of evaluative information that is already available for use in the contracted evaluation.
- The evaluative feedback that the evaluation's intended users currently need.

Even when an evaluation begins, for example, with a proactive process evaluation or a proactive product evaluation, the client and evaluator may agree to conduct retrospective context and input evaluations as well. In the case of the Consuelo Foundation's self-help housing project (see Chapter 3), the contracted evaluation started with proactive process and product evaluations. The foundation had already conducted its own context and input evaluations when it set up the Ke Aka Ho'ona project. The information amassed in these past evaluations provided useful foundational information for the subsequent contracted, 8-year evaluation. Nevertheless, both the foundation and the evaluator agreed that the contracted evaluation should conduct additional context and input evaluations. The foundation needed these evaluations to help assess its Ke Aka Ho'ona project in the context of unfolding housing needs in the project's geographic area and to compare the Ke Aka Ho'ona approach to other area projects concerned with the housing needs of low-income families.

In some cases, it can be appropriate to contract just for conducting one type of evaluation. For example, an organization might seek only a context evaluation in order to decide whether to mount a project in a given area. If the assessed needs do not justify proceeding with a responsive intervention, then there is no need for input, process, and product evaluations. In an evaluation led by Stufflebeam, the U.S. Marine Corps contracted only for a context and input evaluation. The key questions were: What is right and wrong with the Corps' current performance review system? What revised or totally new evaluation framework would meet the Corps' need for improved, fully defensible evaluations of officers and enlisted personnel? After Stufflebeam's evaluation team had completed the context and input evaluations and after the Marine Corps had chosen a new approach to evaluating officers and enlisted

personnel, Stufflebeam presented the Corps with plans for conducting their own process and product evaluations in pilot testing and institutionalizing the new evaluation system.

Table 4.7 helps administrators and evaluators determine the types of evaluation to be employed both at the beginning of an evaluation and at a later time. The table lists items for and against conducting each type of evaluation. In using the table, we suggest that the client and evaluator first independently use their judgments in checking off what items they believe apply to the given evaluation. Then we suggest that they compare their completed checklists to guide their discussion of why they should or should not conduct each type of evaluation. As appropriate, they should engage representatives of the evaluation's stakeholders in this planning exercise. For example, once the client and evaluator have reached agreement on applicable checkpoints, they should meet with other stakeholders to get their reactions to how the client and evaluator have filled out the checklist. Ultimately, Table 4.7 is a tool for clients, evaluators, and other stakeholders in deciding what types of evaluation to conduct.

Guidelines for Engaging Stakeholders

The preceding sections focused on the need for client–evaluator collaboration in launching and implementing a sound project evaluation. Clearly, the client and evaluator are two key stakeholders in any evaluation. However, if an evaluation is to be implemented efficiently, foster project improvement, and meet accountability requirements, an appropriate range of stakeholders must be involved throughout the evaluation process.

Beyond the evaluator, such stakeholders typically include:

- The organization's administrator, who oversees the project
- The board of the organization that houses the project
- The project's director
- The project's staff members
- The project's beneficiaries
- The project's funder
- Members of the project's relevant profession

TABLE 4.7. A Tool for Selecting Types of Evaluation for a Given Assignment

Context Evaluation	Input Evaluation	Process Evaluation	Product Evaluation
	Reasons to conduct this type of evaluation		
— Client group needs evaluative guidance for formulating and validating goals. — A funding organization requires needs assessment as part of a funding proposal. — Client group wants to track relevant, unfolding needs and opportunities. — The evaluator will need additional context evaluation beyond what exists as a basis for judging project outcomes.	— Client group needs to identify and address optional approaches to achieving project goals. — A funding organization requires that a funding proposal clearly defend its proposed approach against assessments of critical competitors. — Client group has found that its selected approach is deficient and needs guidance for fixing or replacing it. — The evaluator will need input evaluation information beyond what exists for use in judging why the project succeeded or failed.	— Project staff needs periodic feedback on implementation issues. — Project supervisor needs documentation and periodic progress reports on the project's implementation. — Outside sponsor requires periodic reports on the project's progress. — Evaluator needs information beyond what exists on the project's implementation for use in preparing the final report. — Although the project has been completed, it failed and there is a need to diagnose why.	— Project staff needs interim feedback on progress in achieving goals and meeting beneficiaries' targeted needs. — Project overseer requires an assessment of final outcomes. — Intended users of the final report are interested in and would use findings on the project's outcomes. — Outside sponsor requires a product evaluation report. — Evaluator needs product evaluation information beyond what the project staff have or will collect in order to produce the final report.
	Reasons not to conduct this type of evaluation		
— Client group has amassed sufficient background context evaluation information. — Goals have been set and validated. — The subject project is mature, progressing according to plan, and clearly grounded in previously collected context evaluation. — Client group decides that additional context evaluation information would not be of interest or used.	— Client group has amassed sufficient information on its approach compared to critical competitors. — The selected approach has been successfully implemented. — Client group decides that additional input evaluation information would not be of interest or use. — Evaluator decides available input evaluation information is sufficient for developing the final evaluation report.	— Project implementation has been fully documented and completed. — Outside funder is satisfied that it has received sufficient information on the project's implementation. — Client group decides that additional process evaluation information would not be of interest or use. — Evaluator decides available process evaluation information is sufficient for developing the final report.	— Project staff have thoroughly and acceptably documented and assessed project outcomes. — Project overseer is satisfied with the staff's product evaluation report. — Outside funder is satisfied with the project staff's final assessment of the project's success. — Evaluator judges that additional assessment of project outcomes would not be worth the cost. — No intended users of an independent product evaluation report are interested in receiving and using such a report.

The client and evaluator should provide stakeholders with opportunities to:

- Help identify or validate the evaluation's key questions.
- Understand and endorse standards for guiding and judging the evaluation.
- Keep abreast of the evaluation's needs for assistance and progress.
- Assist the collection of needed information.
- Comment on the accuracy and clarity of draft reports.
- Learn and use the evaluation's findings.

It is often useful to set up and meet periodically with an evaluation review panel. Such a panel should be representative of the project's stakeholders. We prefer that one of the stakeholders, other than the evaluator, chair the panel. The panel's periodic meetings should coincide with clear points of project decisions and succeeding stages of the evaluation. Accordingly, the panel should be engaged throughout the course of an evaluation.

The previously mentioned evaluation of the U.S. Marine Corps' personnel evaluation system provides an excellent example of an evaluation-oriented leader's effective employment of review panels to engage stakeholders. Lieutenant General George Christmas, second in command of the Marine Corps at the time, established two review panels and engaged them to review evaluation materials and have regular exchanges with the evaluators. General Christmas chaired one of the panels, which included about 30 marines. The membership of this panel included three-star, two-star, and one-star generals; colonels; lieutenant colonels; majors; and the sergeant major of the Marine Corps. The other panel was chaired by a brigadier general and included about 20 enlisted personnel, including all levels of sergeants. These panels met with the evaluation team on a monthly basis. The evaluators sent an agenda and evaluation materials for distribution to the panels at least 10 working days in advance of each meeting. The panel chair opened each meeting by asking the evaluators to brief the panel on the evaluation's progress and key decisions for which the panel's inputs were being sought. Subsequently, the panel's lead general led panelists in a discussion of the materials they had read before the meeting and of evaluation issues needing resolution. To close the meeting, the chair asked each panel member to state what they considered the meeting's most important point. Then the chair summarized what had been discussed, charged his assistant to prepare and distribute minutes of the meeting, and adjourned the meeting. The meetings with both panels helped the evaluation team conduct a sound, useful evaluation and ensure that key stakeholders would make good use of the evaluation findings. The two evaluation-oriented leaders who chaired the two review panels made invaluable contributions to the evaluation's success. Their actions were consistent with what we mean by effective evaluation-oriented leadership

Advice to Evaluators for Developing Evaluation-Oriented Leaders

Evaluation-oriented leaders play a strong role in an evaluation's entire process. Accordingly, evaluators should do all they can to support administrators in their role of evaluation-oriented leader. Evaluators can support administrators to implement the role of evaluation-oriented leader as follows:

- Instruct the administrator in the standards of the evaluation field and work with them to have their organization adopt such standards and employ them for guiding and assessing evaluations.
- School the administrator in the key concepts of evaluation, especially formative and summative evaluation, the types of evaluation included in the CIPP Model, intended uses and users of evaluations, evaluation budgeting, and evaluation contracting.
- Recommend a framework for planning and conducting the organization's evaluations (e.g., the CIPP Model, as explained in Chapter 3).
- Recommend adoption of a common language for evaluation that can be taught, then applied throughout the organization; such a common language should include general and operational definitions of evaluation, standards for evaluations, the main tasks in a sound evaluation, and metaevaluation.
- Stress the importance of stakeholder engagement and instruct the administrator in ways to effectively engage stakeholders.

- Help the administrator discern what constitutes effective communication and use of evaluation findings.
- Educate the administrator as to the staffing and budget needs of an organization's evaluation system.
- Support the administrator in considering the pros, cons, and possibilities for setting up an evaluation office.
- Assist the administrator in planning for meeting organizational needs for evaluation, including drafting a plan for institutionalizing and **mainstreaming evaluation**.
- Identify or develop tools to help the administrator and colleagues to conduct sound evaluation; such tools include checklists for designing, budgeting, staffing, and contracting evaluations and an evaluation procedures manual that provides an organization's staff with a user-friendly exposition of the organization's evaluation framework, standards, policies, procedures, protocols, and forms for use in planning, conducting, reporting, validating, and using sound evaluations.

Summary

Throughout this chapter, we stressed the importance of the role of evaluation-oriented leader, especially in launching and supporting evaluations. We defined the role, listed its key tasks, and provided tools for use in implementing evaluation-oriented leadership. We provided checklists for use in choosing a lead evaluator, setting up an evaluation team, and determining the types of evaluation to conduct. We stressed the importance of stakeholder engagement and identified and illustrated the use of evaluation review panels to engage stakeholders in an evaluation. We concluded the chapter by listing ways that evaluators can help administrators embrace and implement the important role of evaluation-oriented leader.

REVIEW QUESTIONS • • • • • • • • • •

1. Define the role of evaluation-oriented leader.

2. List at least ten tasks that an evaluation-oriented leader would carry out in launching an evaluation.

3. List at least five reasons why administrators should embrace and implement the role of evaluation-oriented leader.

4. List at least five criteria that an evaluation-oriented leader should employ when choosing a lead evaluator.

5. Is it always necessary to engage a team to conduct an evaluation? When and when not?

6. What are at least three possible reasons why a client and evaluator should decide to conduct a context evaluation?

7. What are at least three possible reasons why a client and evaluator could justifiably decide not to conduct an input evaluation?

8. How would you define for an administrator the nature, role, staffing, and operations of an evaluation review panel?

9. What are an administrator's responsibilities in launching an evaluation, distinct from the prospective evaluator's responsibilities?

10. What are joint responsibilities of client and evaluator in launching an evaluation?

11. What are at least five ways an evaluator can help an administrator to embrace and implement the role of evaluation-oriented leader?

Task	Explanation
Foster a climate of support for evaluation.	• Make clear to staff that the organization is committed to systematic evaluation. — Embrace and communicate throughout the organization a clear concept of evaluation, including definitions of evaluation, evaluation standards, and formative and summative uses of evaluations, plus an evaluation framework. — Include evaluation mission and vision statements in organizational documents (e.g., policies and strategic plans). — Provide a flow of opportunities for staff exchanges about evaluation. — Include evaluation in the organization's provisions for continuing education. — Staff and budget the organization's evaluation function.
Determine needs for evaluations.	• Select projects for evaluation for such reasons as the following: — Prospects for significant service to intended beneficiaries — High risk — High cost — Innovative — Controversial — Addressed to important, so far intractable problems — Federal, contractual, accreditation, or other requirements for — evaluation — Intention to disseminate the project or program beyond the local organization
Confirm that evaluation findings would be used.	• Confirm the practical importance of proceeding with an evaluation for reasons such as the following: — Approval of funding depends on evaluation findings. — Policy board expects to be informed of progress and outcomes. — An accrediting organization requires evaluation of the entity to be considered for accreditation. — Staff needs evaluative feedback for planning and executing the project. — Management needs periodic feedback on the project's progress. — Beneficiaries desire that the project be subjected to independent review. — The success or failure and cost effectiveness of the subject project is of interest to the public or other external audiences.

(continued)

Task	Explanation
Choose qualified evaluators or evaluation teams.	• Determine basic considerations for the needed evaluator(s), such as: — Internal or external — Individual or team — Ethnicity preferences or doesn't matter — Credibility to project staff — Credibility to project beneficiaries — Credibility to the organization's board — Credibility to financial sponsors — Credibility to an accrediting organization — Freedom from project-related conflicts of interest — Conveniently located — Availability to concentrate as needed on the assignment • Determine qualifications for individual evaluators, concerning matters such as: — Membership in a professional evaluation organization — Relevant evaluation experience — University degree in evaluation — Awards for past evaluation work — Recommendations from the evaluator's past clients — Knowledge of the project's subject matter — Evaluation-related publications — Expertise in both quantitative and qualitative methods — Proficiency in using information technology — Record of having written clear, credible reports — Demonstrated skills in effectively delivering oral presentations — Evidence of evaluation management proficiency
Focus evaluations.	• Clarify with the evaluator key evaluation parameters, such as: — Particulars of the project to be evaluated, including history, beneficiaries, approach, location, schedule, staff, budget, and so on — The evaluation's main client or client group — Other intended users of findings — Intended uses of findings — Nature of needed evaluation reports — Timing of needed reports — Key evaluation questions — Values and criteria for interpreting findings

(continued)

Task	Explanation
Contract evaluations.	• Consider funding an evaluation planning grant for purposes such as the following: — Acquaint the evaluator with the project's background and status. — Support the evaluator to become acquainted with the project's staff and other stakeholders. — Review available, relevant documentation. — Work out an evaluation plan that reflects the project's realities. • Negotiate a contract for the full evaluation, including provisions such as: — Evaluation standards — Deliverables — Deadlines — Data collection protocols — Local support of data collection — Evaluation staff — Organizational contacts — Funding • Assess and address needs for metaevaluation. — Assure that the evaluator ultimately will attest to the extent that the evaluation adheres to the evaluation field's standards. — As needed, arrange and fund an independent, standards-based metaevaluation.
Engage stakeholders in evaluations.	• Bring organizational staff and policymakers together in embracing and helping apply a common approach to evaluation. — Clearly establish and communicate the organization's commitment to systematic evaluation. — Educate stakeholders about the organization's concept of evaluation, including standards, intended evaluation users and uses, evaluation framework, and importance of stakeholder involvement. — Establish mechanisms for effectively involving stakeholders (e.g., establish an evaluation stakeholders review panel and conduct periodic panel sessions in which the evaluator briefs different stakeholder groups on the evaluation's progress and obtains panel feedback on draft reports).
Help plan responsive evaluations.	• Actively collaborate with evaluators and stakeholders to assure that evaluations are properly focused, feasible for effective implementation, and likely to produce needed answers to high-priority evaluation questions. — Engage stakeholders to examine evaluation plans for their utility, feasibility, propriety, accuracy, and accountability. — Create needed mechanisms to facilitate the evaluator's efforts to collect needed information and report findings to intended users.

(continued)

Task	Explanation
Facilitate the evaluation process.	• Keep apprised of the evaluation's progress, remove barriers to effective implementation of the evaluation process, and facilitate the evaluator's collection of information. — Confirm to project staff and members of the parent organization leadership's full support for the evaluation. — Assure that project staff and the evaluator are well acquainted with each other's roles in the evaluation. — Provide the evaluator with work and meeting space. — Provide the evaluator with clerical and technical support as appropriate. — Provide the evaluator with access to needed project documentation, including expenditures. — Facilitate the evaluator's collection of information from project personnel. — Facilitate the evaluator's collection of information from organizational personnel (e.g., board members).
Foster use of evaluation findings.	• Assure that subject projects and the overall organization receive timely feedback. — Actively engage in face-to-face exchanges with stakeholder groups concerning the evaluation's interim and final reports. — Document and store findings from various project evaluations for later use in organizational improvement efforts. — Assist such organizational groups as the policy board to mine past evaluation reports for information of use in organizational improvement.
Institutionalize evaluation.	• Lead efforts to institutionalize systematic evaluation and mainstream evaluation practices throughout one's organization by: — Creating and adopting organizational policies for evaluation. — Establishing an office or other place for coordinating evaluation efforts. — Staffing essential evaluation operations. — Establishing and mainstreaming funding for the evaluation operations. — Arranging for periodic metaevaluation of the organization's evaluation system.

CHAPTER 5

∙∙

A Second Case Illustrating Application of the CIPP Model to Evaluate a Service-Learning Project

"Those who bring sunshine to the lives of others cannot keep it from themselves."
—Sir James M. Barrie

This chapter describes the application of the CIPP Evaluation Model to an evaluation of a service-learning project. The project involved 25 preservice teachers enrolled in the teacher education program at East Carolina University and 25 response-to-intervention at-risk readers in an elementary school in North Carolina. Zhang and a colleague applied the CIPP Model as a framework for thoroughly evaluating the project. They issued ongoing feedback to help the project task force plan and carry out the needed activities. Ultimately, the evaluators presented the project's full set of stakeholders with an overall assessment of the project's quality and impacts. As this case shows, systematic application of the CIPP Model can help evaluators conduct high-quality evaluations and thereby contribute to a project's success.

Overview

∙∙

Service-learning projects often involve multiple constituencies and aim at meeting the needs of both service providers and community partners. Thus, planning, implementing, and assessing a service-learning project can be especially complex and challenging. This chapter illustrates the use of the CIPP Model in systematically employing evaluation to help educators conceptualize, design, implement, and judge service-learning projects. Such applications of the CIPP Model are focused on providing feedback for continuous improvement and ultimately judging the project's quality and impacts. This chapter delineates the specific utilization of the CIPP Model's four components, analyzes each component's role in helping a service-learning project succeed, and discusses how the CIPP Model addresses the Service-Learning Standards for Quality Practice. The chapter describes how an evaluation team and a faculty service-learning taskforce in a research university used systematic evaluation to successfully carry out a service-learning reading skills tutoring project in teacher education and ultimately take stock of its multifaceted strengths and weaknesses.

Background

Service learning in educational settings involves the integration of community service into the academic curriculum (Koliba, Campbell, & Shapiro, 2006). Service providers achieve curricular goals while providing services that meet a community's needs (Zhang et al., 2008, 2009). As such, successful service learning requires researchers to identify the needs of service providers and community partners, design a project that can effectively address both sets of needs, and successfully implement the project to generate desired outcomes to meet the needs. Each of these steps is vital to the success of service-learning projects. Therefore, each step requires careful monitoring to ensure its effective execution. Moreover, service-learning projects often involve multiple stakeholders and generate intended outcomes as well as unanticipated spillover effects throughout the implementation process. While assessments aiming at a particular impact and focusing on a single stage of a service-learning project can be valuable in answering isolated questions on the merits of service learning, they often fail to employ a comprehensive framework to systematically guide the planning and implementation of service-learning projects and judge their multifaceted impacts on service providers and service recipients.

The CIPP Model can serve as an organized guiding framework for service-learning projects. Its four core components (context, input, process, and product) can systematically guide evaluators, clients, and other stakeholders to pose relevant questions and acquire and use assessments at the beginning (context evaluation and input evaluation), during (input evaluation and process evaluation), and at the end of the project (product evaluation). Specifically, the CIPP Model's context evaluation component can help identify service providers' learning needs and the community's needs for service. The input evaluation component can then help

prescribe a responsive project that can effectively address the identified needs. Next, the process evaluation component monitors the project's process and potential procedural barriers, and identifies needs for project adjustments. Finally, the product evaluation component identifies and judges the project's outcomes and formulates conclusions about its quality, practicality, value to the served community, significance for consideration and use elsewhere, probity, and so on.

Planning, Implementing, and Assessing Service-Learning Projects: A Multifaceted Task in Need of a Guiding Framework

The challenging task of carrying out a service-learning project lies in its complexity resulting from multiple project objectives and multiple stakeholder groups; the task is intensified by the lack of a reliable framework that systematically guides the process (Zhang et al., 2008, 2009). The need for rigorous and authentic assessment of service-learning outcomes has been increasingly recognized, and the many challenges in assessing service learning have been enumerated (Butin, 2003; Gelmon, 2000b; Holland, 2001). Service learning is a complex approach to teaching and learning; it deserves approaches to assessment, evaluation, and reporting capable of capturing and effectively addressing that complexity (Eyler & Giles, 1999; Karayan & Gathercoal, 2005; Mabry, 1998; Moore, 1999; Pritchard, 2002; Steinke & Buresh, 2002; Troppe, 1995).

Although the need for better assessment in service-learning projects has been recognized and a variety of service-learning project assessments have been conducted (Bringle & Kremer, 1993; Hamm, Dowell, & Houck, 1998), no specific model has emerged as a guiding framework (e.g., Baker-Boosmara, Guevara, & Balfour, 2006; Bordelon, 2006; Borges & Hartung, 2007). Researchers have mostly been focusing on the assessment of one or two particular aspects of service-learning outcomes. For example, Marchel (2004) discussed evaluating reflection and sociocultural awareness, and Peterson (2004) discussed assessing performance in problem-based service-learning projects. Even studies that expanded the set of outcomes only used a narrow set of methods, predominantly survey methodology (Kezar, 2002). Other single types of instruments such as portfolios have also been recommended (Banta, 1999).

A few studies have attempted to tackle the complexity behind service learning by focusing on various groups

---

BOX 5.1. The Breakthrough of Service Learning

The breakthrough of service learning at the national level occurred in 1990 when President George H. W. Bush signed the National and Community Service Act. It was reauthorized in 1993 as the National and Community Service Trust Act and signed by President Bill Clinton.

of people involved. A case study model of assessment was developed at Portland State University, Oregon, to measure the impact of service learning on four constituencies: students, faculty, community, and institution (Driscoll, Holland, Gelmon, & Kerrigan, 1996). The follow-up work by Driscoll and colleagues (1998) offers an assessment model for service-learning projects specifically in education that focuses again on the four constituencies of service learning. The approaches described were evaluated and refined in a pilot study with ten service-learning courses. The model provides both quantitative and qualitative measures at three levels of assessment: diagnostic, formative, and summative. Based on this work, Holland (2001) suggested a more comprehensive framework for assessing service learning that was based on a goal-variable-indicator-method design and was focused on four questions regarding the goal, variable, indicator, and method. Its strength is the attention to the complex dynamics behind service learning—the collaborative work of students, faculty, their institutional context, and their community partners. Holland's work represents the first step toward providing a framework for assessing service learning. However, the lack of a sense of sequence and its intertwined nature limits its usefulness in serving as an easy-to-use, systematic guide to a service-learning project's planning and implementation.

The CIPP Model: An Improvement and Accountability Approach

The CIPP Model is configured especially to enable and guide comprehensive, systematic examination of social and educational projects that occur in the real world. It emphasizes learning by doing, along with an ongoing effort to identify and correct problematic project features. As such, it is uniquely suited for evaluating emergent projects in a dynamic social context like the service-learning projects. A fundamental tenet of the CIPP Model is that evaluation's most important purpose is not to *prove* but to *improve*. The proactive application of the CIPP framework can assist decision making and quality assurance; and the retrospective use of the CIPP framework allows the researcher or evaluator to continually reframe and sum up the project's merit, worth, probity, and significance.

The link between the unique features of the CIPP Model and the need for a systematic, comprehensive

guiding framework in service learning is extremely strong. Stufflebeam and Shinkfield (2007) express this relationship in the following way:

> The CIPP Model has a strong orientation to service and the principles of a free society. It calls for evaluators and clients to identify and involve rightful beneficiaries, clarify their needs for service, obtain information of use in designing responsive programs and other services, assess and help guide effective implementation of services, and ultimately assess the services' merit, worth, significance, and probity. The thrust of CIPP evaluations is to provide sound information that will help service providers regularly assess and improve services and make effective and efficient use of resources, time, and technology in order to serve the well-being and targeted needs of rightful beneficiaries appropriately and equitably. (p. 330)

In summary, the CIPP framework can guide needs assessment and project planning, monitor the process of implementation, and provide feedback and judgment of project effectiveness, all for the purpose of continuous improvement. Although the CIPP Model has been widely used in other fields (e.g., Arzoumanian, 1994), it appears that, by 2008, the framework had not been adopted by the service-learning research community itself, where it can be especially useful.

The Four Components of the CIPP Model in the Service-Learning Process

The four components of the CIPP Model are essential in guiding all major stages of a service-learning project. This section analyzes each component's important role in the service-learning process, discusses how the CIPP Model is useful for addressing the Service-Learning Standards for Quality Practice (National Youth Leadership Council, 2008; see Table 5.1, this volume, for a listing of the standards) and describes its application to a particular university-based service-learning assessment project.

Component 1: Context Evaluation

Context evaluation asks the question "What needs to be done?" and assesses needs, problems, assets, and opportunities, as well as relevant contextual conditions and dynamics (Stufflebeam & Coryn, 2014). The objective of context evaluation is to define the relevant context, identify the target population and assess its needs, identify opportunities for addressing the needs, diagnose problems underlying the needs, and judge whether project goals are sufficiently responsive to the assessed needs.

The context evaluation component addresses the important step of needs and goal identification in a service-learning project. An effective project starts with identifying the learning needs of service providers and the community to be served. Many pitfalls are associated with assessments of needs, most of which can be attributed to the failure to adequately identify and articulate, in advance, crucial indicators such as purpose, audience, resources, and dissemination strategies. Application of the context evaluation component of the CIPP Model could potentially prevent these pitfalls.

Component 2: Input Evaluation

Input evaluation asks the question "How should it be done?" and identifies procedural designs and educational strategies most likely to achieve desired results. Its main orientation is to identify and assess current system capabilities, to search out and critically examine relevant approaches, to rank alternative project strategies, and thereby to help plan a project for meeting targeted needs.

The success of a service-learning project requires a good project plan that, if implemented correctly, will produce benefits for both service providers and recipients. Methods used to execute an input evaluation component include inventorying and analyzing available human and material resources, selecting a solution strategy, and converting it to a detailed procedural design, complete with the work plan and budget. Key input evaluation criteria include a proposed plan's relevance, feasibility, superiority to other approaches, cost, and projected cost-effectiveness. Literature searches, visits to exemplary projects, employment of advocate teams, and **pilot trials** are all appropriate tools used to identify and assess alternative project approaches. Once the evaluation client chooses and operationalizes an approach, evaluators employ such techniques as **cost analysis,** scales to assess service providers' relevant knowledge and attitudes, logic models, and the Program Evaluation and Review Technique (PERT) to examine and assess the detailed plan against the input evaluation criteria.

Component 3—Process Evaluation

Process evaluation asks the question "Is it being done?" An effective process evaluation provides a continuous and ongoing check on a project's implementation process and provides feedback regarding the extent to which the planned activities are being carried out as intended. Such assessments inform decisions concerning whether adjustments or revisions of the project's plan are necessary. An additional important purpose of process evaluation is to periodically assess the extent to which participants accept and can carry out their roles.

Methods of use in evaluating a service-learning project's process include identifying and monitoring the service-learning activity's potential procedural barriers and remaining alert to unanticipated defects; regularly interacting with and observing the activities of service-learning providers and recipients as well as other stakeholders; identifying the need for in-process project adjustments; obtaining additional information for determining how best to make needed improvements; and documenting the project's implementation process.

The CIPP Model's requirement for ongoing examination of a project's process is especially valuable to the assessment of service-learning projects because such a review: (1) provides information to make on-site adjustments to the projects (thereby maximizing their potential benefits to both service-learning providers and recipients); and (2) fosters the development of relationships between the evaluator and the client/ stakeholder that are not based solely on expert dependency but on growing collaborative understanding and development of professional competencies. Clearly, a service-learning project staff's systematic receipt of and responses to ongoing feedback on the strengths and weaknesses of a project's implementation can be immensely valuable to them for developing service-learning expertise and, over time, sustaining effective service-learning practices.

Component 4—Product Evaluation

Product evaluation asks the question "Did it succeed?" and identifies and assesses project outcomes. The CIPP Model requires that evaluators examine both intended and unintended outcomes and negative as well as positive outcomes. As has often been demonstrated in the evaluation of pharmaceutical products, it is vitally important to search out and assess an effort's side effects. In both promoting and judging a project's success, a clear-eyed quest must be employed to find both the good and bad aspects of the effort's outcomes. Such balanced assessment is essential for improving an area of service such as service learning. Sometimes such valid evaluations will indicate the need to abandon a failed project before it wastes further time and money—and, more important, before it harms the intended beneficiaries. On the other side, a comprehensive product evaluation that validates a project's merit and worth is invaluable for justifying continuing support and implementation of such a project. The purpose of a product evaluation, as suggested earlier, is to thoroughly assess an enterprise's value by measuring, interpreting, and judging all the effort's outcomes and to determine whether the obtained outcomes justify the cost of producing them. A product evaluation's main objective in evaluating a service-learning project is to ascertain the extent to which the project is meeting the needs of all the beneficiaries in a cost-effective, sustainable way.

Providing feedback is of high importance during all phases of the service-learning project, including its conclusion. The employment of stakeholder review panels and regularly structured feedback workshops can be especially helpful. The communication component of the evaluation process is absolutely essential to ensure that evaluation findings are appropriate, reported on time, and used effectively.

The CIPP Model's Linkage to Service-Learning Standards for Quality Practice

In 2008, the National Youth Leadership Council devised the K–12 Service-Learning Standards for Quality Practice (National Youth Leadership Council, 2008). These standards were vetted through a series of "reactor panels" convened nationwide by the National Youth Leadership Council and RMC Research Corporation (2008). These standards serve as the yardstick for judging the quality of K–12 service-learning practices.

The CIPP Model can serve as an organized, systematic evaluation approach to help service-learning groups meet these criteria for quality service-learning practice. Table 5.1 outlines our assessment of the linkage between the CIPP Model and the K–12 Service-Learning Standards for Quality Practice.

All four CIPP Model components were found to have high relevance to meeting the K–12 Service-Learning Standards for Quality Practice. Context evaluation helped ensure that project goals were aligned with the needs of each targeted beneficiary and the group as a whole. Input evaluation helped ensure that the chosen project approach was superior to other approaches. Ongoing process evaluation provided feedback for keeping the project on track, improving it, and documenting its strengths and weaknesses. Product evaluation assessed both short-range and long-range outcomes and gauged the project's success in relation to its modest cost. Application of the four types of evaluation provided a framework that was very conducive to engaging the full range of project stakeholders in the evaluation process.

The four CIPP Model components are of special value to project staff in providing youth and other project stakeholders with a strong voice in planning, implementing, and evaluating service-learning experiences; engaging participants in an ongoing process to assess the quality of implementation and progress toward meeting specified goals; and using evaluation results for improvement and sustainability.

The East Carolina University Service-Learning Project

During the spring semester of 2008, a special faculty taskforce at East Carolina University (ECU) initiated a service-learning project (1) to identify and address the learning needs of the preservice teachers in the elementary education program at the College of Education, East Carolina University, and (2) to identify and address the needs of at-risk readers in an area local school system. Twenty-five preservice teachers taking a course in Diagnostic/Prescriptive Teaching of Reading completed a service-learning component by tutoring 25 response-to-intervention students (RTI at-risk readers) in kindergarten, first, and second grades at a local elementary school. The evaluation of the service-learning project, explained and described in this chapter, was truly a collaborative effort. Table 5.2 identifies the main roles involved in conducting this evaluation and the persons and groups that carried out the roles.

Contractual Agreements

Learning to Teach, Learning to Serve (LTLS) is a program of SCALE (the Student Coalition for Action in Literacy Education), at the University of North Caro-

TABLE 5.1. Linkage between the CIPP Model and Service-Learning Standards for Quality Practice

Standards for Quality Practice	The CIPP Model's Relevant Components
Service learning actively engages participants in meaningful and personally relevant service activities.	• Context evaluation: help project staff identify intended beneficiaries' needs • Input evaluation: assist project leaders to design a service-learning project that is engaging and targets intended beneficiaries' needs
Service learning is intentionally used as an instructional strategy to meet learning goals and/or content standards.	• Context evaluation: help project staff identify and assess learning goals and/or content standards of service-learning providers • Input evaluation: help staff design a project and assure that the project plan provides an effective instructional strategy for meeting the learning goals of the service-learning providers
Service learning incorporates multiple challenging reflection activities that are ongoing and that prompt deep thinking and analysis about oneself and one's relationship to society.	• Input evaluation: help staff to seriously consider alternative service-learning approaches before choosing the one they will employ, and ensure that the chosen project includes multiple challenging reflection activities • Process evaluation: engage project staff and other participants in an ongoing process of review and assessment of project activities through such procedures as reflective journals, focus group interviews, and surveys on self-perceptions
Service learning promotes understanding of diversity and mutual respect among all participants.	• Context evaluation: assess needs of individual beneficiaries as well as needs of the whole group and thereby provide information of use in providing service-learning activities that serve individuals as well as the total group of beneficiaries • Input evaluation: help design a project that will promote understanding of the beneficiaries' diversity, engender mutual respect among all participants, and individualize service-learning activity as appropriate • Process and product evaluation: formatively and summatively assess whether the project promoted understanding of diversity, mutual respect among all participants, and individualized service-learning activity as appropriate
Service learning provides youth with a strong voice in planning, implementing, and evaluating service-learning experiences with guidance from adults.	• Context, input, process, and product evaluation: meaningfully involve beneficiaries in planning, implementing, and evaluating service learning through such procedures as surveys, focus groups, interviews, and role playing
Service-learning partnerships are collaborative, mutually beneficial, and address community needs.	• Context evaluation: engage representatives of the full range of project stakeholders in assessing beneficiaries' needs and validating project goals • Input evaluation: engage and help stakeholders design a program that is mutually beneficial and allows participants to work collaboratively to address community needs, and identify and assess alternative approaches to the projected service-learning project
Service learning engages participants in an ongoing process to assess the quality of implementation and progress toward meeting specified goals, and uses results for improvement and sustainability.	• Process and product evaluation: engage participants in the ongoing process of assessing the project's implementation and accomplishments, and using results for improvement and sustainability
Service learning has sufficient duration and intensity to address community needs and meet specified outcomes.	• Context evaluation: periodically update the assessment of needs of targeted beneficiaries • Input evaluation: help design a project with sufficient duration and intensity • Process evaluation: provide ongoing update of the project quality, duration, and intensity • Product evaluation: assess whether community needs and specified outcomes are met, and assess the project's cost-effectiveness, impacts, and sustainability

TABLE 5.2. Main Participants in the Evaluation of the Service-Learning Project

Roles in the Evaluation	Key Participants
Client organization	Learning to Teach, Learning to Serve (LTLS) program of SCALE (the Student Coalition for Action in Literacy Education), at the University of North Carolina at Chapel Hill, which was funded by Learn and Serve America, a division of the Corporation for National and Community Service
Top organizational official	Kathy Sikes, Director of Learning to Teach, Learning to Service (LTLS) program, which is part of the Student Coalition for Action in Literacy Education (SCALE) funded by Learn and Serve America
East Carolina University officials overseeing the project	Dr. Rita Gonsalves, East Carolina University's Chancellor of Service Learning and Patricia Anderson, Chair of the Department of Curriculum and Instruction
Funder	LTLS program of the Student Coalition for Action in Literacy Education (SCALE)
Project director	Dr. Christine Shea, a professor in the College of Education of East Carolina University, with expertise in foundations of education
Project implementation team	The service-learning faculty taskforce members
Project staff	The secretary of the Department of Curriculum and Instruction, who kept records and logged project-related decisions to help the taskforce members identify and keep track of decisions and actions related to the service-learning project operation; cooperating teachers at the elementary school, who provided the preservice teachers with guidance and advice related to tutoring the RTI at-risk readers at the elementary school
Beneficiaries	25 participating preservice teachers who provided one-on-one tutoring to RTI at-risk readers
Evaluation contractor	Two faculty members in the College of Education, East Carolina University, with research and evaluation expertise (the second author of this book and Dr. Nancy Zeller)
Evaluation staff	Two graduate students working with the evaluators
On-site traveling observer	Dr. Robin Griffith and Dr. Katherine Misulis, with expertise in reading education, and Dr. Nancy Zeller, with expertise in research and literacy education, traveled regularly to the project site to observe operations, interview participants, and photograph progress
Focus group interviewers and interview data analysts	Dr. Sharon Knight, from the College of Health and Human Performance; the two evaluators; and Dr. Robin Griffith
Other stakeholders	School principal, cooperating teachers, reading specialists, and parents of the RTI at-risk readers
Other interested parties	Service-learning providers and recipients, as well as service-learning researchers and practitioners from throughout the United States and the world; other service-learning foundations

lina at Chapel Hill and funded by Learn and Serve America, a division of the Corporation for National and Community Service. In Fall 2007, as a North Carolina statewide initiative to integrate service learning into teacher education, the LTLS program requested proposals from education colleges in North Carolina to design and implement service-learning projects to improve teacher education and provide evidence for the project's effectiveness.

LTLS was then in its second year, and its network includes faculty, administrators, and students from preservice education programs at 12 universities and colleges across the state of North Carolina. The LTLS was the first program of its kind in the country and provided a network for North Carolina preservice educators committed to making an enduring difference in K–12 education by participating in service learning and learning how to use it in their own classrooms.

Following a review of curriculum vitae and discussions among faculty, Dr. Christine Shea, a professor in the foundations of education, formed a service-learning faculty taskforce. Dr. Shea led the taskforce as the director; the rest of the taskforce consisted of one university administrator, four expert content area faculty members, and two faculty members in research and evaluation methodology. The taskforce submitted a grant proposal and successfully obtained $20,000 in grant funding from LTLS to carry out a service-learning project titled "Learning to Teach, Learning to Serve" in teacher education.

The two faculty members in research and evaluation methodology are Dr. Guili Zhang and her colleague Dr. Nancy Zeller. Besides being on the service-learning taskforce, they also formed an evaluation team and secured a separate $10,000 evaluation grant from LTLS to help the teacher education program prioritize needs, design a project to address the identified needs, and evaluate the service-learning project's effectiveness. LTLS approved the evaluation team's proposal to use the CIPP Model to systematically guide the conception, design, implementation, and assessment of the service-learning project and materially assist its successful completion and attainment of desired outcomes. Therefore, the evaluation contractors became an important component of the project.

LTLS, deeply committed to the protection and **confidentiality** of the program participants, required evaluators to take precautions to increase safeguards for participant-level data. The evaluators agreed to use **Qualtrics,** an online survey system managed by the Odum Institute for Research in Social Science at the University of North Carolina at Chapel Hill, and maintained data behind a firewall; data were accessed only by the owner of the survey (the LTLS Director), who must provide password and user ID. To protect the identities of both LTLS college student and K–12 learner participants, no individual names were linked to the data collected using Qualtrics. Instead, LTLS participating college students were asked to use their college student identification number or an assigned number developed by their campus LTLS team when completing LTLS evaluation forms and surveys. Also, K–12 learners were identified by an identification number linked to their LTLS college student partner's identification number.

LTLS, seeking to streamline its evaluation process, instructed the evaluation teams to submit their evaluation reports by filling out the LTLS's evaluation report forms online using the Qualtrics software system. These online submissions were to be completed by May 9, 2008, when the semester-long service-learning project would end. The evaluators provided those project staff members with process documents that outlined the administration procedures and provided answers to pertinent questions and concerns about participant confidentiality and use of student identification numbers. Because LTLS hoped that its service-learning initiatives would have national impact, the evaluators and LTLS agreed to try to publish the evaluation findings as journal articles, book chapters, and conference presentations.

Budgeting the Evaluation

LTLS offered just $10,000 to conduct the project evaluation. With such a limited amount, frugality was a must. First, $500 out of the $10,000 was set aside to help cover **indirect costs.** Second, each of the two evaluators requested a small percentage of buyout of their spring 2008 semester teaching loads, which totaled $7,029.08 in salary. The evaluators budgeted $500 for a qualitative research specialist from the College of Health Science and Human Performance, Dr. Sharon Knight, to serve as moderator of the evaluation's focus group interviews and to analyze the interview data.

The rest of the evaluation funds were budgeted for conference travel and supplies. Conference travel was a necessary element to be budgeted because they wanted to disseminate the evaluation findings at national conference(s). The supplies included books on service learning and an overhead projector. ECU helped cover evaluation costs by paying two graduate assistants' stipends. As expected, and as it turned out, the evaluation funding was insufficient to cover all of the conference travels, but the evaluators received verbal agreement from the project Principal Investigator, Christine Shea, that the project funding could be used for conference travels for dissemination purposes when needed.

Upon receiving the proposed funding, the evaluators secured the Internal Review Board (IRB) human subjects approval with the university's IRB board, the preservice teachers, the RTI at-risk readers and their parents, prior to the project's implementation. Subsequently, the evaluation team methodically conducted the four CIPP evaluation components using a variety of assessment techniques, as outlined in Table 5.3 and described in the following sections.

Context Evaluation

This evaluation began with an extensive set of context evaluations. These evaluations were conducted to identify relevant needs within ECU's College of Education, associated needs in ECU at large, the involved

TABLE 5.3. Using the CIPP Model to Guide the Service-Learning Reading Skills Tutoring Project

CIPP Model Components	Methods Used in Evaluating the Service-Learning Project
Component 1: Context evaluation—Assess needs and identify assets and opportunities for addressing the needs.	• Assess the setting for the intended service. • Interview school principal, teachers, and reading specialists. • Review school records. • Identify at-risk readers and their needs. • Administer diagnostic tests to at-risk readers. • Conduct initial quantitative assessment of at-risk readers. • Conduct preservice teacher focus group interviews. • Conduct initial quantitative assessments of preservice teachers.
Component 2: Input evaluation—Help prescribe a project to meet the identified needs and identify and assess project strategies and procedural designs.	• Review relevant literature. • Interview school principal, teachers, and reading specialists. • Consult university reading faculty and other experts. • View exemplary projects. • Consult Learn and Serve America. • Form and employ advocate teams. • Meet with service-learning taskforce members on a biweekly basis. • Conduct preservice teacher focus group interviews.
Component 3: Process evaluation—Monitor the project's process and potential procedural barriers and identify needs for project adjustments.	• Identify what activities should be monitored. • Receive biweekly updates from the service-learning taskforce. • Observe service-learning activities. • Keep a log of the activities. • Interview at-risk readers. • Interview preservice teachers. • Interview school principal, teachers, and reading specialists. • Review preservice teachers' self-reflections. • Review students' work samples. • Conduct debriefing with preservice teachers.
Component 4: Product evaluation—Measure, interpret, and judge project outcomes and interpret their merit, worth, significance, and probity.	• Conduct postproject quantitative assessments of the preservice teachers. • Conduct a postproject focus group interview of preservice teachers. • Conduct postproject quantitative assessments of at-risk readers. • Administer at-risk readers survey. • Interview or survey other stakeholders, including faculty instructor, principal, teacher, reading specialist, and parents of at-risk readers.

school district, and the selected school where the main service-learning project would be carried out.

The evaluators, along with the service-learning taskforce, first assessed ECU's needs for the service-learning project and its capability to carry out the project. ECU's College of Education offers both undergraduate and graduate programs of study in teacher preparation. All of its programs incorporate internship opportunities or capstone projects in collaboration with K–12 school professionals and community partners. Service learning had become part of the culture at the university. The creation of a new position, the vice chancellor for service learning, held by Rita Gonsalves

at the time, had generated great interest in service-learning projects and opportunities on and off campus. The university has a well-established infrastructure for service-learning research activities. There were well-integrated projects within the university where students spent a semester or more in a connected series of courses linked to service-learning projects in the community.

The evaluators and the service-learning taskforce next examined the university's mission, curriculum, professional teaching standards, class experiences, relevant literature, and feedback from school systems and also identified the critical need within the College of

Education to work toward improving teacher retention. They further posited that preexposure to school environment will decrease teacher attrition and thereby improve teacher retention. That is, if preservice teachers have a better understanding of the teaching profession and the reality of working with diverse student populations through hands-on practice in schools, they will be more likely to actively acquire needed professional pedagogical skills in the teacher education program and stay in the teaching field once they enter it.

To identify needs within the involved local school system, the taskforce communicated with and interviewed Debbie Metcalf, a part-time faculty member in our College of Education and also a teacher in the project's involved school district. With her help, the evaluators identified assistance to elementary level at-risk readers as the most important need to be addressed by the project.

The evaluators then designed further assessments and discussed them with Kathy Sikes, the director of the LTLS/SCALES project. The evaluators noted that they would examine whether the project activities were keyed to LTLS/SCALES' values to ensure that the evaluations of the taskforce's effectiveness would be grounded in explicit values.

SCALE's mission is to mobilize and support college students and campus-based programs in order to address the United States' literacy needs. Through a dynamic partnership between campuses and communities, SCALE develops leaders who are agents of social change (*http://readwriteact.org/about/*). Sikes concluded that the project activities and evaluation efforts were well keyed to the values of LTLS/SCALES, and fully supported the proposed project activities.

The taskforce then began to ask, "What kind of service-learning project will best meet both the needs of the elementary level at-risk readers and our preservice teachers' needs to gain first-hand experience with diverse student populations?" "Which school has the greatest needs?" The taskforce looked for a school situation that provided the best fit between the preservice teachers' needs and the needs of children.

Once a potential site was identified, the taskforce met with the principal and discussed their proposal. Students in the Response-to-Intervention process (RTI at-risk readers) were selected to be the service-learning recipients because they were working below grade level in reading and writing, were considered at-risk readers and writers, but were not receiving special education services. This target population of at-risk readers need-ed, but had not been receiving, individual assistance in reading.

The service site was an elementary school representative of a typical elementary school; the school's racial and socioeconomic balance was the result of county-wide school district equity policies, achieved through busing—assigning and transporting students to schools so as to redress prior racial segregation of schools, or to overcome the effects of residential segregation on local school demographics. The principal was very receptive to the proposed service-learning project. The elementary teachers to be involved were positive about the potential benefits of the project for their students and were pleased to work with the preservice teachers and ECU service-learning faculty taskforce members.

The evaluators began to design the evaluation based on the available resources and project-related conditions. A true experimental design was not feasible because random assignment of subjects into experimental and control groups was not practical and a relatively equivalent comparison group was not available. The evaluators chose to use a one-group pretest—posttest evaluation design to evaluate the impacts of the service-learning project on the preservice teachers and elementary at-risk readers. This design provides good structure. There is a single selected participating group under observation, with careful measurements performed both before and after applying the intervention.

In continuing the context evaluation (and for later product evaluation using before and after project comparison), the evaluators conducted initial assessments of the preservice teachers in January, before the service-learning intervention. They used multisession focus group interviews to explore their initial attitudes and dispositions about this project and about working with students from diverse backgrounds. The interviews revealed that the preservice teachers were equipped with the knowledge and skills needed to provide effective service to the at-risk readers. More importantly, the teachers expressed strong curiosity and desire to participate in this project.

In an effort to more fully gauge the pre–post changes in preservice teachers associated with the project, the evaluators utilized quantitative instruments prior to project implementation to assess these teachers' initial entry level regarding community service self-efficacy, motivations regarding volunteer activity, self-esteem, and confidence in making a significant contribution to the community through service. The following research instruments were used:

- Self-Esteem Scale (Rosenberg, 1965)
- Community Service **Self-Efficacy Scale** (Reeb, Katsuyama, Sammon, & Yoder, 1998)
- Volunteer Functions Inventory (Clary et al., 1998)
- Personal Social Values Scale (Mabry, 1998)

Similarly, the evaluators completed additional context evaluation-related assessments on the initial status of elementary school students' self-esteem, steps toward independence, and academic achievement in reading and oral and written language skills. The preservice teachers administered literacy assessments, including running records (Clay, 1993), the Qualitative Reading Inventory–4 (Leslie & Caldwell, 2006), the Elementary Reading Attitude Survey (McKenna & Kear, 1990), and the Burke Reading Interview (Burke, 1980). Based on these assessments, the preservice teachers later designed and taught lessons that targeted the students' assessed needs while building on their strengths during the service-learning project. They also shadowed their assigned students during reading and writing instruction.

Input Evaluation

The evaluators completed input evaluation in order to help the taskforce prescribe a sound service-learning project. They conducted meetings with ECU College of Education reading faculty Robin Griffith and Katherine Misulis, several reading specialists in the elementary school, and potential collaborating classroom teachers to discuss what kind of service-learning projects would best meet the students' needs. Based on information gathered in this process, the project taskforce designed and prescribed a reading skills tutoring intervention that would join preservice teachers in a reading methods course with a selected cohort of RTI at-risk readers. Each week during the 15-week semester course, the preservice teachers would be assigned to spend 3 hours and 30 minutes in preparing to tutor a selected RTI at-risk reader, followed by 1 hour and 30 minutes in providing direct tutoring service to the at-risk reader.

Next, the taskforce conducted an extensive literature review on best practices for working with at-risk readers. The taskforce members talked with faculty at ECU and other universities in the area of reading education. They also discussed the plan with and sought feedback from reading specialists in the targeted elementary school. Finally, the taskforce watched videos of exemplary service-learning projects, visited leading service-learning websites, and discussed elements that would be important to include in this project.

As an important part of the input evaluation, expert input was sought to judge the feasibility of the service-learning reading skills tutoring project before its implementation, and adjustments were made to improve the project's design. The queried experts included service-learning specialists at Learn and Serve America; director of LTLS/SCALES, Kathy Sikes; several nationally recognized experts in the area of service learning, including Robert Bringle and Patti Clayton; ECU's vice chancellor for service-learning, Rita Gonsalves; and the chairperson of the Department of Curriculum and Instruction, Patricia Anderson. Based on the input received, the taskforce conducted face-to-face discussions as well as Delphi studies to refine the project plan. The improved plan was then shared with the principal and cooperating teachers for their input. Finally, the project taskforce adopted the refined project plan for implementation.

Process Evaluation

To assess the project's process, the taskforce members and the evaluators held biweekly meetings to give updates on the project's implementation. They also shared positive stories and discussed any potential problems that needed to be addressed. The evaluators held regular discussions with the collaborating teachers, the principal, and the reading specialists.

With the help of Robin Griffith, the university faculty member who was teaching the reading course and her graduate assistant, the evaluators observed the service-learning activities regularly. They compiled the obtained information and presented feedback to the project taskforce during their biweekly meetings. In turn, that group often acted on the evident needs to strengthen project activities. For example, project staff promptly addressed needs for guidance on administering an assessment and modifying instruction for English learners. The evaluators also held weekly in-class debriefings with the preservice teachers on the service-learning project.

The evaluators used the preservice teachers' self-reflections as an important window to look into the operation of the project and its impact on them. Self-reflection has been recognized as an essential link between community experience and academic learning (Ash & Clayton, 2004; Felten, Gilchrist, & Darby, 2006). Reflection can also serve to reveal the inner changes in preservice teachers and make these changes visible. Following each tutoring session, the preservice teachers spent 15–20 minutes reflecting on what they had gained from the tutoring session and what they had contributed to the students and the cooperating teacher.

To monitor and assess the ongoing delivery of tutoring to the RTI at-risk readers, the evaluators, along with the university instructor and the cooperating teachers, conducted formal and informal academic assessments (e.g., **content analysis** of samples of student work), structured observations, and curriculum-based measures during the project. They regularly observed the service-learning tutoring activities and provided oral and written feedback and updates to the preservice teachers.

Product Evaluation

The evaluators conducted product evaluation centered on two overarching questions:

1. What impacts did the service-learning reading skills tutoring project have on the preservice teachers?

2. What impacts did the service-learning reading skills tutoring project have on the RTI at-risk readers and other stakeholders?

The evaluators assessed the impact on preservice teachers from the following perspectives: preservice teachers' own reflections; direct quantitative assessments using survey research scales; focus group interviews of preservice teachers; responses to key course assignments; faculty observations of tutoring sessions; and input from university faculty advisors, the elementary school principal, cooperating teachers, reading specialists, and RTI at-risk learners. The assessment of other impacts generated by the delivered services attempted to uncover all noteworthy impacts on involved community partners, with an emphasis on the RTI at-risk readers being tutored.

Assessing Impacts on Preservice Teachers

REFLECTION

The university instructor collected the preservice teachers' reflective journal entries and entered their entries into NVivo 8. Three experienced researchers, Robin Griffith, Guili Zhang, and Nancy Zeller, conducted qualitative analyses of the journal entries. They adopted a codebook structure and the iterative process

of discussing each code until agreement was reached. One group member was assigned the role of *code keeper* and another, the role of *note taker*. The team members, working both independently and collaboratively, helped the *code keeper* give each code a definition, set inclusion and exclusion criteria, and identify sample text references from the entries. Each journal entry was independently coded by all three members of the team. Disagreements were resolved through discussion at our weekly meetings so that the codes were further refined. This process enhanced intercoder consistency (Fonteyn, Vettese, Lancaster, & Bauer-Wu, 2008).

FOCUS GROUP INTERVIEW

The evaluators and Sharon Knight conducted multi-session focus group interviews of the service-learning group before and after the service-learning intervention to explore whether the service-learning tutoring experience had made a difference in their attitudes and dispositions toward working with students who came from diverse backgrounds.

These focus group interviews were video-recorded directly to DVD, transcribed, and analyzed using NVivo 8 (Zeller, Griffith, Zhang, & Klenke, 2010). NVivo 8 enabled them to code each focus group interview participant, as well as group and individual responses to each question, and thus track comments and attitude changes from January to April (before and after the service-learning project). The Constant Comparative data analysis method was used to analyze the focus group interview data. It allowed examination of the evaluation questions from different vantage points. According to Krueger and Casey (2009), analysis of focus group interview data is "a deliberative, purposeful process consisting of four distinct and critical qualities. It is systematic, uses verifiable procedures, is done in a sequential manner and is a continuing process" (p. 128), all of which fit within the scope of the constant comparative method. And the basic, defining rule for the constant comparative method is that "*while **coding** an incident for a category, compare it with the previous incidents in the same and different groups coded in the same category*" (p. 106, emphasis added).

The evaluators examined the attendance and extent of participation (the amount of what was said) in the focus group interviews in January versus April. In addition, they observed the extent of synergy in the focus group interviews (number of incidents of students' responding to each other, asking each other questions, or referring to another group member's contribution). Finally, *and most important,* they compared and analyzed the January versus April quality, content, and level of nuance in responses. While examining students' responses, especially to the questions about diversity, the evaluators took note of the length of responses as well as the effort students appeared to make in answering the questions—for example, their searching for words to express their ideas, changing gears while talking, or hesitating to assert their opinions as fact. They also observed the number of times students responded to the same question and commented on other students' experiences.

The study found that the preservice teachers made significant positive changes from the beginning of the project to the end in terms of their attitudes toward students from diverse populations, level of engagement in the focus group interviews, group synergy, and quality and level of nuanced responses to key questions about diversity.

QUANTITATIVE ASSESSMENTS OF AFFECTIVE LEARNING USING STANDARDIZED RESEARCH SCALES

The evaluators utilized quantitative instruments before and after the service-learning project to assess changes in preservice teachers regarding the following constructs: community service self-efficacy, motivations regarding volunteer activity, self-esteem, and confidence in making a clinically significant contribution to the community through service. They used the following research instruments: the Self-Esteem Scale (Rosenberg, 1965), the Community Service Self-Efficacy Scale (Reeb et al., 1998), the Volunteer Functions Inventory (Clary et al., 1998), and the Personal Social Values Scale (Mabry, 1998). The quantitative data were collected and entered into the **Statistical Package for the Social Sciences (SPSS)**. The evaluators then utilized correlated *t*-tests to statistically compare the preservice teachers' responses on these research scales before versus after the service-learning project, and found statistically significant positive changes associated with the service-learning project.

OTHER ASSESSMENTS OF PRESERVICE TEACHERS' LEARNING

The course-related academic performances of preservice teachers should not be compromised by the service-learning component; rather, they should be enhanced. Preservice teachers' academic performances were monitored throughout the process. University fac-

ulty advisors Robin Griffith and Katherine Misulis and the two evaluators regularly conducted nonparticipatory observations of the tutoring sessions. They collected and assessed samples of preservice teachers' coursework, faculty observation field notes, curriculum-based measures, and reflective journals to explore the preservice teachers' understandings and mastery of the reading process and reading instruction. Additionally, the evaluators interviewed the community partners working closely with preservice teachers, including the principal, the cooperating teachers, and reading specialists, regarding their feelings about these preservice teachers.

Assessing Impacts on At-Risk Readers

Using an approach similar to the assessment of the preservice teachers, the evaluators continuously assessed the project's impacts on the elementary at-risk readers. To document and assess the effect of the project on the at-risk readers' self-esteem, independence and growth, and academic achievement in reading and oral and written language skills, the evaluators employed formal and informal academic assessment, structured observations, curriculum-based measures, and students' reflective journals both during and at the end of the project. They assessed the elementary at-risk readers' perceptions of themselves as readers, oral communicators, and writers—pre and post—through student interest inventories and the Elementary Reading Attitude Scale (McKenna & Kear, 1990). They also conducted a survey of the cooperating elementary school teachers to measure their beliefs about the project's impacts regarding each of the RTI at-risk readers who participated in the reading skills tutoring project. The outcomes measures obtained indicated that the RTI at-risk readers had greatly benefited from the service-learning experience provided by the preservice teachers.

BOX 5.2. After the Service-Learning Project

Two years after the service-learning project, one of the preservice teachers, Jessica, showed up at the door of Guili Zhang's office and told her (with much enthusiasm) that she had already entered the teaching profession, the project had a profound and long-lasting impact on her, and she was still in touch with the at-risk reader, the little girl she tutored 2 years earlier.

Client Group Response to the Evaluation

The project's client group reported to the evaluators that information derived from the evaluation had proved to be indispensable to the project's success. They said use of the evaluation's timely feedback helped keep the service-learning project's operation on track and headed for its eventual success. Cited examples of the evaluation's important contributions included identification of student, teacher, and school system needs on which to focus the project; early detection of and attention to implementation problems that could have derailed the project; and a rich array of outcome measures for use in judging the project's accomplishments. Through the conduct of context, input, process, and product evaluations, the evaluators assisted the project's staff in effectively carrying out the many requirements of this complex project, meet challenges that emerged along the way, and ultimately issue informative reports on the project's goals, structure, operations, and outcomes.

Sustainability and Transportability Evaluation

As part of the evaluation agreement between the evaluators and the LTLS/SCALE, the evaluators adopted the Service-Learning Sustainability Checklist to evaluate the sustainability of the service-learning reading skills tutoring project. This checklist was adapted from the Self-Assessment Rubric for Institutionalization of Service Learning in Higher Education developed by Andrew Furco. The evaluators used the adapted checklist to assess ECU's level of institutionalization of the service-learning project for its projected use in future years. Per LTLS's request, the checklist was completed online by ECU's service-learning taskforce. The taskforce downloaded and printed the checklist from the LTLS Faculty and Administrator Resource webpage and then met to complete it as a group. The taskforce designated one team member to submit the LTLS team responses online using the web link e-mailed to the campus project PI.

To reach a bottom-line conclusion about the project's potential for institutionalization and long-term use, the evaluation team conducted a series of interviews of the taskforce members, preservice teachers, the principal, at-risk readers, cooperating teachers, and reading specialists. The evaluation team's bottom-line conclusion regarding sustainability was that the service-learning reading skills tutoring project is an important part of learning for both the preservice teachers and the at-risk readers and is mutually beneficial; that it should be institutionalized as part of the teacher education program; and that the prospects for sustaining the service-learning process appeared promising.

Regarding transportability, the evaluation team judged that other teacher education programs and co-operating schools could meet the requirements for successfully applying the elements of this project to engage and instruct teachers in the process of service learning and subsequently identify and serve the needs of a selected group of elementary school at-risk learners. The evaluators concluded that adopters of this project's approach would need to incorporate the following key elements of the project:

- A base level of funding of approximately $20,000.
- A teacher education program that is or can become engaged in collaborating with one or more local elementary schools to serve needy students and that desires to adopt and apply concepts and procedures of service learning.
- Faculty in the adopting teacher education program who know or are willing to learn how to implement the concepts and procedures of service learning.
- A taskforce of university and elementary school educators who are capable and committed to leading the project.
- Strong support for the project from university and school district administrators.
- Parents of involved elementary school students who are supportive of the intervention and willing to cooperate with it.
- An elementary school that agrees and makes the necessary arrangements to collaborate with the adopting teacher education program to test the service-learning approach's ability to improve the education of at-risk learners.
- Willingness of the involved university educators and elementary school teachers to respond to evaluation instruments and procedures.
- Abilities of the teacher education program and participating elementary school to meet relevant human subjects' institutional review requirements.
- An evaluation team that would conduct proactive processes of context, input, process, and product evaluation and disseminate the evaluation findings.
- A willingness by the participating teacher education program and elementary school to build on

lessons learned from this collaboration and sustain positive aspects of the project.

Although the evaluation of the ECU service-learning project did not confirm the project's transportability by assessing the approach's actual adoption at other sites, the evaluators firmly concluded that the project approach had proved it to be worthy of consideration for adoption and testing elsewhere and that its elements were amenable to application in a wide range of teacher education programs and elementary schools. The evaluators offered the above bullet points as a kind of checklist that interested teacher education programs and partner school districts could employ in evaluating their readiness to engage in a cooperative service learning project.

Metaevaluation

Unfortunately, because of the limited evaluation funding, a metaevaluation was not part of the evaluation of the service-learning reading skills tutoring project. However, with both evaluators being specifically trained in evaluation, and having substantial experience in conducting research and evaluation in education, they were fairly confident about the quality of this evaluation work. Moreover, to further ensure that the evaluation closely reflected the CIPP Model and met the evaluation field's standards, the evaluators sent a detailed summary of their work to Stufflebeam. Although he did not conduct and report a standards-based metaevaluation, he did congratulate the evaluators on their systematic application of the CIPP Model. Notably, this exchange about the evaluation of the service-learning project was the original basis for Stufflebeam's subsequent invitation to Zhang to join him in coauthoring this book.

Reporting and Disseminating Evaluation Findings

As requested by the funder, the evaluators completed the evaluation report by filling out the LTLS's online survey and worked hard to strengthen the more heavily emphasized aspect of evaluation reporting for this project—research dissemination. The evaluators ensured that all the reports protected the privacy of the project participants. Different aspects of the evaluation report were presented at national conferences (Griffith, Zhang, Metcalf, & Heilmann, 2008; Zhang et al., 2008, 2009, 2010, 2011; Zeller, Griffith, & Zhang, 2009; Zeller, Griffith, Zhang, & Klenke, 2009).

The evaluators also published different aspects of the evaluation report, and some adapted portions of the report as research in journals and books:

- Article titled "Using the Context, Input, Process, and Product Evaluation Model (CIPP) as a Comprehensive Framework to Guide the Planning, Implementation, and Assessment of Service-learning Programs," published in *Journal of Higher Education Outreach and Engagement* (Zhang et al., 2011b).
- Article titled "Service Learning in Teacher Preparation: Returns on the Investment," published in *The Education Forum* (Griffith & Zhang, 2013).
- Article titled "From Stranger to Friend: The Effect of Service Learning on Preservice Teachers' Attitudes towards Diverse Populations," published in *Journal of Language and Literacy Education* (Zeller, Griffith, & Zhang, 2010).
- Article titled "Connecting, Listening, and Learning to Teach," published in *The Community Work Journal* (Griffith, Zeller, & Zhang, 2010).
- Book chapter titled "Toward a Better Understanding: A 360° Assessment of a Service-Learning Program in Teacher Education Using Stufflebeam's CIPP Model," published in the book *Transforming Teacher Education through Service-Learning* (Zhang et al., 2013).

Discussion

Service-learning projects involve multiple stakeholders and aim at meeting the needs of both service providers and community partners. Their complex and dynamic nature calls for an evaluation framework that can help *operationalize* the process and provide step-by-step systematic feedback and guidance. Effectiveness is essential to the continued viability and growth of service-learning projects throughout the United States. Poorly planned, unsatisfactorily conducted, and ineffective service-learning projects are not only unbeneficial, but can also be wasteful. Without the guidance of a comprehensive evaluation framework, evaluators, researchers, and other stakeholders will be constantly challenged by a service-learning project's complexity; without an ongoing improvement-oriented evaluation of the project, they will not systematically be kept informed of the effort's strengths and weaknesses.

The issue of multiple goals and multiple constituencies is a major challenge in evaluating service learning. Without a guiding evaluation framework that is well aligned with the unique features of each service-learning project, assessing these projects will likely remain formidable to many researchers. The lack of effective evaluation can be detrimental to the future of service learning. Service providers cannot improve their projects and services until they learn their areas of strengths and weaknesses. Service providers cannot be sure their goals are worthy unless they validate the goals' consistencies with sound values and a structured responsiveness to the needs of service recipients. Service providers cannot plan effectively and invest their time and resources wisely if they do not identify and assess options. Service-learning providers cannot earn continued respect and support if they cannot show that they have responsibly carried out the project plan, produced beneficial results, and met the needs of those they served.

The CIPP Model can provide a useful framework for the service-learning community in guiding the planning, implementation, and assessment of service-learning projects. All four components of the CIPP Model used together are important and can be conducted to systematically address all elements of a service-learning project. The CIPP Model not only provides guidance for assessing the impact of the service-learning activity, but also helps identify community needs by working *with* the community organization to identify needs and goals to be addressed through the service-learning project. The model also helps formulate a project targeted to best meet community needs, monitor project implementation, evaluate project outcomes, and provide recommendations for project improvement.

Because the CIPP Model is a social systems approach to evaluation, evaluators, in collaboration with stakeholders, help design service-learning projects to most effectively meet the articulated needs of the service providers and service recipients. Consistent with the Joint Committee's Program Evaluation Standards (1994, 2011), the evaluator should identify all relevant stakeholder groups and engage at least their representatives in hermeneutic and consensus-building processes. Involving all stakeholder groups is essential because sustained, consequential involvement positions them to contribute information and valuable insights and inclines them to accept and act on evaluation reports. This social systems approach fosters an understanding and connection among service providers, community partners, and other stakeholders and can promote the long-term sustainability of service-learning projects.

Systematic evaluation of a service-learning project is required from its initial conceptualization to its activation, throughout its implementation, and beyond. To succeed, a project team requires an ongoing flow of sound evaluative information, including needs assessment, assessment of plans, assessment of implementation, and evidence of positive and negative outcomes. The snapshot type of evaluation that assesses only project outcomes, after the project has been concluded, is useless for guiding project planning and execution and is unlikely to give educational policymakers the information they need to decide whether or not to adopt the assessed project approach. As shown in this case study of an evaluation of a service-learning project, the CIPP Model can guide evaluators to systematically gather and report the evaluative information that a project's staff needs in carrying through all stages of a service-learning project and ultimately assessing its merit and worth.

Summary

In contrast to the multiyear large-scale CIPP evaluation case illustrated in Chapter 4, this chapter describes the application of the CIPP Model to a small-scale, one-semester service-learning project titled "Learning to Teach, Learning to Serve," contracted by Learn and Serve America, a division of the Corporation for National and Community Service. The project involved 25 preservice teachers tutoring 25 RIT at-risk readers in kindergarten through second grade at a local elementary school.

The CIPP Model was used as a framework to guide the systematic planning, implementation, and evaluation of the project, and both measured the project's success and improved its quality. Utilizing the context, input, process, and product components of the CIPP Model, the evaluators helped the university service-learning faculty taskforce systematically identify the needs of the preservice teachers and the at-risk readers, plan the service-learning reading skills tutoring project, monitor the project's implementation, assess its interim and longer-range outcomes, and assess its potential for sustainability and use in other settings.

The chapter also discussed the CIPP Model's linkage to Service-Learning Standards for Quality Practice and delineated a wide variety of research methods and data collection and analysis techniques used in evaluating the service-learning project within each CIPP component. Overall, the project gave the preservice teachers firsthand experience of working with elementary students and improved their appreciation and understanding of students from diverse backgrounds. The project also produced both cognitive and affective outcomes in the elementary at-risk readers.

REVIEW QUESTIONS • • • • • • • • • • •

1. What elements of the CIPP Model were shown to be especially appropriate for evaluating the service-learning project?

2. What were the key steps in carrying out the context evaluation for the service-learning reading skills tutoring project?

3. What were the key steps in carrying out the input evaluation for the service-learning reading skills tutoring project?

4. What main elements were involved in carrying out the process evaluation for the service-learning reading skills tutoring project?

5. What main elements were involved in carrying out the product evaluation for the service-learning reading skills tutoring project?

6. What were this chapter's reported linkages between the CIPP Model and the K–12 Service-Learning Standards for Quality Practice?

7. Who needed the process evaluation reports, why did they need them, what were examples of the process information that was provided, and what examples can you cite of how the intended users of the process evaluation feedback actually used the feedback?

8. What assessments were conducted to evaluate the impact of the service-learning reading skills tutoring project on the participating preservice teachers? Please give your assessment of the utility of these assessments for helping the project to succeed and for judging its merit and worth.

9. What assessments were conducted to evaluate the impact of the service-learning reading skills tutoring project on the participating at-risk readers? Please comment on the choice of these assessments, with regard to their usefulness for the participating elementary school.

10. How well did the evaluation, as described in this chapter, effectively engage the full range of project stakeholders in the evaluation? If you found the evaluation wanting in this regard, what might you have done to strengthen stakeholder engagement in the evaluation process?

11. Describe a project that you might propose to evaluate, and explain how you would use the CIPP Model to accomplish the evaluation.

12. For the project evaluation you identified in response to question 11, what purposes might the context, input, process, and product components serve in the project's success?

13. Download the Program Evaluations Metaevaluation Checklist available online; see the box at the end of the table of contents. Then conduct and summarize the results of your metaevaluation of the service-learning evaluation presented in this chapter.

CHAPTER 6

Designing Evaluations

"A good evaluation design is the blueprint for effective evaluation."

A sound evaluation design is essential to ensure that an evaluation meets evaluation standards, is grounded in a defensible budget, is carried out systematically, validly appraises the project's quality and worth, and effectively reports its findings. This chapter provides practical guidelines and tools to help evaluators and their clients collaborate in designing an evaluation to maximize its fiscal viability, quality, credibility, and utilization. We provide 11 prompting questions to help evaluators and their clients reach basic evaluation design agreements; a detailed checklist to help evaluators make specific design decisions; a shorter checklist that was used to design an evaluation of a National Science Foundation supported project; explanations of how that checklist's key checkpoints were applied; and suggestions for synthesizing design decisions into an action plan.

Overview

This chapter delineates and illustrates the substance and process of developing and periodically updating sound evaluation designs. We begin by discussing the general nature of evaluation design. We next list general questions that can help start a small, usually internal evaluation. Subsequently, we present a detailed checklist for evaluators to reference when they must start an evaluation assignment by presenting a comprehensive, specific evaluation design. We next present the evaluation design checklist that was used to design a National Science Foundation–supported evaluation of a University of Florida Integrative Graduate Education project, and we explain how each of that checklist's main

checkpoints was applied. We conclude the chapter by discussing the creative process of synthesizing design decisions into a coherent plan of action.

The General Nature of Evaluation Design

A technically sound evaluation design is absolutely critical to an evaluation's success. How do we judge an evaluation design's quality? A sound evaluation design should clearly identify the project; be keyed to professional standards for evaluations; provide for meaningful engagement of the evaluation's stakeholders; focus on the target audience's information needs; list the evaluation questions to be addressed; identify the criteria for judging the project's merit and worth; delineate the needed data collection, analysis, synthesis, and reporting procedures; and outline the evaluation's staffing requirements.

Situations calling for evaluation designs range from internal, relatively informal evaluation assignments that begin with a general evaluation plan to contracted, externally funded evaluation assignments that require advance specification of all the tasks to be carried out. In the former situation, an evaluator may start the evaluation with a general outline of needed evaluation tasks and then add specificity as the evaluation unfolds. In the case of evaluation assignments that are large scale, external, and contracted, usually, the evaluator must immediately provide a comprehensive, specific evaluation design that enables the development and justification of the evaluation's budget.

In many large, specifically designed evaluations, the evaluation design will be updated throughout the evaluation based on exchanges with project stakeholders and the evolution of the subject project. The exception is the case in which the evaluation is to be conducted according to the canons of controlled, **variable manipulating experiments.** In such evaluations, the design is set in stone because when **randomized true experiments** are involved and outcome measures on experimental and control groups are compared to judge treatment effects, the treatment and control conditions must be held constant to avoid introducing any threats to the study's internal validity. In such cases, the initial evaluation design is considered to be fixed and must be laid out very specifically. Nothing should be changed in the middle of project implementation because changes might contaminate the outcomes. In our experience, fixed project evaluation designs—as in the case of controlled, variable manipulating experiments—are rarely used, have often been shown to thwart rather than assist project improvement, and usually are not feasible in real-world development projects.

Evaluation design is both process and product. However detailed it may be, an evaluator's initial evaluation design typically is only a starting point. Because many evaluations deliver an ongoing flow of evaluative feedback to the client group, the client group is likely to generate new questions for the evaluator to address. Thus, evaluators should continuously revisit, reexamine, and update the evaluation design in response to the client group's evolving needs and changes in the project being evaluated.

In large-scale, externally funded evaluations, the evaluator should make the initial evaluation design as complete and specific as is practicable. This is necessary to develop a sound evaluation budget and often is a requirement for negotiating an evaluation contract. Nevertheless, as the evaluation unfolds, the evaluator, in consultation with the client, should regularly update the evaluation design to keep the evaluation maximally responsive to the client group's evolving needs for evaluative feedback. This is especially important in evaluations that are for formative uses as opposed to evaluations used only for summative/accountability purposes.

General Questions for Designing Relatively Small-Scale, Internal Evaluations

The following 11 questions are designed for those evaluators and clients who need to begin an evaluation with just a general notion of the work to be done. Basically, these questions refer to what the client group likely will consider the essential elements of the needed evaluation. Whereas these general questions are targeted to uses in designing internal, relatively small evaluations that require little specificity from the evaluation's beginning, they are also part and parcel of the detailed evaluation checklists presented later in this chapter. Moreover, even in small, internal evaluations, the evaluator and client will need to interact throughout the evaluation to add appropriate detail or to make adjustments to the evolving evaluation design.

Here, then, are questions an evaluator needs to go over with the client as they reach general agreements on what the evaluation will entail, and it is assumed that detail will be added as the evaluation evolves. In effect, the following 11 questions are an interview guide for the evaluator as he or she reaches initial agreement with the client.

1. What is to be evaluated?
2. What are the time limits for conducting the evaluation?
3. What standards should the evaluation meet?
4. What evaluation framework will guide the evaluation?
5. Who are the intended users of the evaluation, and what are the intended uses of findings?

6. How should the project's stakeholders be engaged in the evaluation?

7. What values should be invoked to judge the project?

8. What key evaluation questions should be addressed?

9. What main reports will be needed and at what times?

10. What protocols should be observed in collecting and managing information and issuing reports?

11. Will the client group need the evaluator's assistance in applying evaluation findings following delivery of the final report?

A Comprehensive, Generic Checklist for Evaluation Designs

Following initial deliberations with the client to answer these questions, the evaluator needs to draw a blueprint for the evaluation, that is, a fully functional evaluation design. An evaluation design is a set of specific decisions required to carry out an evaluation. Designing an evaluation involves making a wide range of decisions that include agreements with the client on answers to the above 11 questions, plus a considerable amount of added technical detail. Checklist 6.1 (at the end of this chapter) presents a comprehensive, generic checklist for reference as a detailed evaluation design is being prepared. Whereas we advise evaluators to consider all of the checkpoints, the evaluator should address only those that are germane to the particular evaluation assignment.

To address the extensive list of checkpoints in the checklist, the evaluator will need to interview stakeholders, review a wide range of relevant documents, and apply technical expertise in deciding on the required evaluation tasks. During the course of applying the checklist, the evaluator should make an extensive list of the design decisions that were reached. Subsequently, the evaluator will need to exhibit creativity and responsiveness in synthesizing the long list of design decisions into a coherent plan of action (the topic of this chapter's concluding section).

Next, we turn from theory to a real-world example of using an evaluation design checklist to design an evaluation. The checklist applied in the following real-world case is shorter, and somewhat different from, the comprehensive Checklist 6.1, though it is largely consistent with it. By presenting the two somewhat different, but compatible, checklists, we stress that evaluators should avail themselves of checklists that best fit their particular assignment.

An Evaluation Design Used to Evaluate an Integrative Graduate Education and Traineeship Project

To make the evaluation design topic tangible, we discuss an example of an evaluation design that is based on an actual evaluation of an Integrative Graduate Education and Research Traineeship (IGERT) project funded by the National Science Foundation (NSF). The example given is typical of evaluations encountered in practice, and it provides an advance organizer for recounting the wide assortment of the essential elements of an evaluation design employed in the IGERT evaluation.

IGERT is the NSF's flagship interdisciplinary training project, educating U.S. PhD scientists and engineers by building on the foundations of their disciplinary knowledge with interdisciplinary training. The IGERT project was created in response to the 1995 National Academy of Science's Committee on Science, Engineering, and Public Policy report, and the Graduate Education and Postdoctoral Training in the Mathematical and Physical Sciences report (NSF 96-21). Both reports recommended that graduate science and engineering projects should: (1) be more flexible and provide more interdisciplinary options for students; (2) include options for education and training grants; (3) increase participation of women and underrepresented minorities in science and engineering research and training; and (4) provide students with broad-based professional and ethical skill training and career information.

In 2006, a professor in the Biology Department of the University of Florida (UF) presented a plan to apply for a NSF grant for an IGERT project that would provide interdisciplinary training to PhD students in four departments (Biology, Mathematics, Geography, and Statistics) and involve faculty from these departments. The project was named the QSE³ IGERT, which stands for **Q**uantitative **S**patial **E**cology, **E**volution, and **E**nvironment IGERT.

This example evaluation design was set in motion when the primary investigator of the QSE³ IGERT grant invited the evaluator (Zhang) to become a member of the grant application team as an external evaluator. The evaluator's key responsibilities were to design and write up the evaluation-plan part of the grant application and if/when the project was funded, to conduct the evaluation that would judge the impacts of the QSE^3 IGERT project.

To evaluate the impacts of the QSE^3 IGERT project and meet the information needs of its right-to-know audiences, the evaluator designed an evaluation grounded in the Joint Committee on Standards for Educational Evaluation (1994) and the CIPP Evaluation Model (see Chapters 1, 2, and 3). In the following sections, we offer a generic checklist for designing evaluations that evaluators and their clients can use to plan evaluation activities at their desired level of detail (see Checklist 6.2 at the end of this chapter). Then, we use the QSE^3 IGERT project example to discuss the key components of the evaluation design used for evaluating the QSE^3 IGERT project, where you will find detailed information and advice on the approaches needed to design a project evaluation. We provide advice on planning and executing such a design, while carrying out an iterative process to keep everything in sync. This list enables one to define specific evaluation aims and actions, while ensuring access to the necessary resources and tools to complete the work going forward.

A. Focusing the Evaluation

The first step in evaluation is to clarify the project. At first glance, it might sound strange that the evaluator has to determine the project inasmuch as when evaluators are approached by the clients, they are always told by the clients what to evaluate. The truth is that the clients are not always clear about exactly what is to be evaluated; sometimes they need the evaluator's help in identifying the project, and especially in determining what aspects of the project should be evaluated. Sometimes, too, the evaluator needs to conduct an input evaluation to help the client determine what project approach should be followed to address assessed needs and the client's goals.

Such was the case with the QSE^3 IGERT project. The clients contacted the evaluator with a basic plan for the project and expressed their hope to flesh out the project plan with the evaluator. Using the clients' own words, "we will recruit a group of students from different disciplines; bring them together with interested students at UF under the direction of energetic, creative

faculty who will work together to train them; and present them with research challenges that require them to collaborate and learn a wide variety of tools." Evaluators, especially those who use the CIPP Evaluation Model, should welcome such a chance to be involved from the get-go. The evaluators are well positioned to better align the evaluation with the project and maximize the "improvement" function of evaluation.

Upon receiving the evaluation request from the QSE^3 IGERT project's Principal Investigator (PI), the evaluator referenced and examined the bigger, relevant social context within the nation and across the world. The evaluator opined that, as economies become increasingly more global, tomorrow's scientists must be able to communicate and collaborate across disciplinary boundaries to address exigent problems. To succeed in 21st-century careers, they need to obtain the requisite personal and professional skills.

The evaluator then explored the context within UF and determined that there was a need for the university to prepare future scientists equipped with interdisciplinary knowledge and skills, by providing graduate students with interdisciplinary education and training. Collaborative education and training can transcend traditional disciplinary boundaries and provide students with the tools to become future leaders in science and engineering. Diversity among the students contributes to their preparedness to solve large and complex research problems important at national and international levels.

The evaluator continued in this vein of context evaluation and further determined that resources within UF could be used to meet the identified needs of the graduate students with regard to interdisciplinary education and training. The PI was an interdisciplinary national expert with a strong background in both biology and statistics. More than ten faculty members from multiple departments expressed enthusiasm about becoming involved in the work, including those whose areas of expertise included biology, wildlife ecology and conservation, statistics, mathematics, geography, and fisheries and aquatic sciences.

Once the needs and resources were identified and recorded, the evaluator conducted an input evaluation to review the existing literature on the IGERT project and find exemplar projects that best addressed graduate students' interdisciplinary education and training needs. The evaluator determined that the audience included the PI, the project coordinator, the eight faculty members who made up the IGERT council, and the participating IGERT fellows. The evaluator requested input from the faculty members to help the client group design a responsive IGERT project, as well as from national experts to adjust and improve the project plan formed by the faculty members.

The QSE[3] IGERT project took shape and became the "project." It was to start in Fall of 2008 and would involve students and faculty from at least three departments. Later on, as the QSE[3] project gained increased popularity, students and faculty joining the project encompassed ten program areas and departments at UF (Biology; Mathematics; Statistics; Wildlife Ecology and Conservation; Geography; Fisheries and Aquatic Sciences; Forest Resources and Conservation; Agricultural and Biological Engineering; Infectious Diseases and Pathology [Veterinary Medicine]; Computer and Information Science and Engineering). Additionally, outside clients from state, federal, and international agencies also became part of the project. The project focused on the critically important and conceptually unifying theme of spatial dynamics, covering topics such as the evolution and spread of emerging pathogens; the causes and consequences of shifting species distributions; and conservation of species in patchy habitats. To tackle these critical issues, graduate students must acquire an arsenal of tools from the disparate fields of mathematics, biology, geography, and statistics.

The project's goal was to train scientists and engineers to address the global questions of the future. By using innovative curricula and internships, and by focusing on problem-centered training, these projects give their graduates the edge needed for them to become leaders in their chosen fields. The project team sought to train scientists who embraced a new philosophy about quantitative tools, who could speak to colleagues from different disciplines, and who could function as part of intellectually diverse teams by bringing different tools to bear on shared problems.

The QSE[3] project was slated to admit five students per year to the project, called IGERT fellows, distributed among biology, geography, mathematics, and statistics. The IGERT would provide support to the IGERT fellows in their second and third years; other support (teaching or research assistantships) would come from mentors and home departments. The university would provide additional funds to support some IGERT fellows to work on continuing, or new, research or educational projects in years 4 and 5 of their projects. All IGERT activities would be open to students with other sources of support. Faculty from two different disciplines would co-advise IGERT fellows. Table 6.1 summarizes the education plan of the QSE[3] project.

To increase its broader impact, other students at UF could become part of the QSE[3] IGERT project through a number of avenues. The weekly colloquium would be open to all students and would feature guest speakers, student-led discussions, and hands-on mini-workshops for learning mathematical and statistical techniques related to analyzing spatial data. By filling out a short online application, students could become QSE[3] affiliates and would be eligible to submit proposals for annual research funds, attend some IGERT activities such as field trips, and enroll in IGERT classes when space allowed.

The QSE[3] Annual Symposium would be held during spring semester of each year. The Symposium would include a variety of activities, including guest speakers, student and faculty presentations, discussion pan-

TABLE 6.1. Education Plan of the QSE[3] Project

Year	Semester 1	Semester 2	Summer
1	Spatial colloquium; disciplinary coursework	Spatial colloquium; disciplinary coursework	Disciplinary coursework
2	Spatial colloquium; gateway courses	Spatial colloquium; gateway courses	Cross-disciplinary rotations; modular courses
3	Spatial colloquium; workshop in spatial dynamics (WSD): tools	Spatial colloquium; WSD: research	WSD: research and field visits; modular courses
4–5	Dissertation research; continuing research and training projects		

Note. "Year" and "semester" refer to timing of participation in the IGERT project; timing within students' overall PhD project will vary.

els, and workshops. The Symposium would be open to all interested in learning about spatial ecology and the activities of the QSE[3] IGERT.

Carefully focusing the proposed evaluation work laid an important foundation for the evaluator to design the evaluation. It gave the evaluator a good understanding of project and evaluation responsibilities, and helped her make informed decisions regarding the proposed evaluation assignment. The evaluator could "take it" if everything made it seem wise to proceed, "leave it" if it was not in the cards to conduct a professionally responsible evaluation, or "negotiate" if certain elements stuck out as inappropriate or beyond the evaluator's abilities. It was important to negotiate matters that were critical to the evaluation's success before signing a contract. Even after signing the contract, some design issues needed to be renegotiated as the work unfolded.

B. Clarifying the Values and Standards

The values applied to this evaluation were based on the mission of the IGERT project: the Integrative Graduate Education and Research Traineeship (IGERT) project had been developed to meet the challenges of educating U.S. PhD scientists and engineers who were pursuing careers in research and education, with the interdisciplinary backgrounds, deep knowledge in chosen disciplines, and technical, professional, and personal skills to become, in their own careers, leaders and creative agents for change. The project was intended to catalyze a cultural change in graduate education, for students, faculty, and institutions, by establishing innovative, new models for graduate education and training in a fertile environment for collaborative research that transcended traditional disciplinary boundaries. It was also intended to facilitate diversity in student participation and preparation and to contribute to a world-class, broadly inclusive, and globally engaged science and engineering workforce.

The evaluator put forward the CIPP Model as the evaluation framework to be followed, explained its features to the client, and received his agreement. Importantly, at the outset of planning an evaluation, the evaluator should reach an agreement with the client on the standards that will guide the evaluation. The evaluator proposed to have the evaluation keyed to professionally developed standards for sound evaluations—the Joint Committee on Standards for Educational Evaluations (1994), which was, at that time, the most up-to-date

version of the standards—and reach a consensus with the client.

In this book, we advise evaluators to seek advance agreements with their clients that the Joint Committee on Standards for Educational Evaluation (2011) *Program Evaluation Standards* be adopted, and used to guide and judge the evaluation. (These standards are summarized in Table 2.7 in Chapter 2.)

C. Formulate Evaluation Questions

It is important to formulate a list of evaluation questions that will meet the information needs of the client, the evaluation audience, and society, in general. Evaluation questions can also guide the evaluation work, especially regarding what kind of technical design to use, what information to collect, and how information should be analyzed. Once the evaluator has clarified the information needs of the project staff and other stakeholders, evaluation questions should be formed to guide what information to collect and how to look at the information collected.

Evaluations that focus on a project that is under way should answer two broad categories of questions:

1. *Process-focused questions*: How is the project operating?
2. *Product-focused questions*: What is the project accomplishing?

Process-focused questions ask how a project functions, such as the types of activity the project offers, the number and types of people who are served by the activities, how individuals gain access to the activities, and how activity participants experience the activities. Process-focused questions should be probed throughout the project process and should not be neglected at the beginning stages. The answers to process questions should be reported continuously so that the information can be used to adjust and improve project implementation.

Product-focused questions ask about the outcome brought about by the project, including whether the project benefits recipients in the intended way. The best time to ask product-focused questions is when a project is fully implemented or has been in place for a while.

The questions evaluators generate should reflect the priorities of the project client and stakeholders. These questions could be adjusted as needed over time. For example, as the project and evaluation evolve, evaluators need to revisit and modify the evaluation questions, if needed, especially as the evaluation results are used to guide future activity planning.

To monitor the project process, a series of questions were asked in relation to the IGERT project components, activities, and whether they were carried out effectively. With regard to product evaluation, the main evaluation questions were:

- Were the IGERT fellows' critical thinking skills improved over the course of the QSE^3 project?
- Were the IGERT fellows' problem-solving skills improved over the course of the QSE^3 project?
- Were the IGERT fellows' self-efficacy levels improved over the course of the QSE^3 project?
- Were the IGERT fellows' interpersonal reactivity improved over the course of the QSE^3 project?
- How well did the QSE^3 project prepare the IGERT fellows to conduct high-quality research in spatial ecology and evolution?
- Did the QSE^3 project improve the IGERT fellows' ability to work in multidisciplinary teams?
- Did the QSE^3 project improve the IGERT fellows' ability to communicate inside and outside their fields?

D. Determining the Technical Design

When the evaluator began the dialogue with the client regarding the technical design for the evaluation, the client group expressed their desire to use a highly controlled, true experimental design with double control groups. The first set of controls would be randomly selected from the cohort of graduate students at UF who entered the department of a given IGERT student in the same year, matched by gender. The second control group would be randomly picked from the pool of students who applied for an IGERT fellowship in the same year, and who were competitive, but were denied acceptance. The intention was to use comparisons to the first control group to assess the general impact of IGERT training on an "average" graduate student in a given department. Use of the second control group would minimize the selection/motivation bias because it would constitute students who expressed strong interest and evidenced qualifications to participate in the IGERT program.

Given the fact that the client group is very concentrated in the "hard science" disciplines (and some were even proficient in very sophisticated statistical methods), the evaluator was not surprised by the proposed true experimental design. She entertained the thought of using such a design but subsequently guided the client team to think through its feasibility.

Both sides realized quickly that such a design would not be feasible and would not meet the NSF IGERT program's mission and needs. First, the QSE^3 project was new and evolving; it would be difficult and essentially wrong to hold the "IGERT treatment" constant. Holding treatment and control conditions constant would have stifled, rather than assisted, ongoing project improvement. Second, this approach was not feasible because the project would not allow random assignment of subjects to comparison groups and differential treatment of the groups, and it would be virtually impossible to form a fair control group through matching. For each IGERT fellow, to look for another PhD student entering the same program during the same year with similar background characteristics as a matched comparison would prove fruitless. Third, the exclusive employment of the experimental design approach would yield only a narrow set of outcome information. Lastly, and perhaps most importantly, by shutting the door in the face of those who try to benefit from the IGERT program, the project would have defeated NSF's mission to foster institutional and cultural change toward integrative education.

The evaluator and the client consulted the IGERT program officers regarding the evaluation's study design and were confirmed in their belief that the "experimental design with double controls" should not be used. In particular, there would be no control available because the project would welcome students who were not "IGERT fellows" to be involved as much as they could and become "IGERT affiliates." Therefore, conducting a randomized, highly controlled, and variable manipulating experiment was out of the question.

The evaluator proposed to employ a qualitative–quantitative mixed design for data corroboration and triangulation to enhance the trustworthiness of the evaluation findings. The quantitative investigations would focus on project impacts and compare the IGERT fellows' performance measures before the project and at the end of each grant year to monitor growth in problem solving, critical thinking, interpersonal reactivity, and self-efficacy. The qualitative investigations would complement the quantitative investigation and focus on both project operation and impacts. Qualitative approaches included focus group interviews of the IGERT fellows, one-on-one interviews of the IGERT faculty council members, observations of the weekly colloquium and annual symposium, and case studies of a few representative IGERT alumni after they entered the workforce. The mixed-methods evaluation approach combined the strengths of both qualitative and quantitative methods, was responsive to the audience's request for a holistic evaluation of the IGERT project, and was embraced by the client as a viable study design.

E. Collecting Information

Competent information collection is essential to an evaluation's success. Incomplete or inaccurate information can negatively impact an evaluation's utility and integrity by leading to invalid conclusions. Information collection methods for evaluation vary along a continuum from quantitative methods to qualitative methods. The evaluator in the QSE[3] project collected a wide range of rich information about the project from a variety of sources at the appropriate time points. These information collection methods included:

- A review of publications describing other, previous IGERT projects.
- Administering the California Critical Thinking Skills Test (CCTST) before, during, and at the end of the project to detect growth in the IGERT fellows' critical thinking skills.
- Administering the Interpersonal Reactivity Index before, during, and at the end of the project to detect growth in the IGERT fellows' interpersonal skills.
- Administering the **Problem Solving Inventory** before, during, and at the end of the project to detect growth in the IGERT fellows' problem-solving ability.
- Administering the Self-Efficacy Scale before, during, and at the end of the project to detect growth in the IGERT fellows' self-efficacy.
- Interviewing IGERT faculty council members prior to the project and annually during the project to obtain their feedback regarding project operation and impacts on IGERT fellows, faculty, and the university.
- Conducting focus group interviews of IGERT fellows' annually during the project to obtain their feedback on the project's activities, operation, and impacts.
- Observing the weekly colloquium throughout the project's implementation to document the project's operation and effectiveness.
- Conducting annual symposiums throughout the project implementation process to secure feedback on the project's operation and effectiveness.
- Conducting content analyses of IGERT fellows' coursework throughout the project's implementation and at its end.
- Conducting content analyses of IGERT fellows' conference presentations and research publications throughout the project's implementation and at its end.

The entire populations of IGERT fellows, administrators, and faculty council members were used to collect information from these sources because their sizes were deemed manageable. The evaluator ensured that each main question was addressed with multiple methods and data points. For example, to answer the question regarding IGERT fellows' growth in problem solving skills, four sources of information were incorporated to corroborate the findings: the Problem Solving Inventory score change, the IGERT fellows' feedback during focus groups, IGERT faculty council members' feedback during the one-on-one interviews, and the analysis of IGERT fellows' sample coursework, presentations, and publications.

A detailed plan was created that included an information collection time line, personnel assignments, and information collection protocols. The CCTST required special training, and the evaluator agreed to undertake the training provided by the test developer, Insight Assessment. The project coordinator agreed to facilitate the data collection process and handle such matters as scheduling interviews and sending out online test reminders. The evaluator discussed the rationale for the information collection plan with the client, reviewed the plan's details with the client, and subsequently reached accord on the plan's appropriateness and feasibility.

F. Organizing Information

The amount and types of evaluation information collected for an evaluation can be vast in quantity and will thus require careful and methodical organization. Although the IGERT evaluation was fairly small, its information requirements were considerable. The evaluator developed an information management plan and arranged to process, update, and control the collected information.

The evaluator ensured that the confidentiality requirement was met at all times. The respondent's confidential information would be removed or replaced with an identifier. The electronic information was only to be kept on the evaluator's laptop and desktop. The physical files were to be kept in her office, in locked file cabinets. Under the evaluator's regular guidance, a graduate assistant (GA) would be responsible for organizing, processing, entering, and updating the data. Both the evaluator and the GA were IRB trained and fully understood the confidentiality requirements for the project's information. The commercial tests would be scored by the test developer, and scores would be password protected.

When making information organization decisions, the evaluator kept data analysis needs in mind. Quantitative data would be entered, organized, updated, and analyzed using the SPSS statistical tool. For information to be measured repeatedly over time, an identifier was assigned to each participant so that subsequent responses could be linked to the same person. The evaluator established a functional system to file, control, and retrieve information that directly reflected the structure of the evaluation. The following general categories were used:

- *Focusing the evaluation category*: task order, the proposal, the contract, the budget, IRB records, evaluation standards and criteria, key participants' correspondence records, relevant background reports, literature, and evaluation schedule.

- *Information collection category*: methods and information collection instruments, sampling plans, information sources and their protocols, information collection assignments, information collection personnel training, and information collection schedules.

- *Information analysis category*: analysis plans, synthesis plans, analysis assignments, rubrics, instruments, and users' manuals.

- *Reporting category*: reporting plans, reporting schedule, draft reports, final reports, stakeholders'

feedback on draft reports, technical appendices, and multimedia materials for presentations.

The evaluator planned and followed systematic steps of information organization and management to ensure the obtained information's accuracy and security. She created a longitudinal database and tracked project participants for 5 years during the project and 5 more years after the project to assess the project's short-term and long-term impacts. Quantitative data collected through Qualtrics were imported into the IGERT database in SPSS. The GA was trained for data entry, and the evaluator regularly checked the work for accuracy. Field observation notes, video recordings of focus group interviews, and audio recordings of individual interviews were to be transcribed and kept as Word files for later qualitative data analysis.

G. *Analyzing Information*

The evaluator planned to conduct quantitative and qualitative data analyses to address the evaluation questions. An **analysis of variance (ANOVA)** procedure with post-hoc tests was used to compare the IGERT fellows' scores on each set of the quantitative measures over the 5 years (critical thinking, interpersonal reactivity, problem solving, and self-efficacy) to detect growth. Line graphs were also used to visually depict the trends over the five years. The ***p*-values** were supplemented for the ANOVA *F*-tests with effect sizes, as significant testing results could be greatly impacted by sample size, while effect sizes were not (Zhang & Algina, 2008, 2011). This was especially important when dealing with a small number of subjects.

The process of qualitative data analysis involves making sense out of text and image data. The evaluator planned the following qualitative analyses to address the evaluation questions:

- Content analysis of publications describing other IGERT projects to help the client plan the QSE[3] project.

- Analysis of the IGERT council member interview information over the years to examine their opinions regarding the operation and impact of the QSE[3] project.

- Analysis of the IGERT fellows' focus group interview information to explore their appraisal of the

QSE[3] project activities and operation, plus its impacts on the IGERT fellows.

- Analysis of the observation notes and photos of the IGERT weekly colloquiums to appraise the project's implementation and effectiveness.
- Analysis of the observation notes and photos of the annual symposium to evaluate the project's implementation and effectiveness.
- Content analysis of IGERT fellows' coursework completed throughout the project and at the end to identify changes.
- Content analysis of IGERT fellows' conference presentations and research publications completed throughout the project and at the end to identify changes.

H. Reporting Information

Communicating evaluation findings effectively to members of the audience and securing their appropriate utilization of these findings is undoubtedly a fundamental goal of evaluators. Therefore, it is critical that, at the evaluation planning stage, as well as throughout the evaluation process, evaluators carefully consider all steps that can be taken to promote and secure effective use of evaluation findings.

The first step in the evaluation reporting effort is to determine the audience to whom the evaluators will furnish the evaluation reports. The client is an obvious member of the audience; however, an evaluator typically should reach a much broader group of the evaluation's stakeholders. Such persons include those who can use findings to improve their work, those who have a right to know how the project proceeded and what it achieved, and those who are entitled to be informed about the project's accountability, especially its use of funds. Effectively informing all such stakeholders is in the interest of maximizing the evaluation's influence and impact. In the IGERT project, the audience identified by the evaluator included the primary investigator, the faculty council members, the other faculty members in the ten involved departments, the IGERT fellows, the IGERT affiliates, the project staff, the industry partners, the external advisory board members, the funder (i.e., NSF), and the IGERT research community.

In communicating with the client, the evaluator learned that the client needed to complete and submit NSF's annual reporting form online at the end of each funding year. A question on the form requiring the evaluator's response was: "Please describe a key insight that has been identified through assessment and evaluation during this reporting period (1000 characters)." In addition to including this question in her reporting plan, the evaluator projected the following reports in a variety of formats (Stufflebeam & Coryn, 2014):

- Prompt feedback to the PI and project coordinator on issues that need timely attention.
- Prompt feedback to individual IGERT council members regarding their IGERT fellows' thoughts and needs.
- Brief oral report to IGERT fellows regarding the evaluation procedures and progress, and summary of feedback from IGERT council members.
- Regular oral or email reports to the PI and project coordinator regarding project implementation and progress.
- Annual project progress report.
- Final report separated in three subreports: **project antecedents, project implementation,** and **project results** to suit different audience's needs. A technical appendix is included at the end.
- An executive summary report.
- Conference presentations of evaluation findings.
- Possible journal publication of evaluation findings.

While constantly interacting with stakeholders to obtain their feedback, the evaluator took good measures to maintain independence. Feedback was welcomed from all interested stakeholders; but the evaluator carefully judged the feedback's relevancy and dependability, and used it only when deemed appropriate for producing evaluation findings. More importantly, the evaluator always ensured that the privacy rights of human subjects were well protected, regardless of report type and/or delivery format.

I. Administering the Evaluation

A good evaluation design must be well executed for the evaluation to reach its greatest potential. Effective execution of a good evaluation design is central to an evaluation's success. To effectively carry out an evaluation, the lead evaluator often plays a role similar to that of the conductor in a concert. The primary duties of the conductor are to unify performers, set the tempo, execute clear preparations and beats, and listen critically in the process of shaping the sound of the ensemble. The lead evaluator develops an evaluation plan, assembles an evaluation team, specifies staff responsibilities, works out a schedule of activities and executes them systematically, pays close attention to the implementation process, and intervenes and makes adjustments as necessary.

The evaluator should include a schedule of evaluation activities and staff assignments in the evaluation design. The schedule and staff assignment should be examined by the client to ensure their feasibility, in terms of time, personnel availability, costs, and all other related factors. The evaluation activity schedule and staff assignments need to be updated on an as-needed basis as the evaluation unfolds. Having a graphic representation or flowchart to depict key aspects of the evaluation design's components and process may also prove helpful.

Budget availability and a sound advance contract are essential ingredients in an evaluation's successful execution. The evaluation's design should be fully reflected in the evaluation's budget, with its key cost items including evaluation personnel, consultants, equipment, materials, facilities, travel, communication, incentives, and indirect costs. The evaluator should negotiate a contract with the client that guarantees the evaluation's **fiscal viability** as well as its integrity. Chapters 7 and 8 address the budgeting and contracting issues, respectively, in considerable detail.

The quality of human resources is an essential ingredient in any project's success. Accordingly, staffing the evaluation is an important administrative task for the evaluator. The evaluator should recruit, assign, train, and coordinate staff members who collectively can carry out all aspects of the required evaluation activities smoothly, effectively, and credibly. In implementing their assignments, the evaluation's staff members need competence to establish rapport with the client and stakeholders and earn their trust and confidence. When staffing the evaluation team, the evaluator should seek such important competencies and areas of expertise as the following: research design, measurement, and statistical analysis; qualitative research and analysis methods; computer technology; interpersonal skills; knowledge of the project; and oral and written communication skills. Often it is also important to include, within the evaluation team, perspectives that the evaluation's audience consider important, especially gender, ethnicity, and familiarity with the subject project's environment.

Since the IGERT evaluation project was small, staffing the evaluation was almost effortless. Because the evaluator was proficient in research design as well as quantitative and qualitative research, the only evaluation personnel needed to carry out the main evaluation tasks were the evaluator and a graduate assistant. There were no issues of the evaluators' credibility to the client group, associated with such factors as familiarity with the project's context or gender and race, because the client chose the evaluators. In addition, the lead evaluator was well known and respected within the university that housed the project. She had earned her PhD in Research and Evaluation Methodology in that university and had successfully carried out the evaluation work of several NSF-supported projects in the Science, Technology, Engineering, and Mathematics disciplines. The budget and contract processes were both quite straightforward.

One particular element that proved to be especially challenging, but was anticipated and addressed in the research design, was scheduling. Because the evaluator lived several states away and the funding limited the number of trips she could make, many events had to be scheduled within a few days during the evaluator's trips to the UF campus. The events included observing the weekly symposium and annual colloquium, conducting focus groups, interviewing project personnel, and making presentations to update stakeholders. Weaving all of these events together in only a few days was made possible by starting the scheduling early and working collaboratively with the project coordinator.

J. Promote Evaluation Utilization

The ultimate goal for an evaluation is that its findings will be read and utilized, and will make an impact. Unfortunately, this is not the case for many evaluations. Too often, an evaluation and an evaluator's service end with the delivery of the final evaluation report. In such regrettable cases, both the client group and the evaluator miss an important opportunity to work toward maximal, beneficial use of findings and to secure the evaluation's impacts. Such impacts may include project improvement, dissemination, and even additional funding. With adequate forethought and advance budgeting, the evaluator and client can follow up the completion of a final evaluation report with a number of practical steps to promote and support the use of evaluation findings.

In planning the evaluation, the evaluator should engage the evaluation client to set goals for applying the evaluation's findings and design, budget, and contract the evaluation work accordingly. Provisions should be made for potential beneficiaries to study, assess, and soundly interpret and apply the evaluation's findings. Such evaluation users often need some prompting and some motivation, as well as some structure and assistance to do so. The following are steps an evaluator can follow to meaningfully engage an evaluation's stakeholders in the process of assessing and using evaluation findings.

First, evaluators may form a **stakeholder review panel** and regularly engage it in reviewing draft plans and reports and offering inputs throughout the evaluation process. This will generate a sense of ownership in the stakeholders toward the evaluation's findings and engage them in a process through which they can help assure the evaluation's quality and impacts.

Second, evaluators should take steps to make evaluation reports both easily understandable and helpful. Evaluation reports should be written using clear, unambiguous language and should be free of technical jargon, if possible. If some technical jargon is inevitable, it should be supplemented with plain language explanations. Acronyms should be avoided or used sparingly; if needed, they should be spelled out completely the first time they appear. Writing should be clear, coherent, and with enough needed details but still succinct, so as not to discourage the potential reader. Again, separating the final reports into three main parts (project antecedents, project implementation, and project results) will allow the audience to read just the part(s) of interest and potential benefit to them. As relevant, the evaluation report can generate interests in an audience by including material of use in institutionalizing or disseminating successful aspects of the subject project.

Beyond what can be done with the contents of the reports, evaluators can take the initiative to provide valuable assistance to the client group by meeting with them to support their study and application of evaluation findings and by employing structures and procedures to foster and support sound use of findings. The evaluators may conduct follow-up focus group sessions, meet with the parent organization's board, conduct workshops with stakeholders focused on use of findings, or jazz things up by developing a sociodrama by

which stakeholders can role-play consideration and use of evaluation findings, and so forth. Such follow-up assistance will need to be enabled by appropriate, advance provisions in the evaluation's budget and contract.

The IGERT evaluation was designed to promote its use. During the project, the evaluator kept close communication with the project team and provided prompt feedback and timely reports. Such an approach made it possible for the project team to act on the information and make adjustments to the project as needed. For example, during a focus group session, the IGERT fellows indicated that they were not in favor of the workshop format, where the faculty advisor was in total control of the project topic and dictated the research approaches. The fellows expressed their desire to take more control over the research topic, as well as how the team tackled it. The evaluator relayed this information to the project team, who found the suggestion of great merit and immediately made the adjustment. The end result was that the faculty advisor was relieved of the huge decision-making burden, and the IGERT fellows chose and worked on a project of great interest to them, gaining a great deal of leadership and interdisciplinary skills in the process.

To promote evaluation utilization, regular and effective interaction between the evaluator and the audience throughout the evaluation process was essential. It was an effective way to discern the audience's information needs, motivate them to request and use the evaluation findings, obtain their help when collecting data, and receive their feedback on the reports. In particular, providing a draft report to the audience and obtaining their feedback not only increased the clarity and correctness of the final report, but also made the audience an engaged part of the evaluation reporting.

After the reports were delivered, the evaluator and evaluation audience had "a celebration party" during the IGERT annual symposium. The evaluator gave an organized, fun, and dynamic presentation summarizing the project history, background information, implementation, and evaluation findings. Then, a dialogue ensued on a variety of topics, including:

- What do you think of the effectiveness of the IGERT project?
- How can we make the project better?
- When the funding ends, how can the project activities be sustained?

- How can we make the outside world know the benefit of such a project as well as the lessons we learned?

The audience was fully engaged with highly interactive discussions and was motivated to read the reports and keep the dialogue going after the event. A year later, the PI took a faculty position in another university but has been communicating with the evaluator about the IGERT project. He is getting ready to start a "new and improved" IGERT project in the new university based on the evaluation findings from the QSE[3] project. As the evaluator was writing this chapter, an invitation from one of the IGERT faculty council members was extended to her to participate in an updated integrative education project designed to train 66 graduate students at UF and 100 more nationwide as future coastal scientists.

To increase the evaluation's broader impacts, the evaluator presented the evaluation findings at the 2010 annual conference of the American Educational Research Association (Zhang et al., 2010). The findings will also be used to prepare a manuscript for journal publication. The IGERT alumni established professional connections with the evaluator on LinkedIn, are putting their IGERT experience, knowledge, and skills to work, and are becoming scientific leaders in their fields.

Synthesizing Design Decisions into a Coherent Plan of Action

After an evaluator has listed all the key elements of an evaluation design, there remains the complex and challenging task of converting the listed elements into a coherent plan of action. In addressing this task, the evaluator must be creative in producing a fully functional design. Such a finished design should provide for efficiently guiding the evaluation work, developing an appropriate budget, producing a detailed management plan, and responding to what the evaluation's funder (if there is one) wants to see in the evaluation design. There is no one format for a finished evaluation design that will be suitable in all evaluation situations. In the case of responding to a published request for an evaluation proposal (RFP), it is a very good idea to organize the evaluation design in accordance with the RFP's structure. The benefits of doing so are that the potential sponsor will readily see that the evaluation design is responsive to what the client group needs from the projected evaluation and that the design provides a sound basis for the evaluator's proposed budget. Of course, in preparing a design in this way, the evaluator must ensure that the design includes all the key elements needed to conduct an evaluation that fully meets not only the client's requirements but the standards of the evaluation field as well.

Summary

An evaluation design is a set of decisions required to carry out an evaluation. A technically sound evaluation design is an indispensable blueprint for effective evaluation. The essential components of a project evaluation design include: identifying the project to be evaluated, keying the evaluation to standards for evaluations, clarifying values for judging the subject project, determining the intended users and uses of the evaluation, engaging stakeholders in the evaluation process, choosing an appropriate framework for the evaluation, formulating evaluation questions, collecting information, organizing and managing information, analyzing information, reporting information, administering the evaluation, and promoting evaluation utilization.

This chapter provides detailed checklists for use in designing evaluations and illustrates the use of one of the checklists to design an evaluation of a NSF project. In applying these or other checklists, the evaluator will first list all the elements of the needed evaluation design and then synthesize them into a plan of action that is both functional for carrying out the needed evaluation work and responsive to what the client wants to see in the evaluation design. Initial designs may be relatively general for small, internal evaluations but should be highly detailed for large-scale, externally funded evaluations. In either case, the evaluator should regularly revisit and update the initial design as needed throughout the course of the evaluation. The exceptions are the rare project evaluations that employ controlled, randomized, variable manipulating experiments as the framework for the evaluation, and require constancy of treatment and control conditions throughout the course of the study. The overall goal of designing an evaluation is to systematically delineate and guide all aspects of the needed evaluation to help evaluators efficiently orchestrate the evaluation activities and ensure the evaluation's utility, feasibility, propriety, accuracy, accountability, and beneficial impacts.

REVIEW QUESTIONS • • • • • • • • • •

1. How would you define evaluation design? What is the role of evaluation design?

2. What main components should be included in an evaluation design?

3. Why should the evaluator make design decisions before the evaluation commences?

4. Why is planning an evaluation design an ongoing process?

5. Why is it important to understand the audience's information needs when designing an evaluation?

6. In the QSE[3] IGERT evaluation example, what types of information were collected and from what sources? Why is it important to collect multiple types of data from multiple sources?

7. What steps would you take to organize information?

8. What needs to be included in an evaluation design to ensure successful administration of the evaluation?

9. What types of project evaluations require very specific evaluation designs before the evaluation begins, and why is this so?

10. What elements should be included in an evaluation design to ensure that the evaluator will promote evaluation utilization and impact?

SUGGESTIONS FOR FURTHER READING

Davidson, E. J. (2005). *Evaluation methodology basics: The nuts and bolts of sound evaluation.* Thousand Oaks, CA: Sage.

Stufflebeam, D. L. (2004). *Evaluation design checklist.* Kalamazoo: Western Michigan University, The Evaluation Center. Retrieved from *https://www.wmich.edu/sites/default/files/attachments/u350/2014/evaldesign.pdf.*

Focusing the Evaluation

____ Determine the evaluation assignment and client.

____ Identify the major levels of evaluation audiences (e.g., project leaders, staff, and recipients).

____ Identify each audience's questions, information needs, and concerns about the evaluation.

____ Identify parties who might be harmed by the evaluation, and obtain their input.

____ Examine the background of the request for the evaluation and its social and political contexts.

____ Clarify the values to be invoked in judging the subject project.

____ Identify and address potential barriers to the evaluation, for example:

____ Need to gather sensitive information	____ Client's hedging on decisions to release reports to all right-to-know audiences
____ Limited access to all the relevant information	
____ Human subject review requirements	____ Opponents of the evaluation
____ Requirements for confidentiality or anonymity	____ Conflicts of interest
	____ Issues of race and language
____ Restrictions on the evaluator's authority to edit reports	____ High indirect cost rate
	____ Lack of needed funds

____ Identify and review relevant information (e.g., previous evaluations of the project, evaluations of similar projects, pertinent literature, and relevant needs assessments).

____ Reach agreement with the client on the evaluation model or approach to be applied.

____ Decide whether to conduct context, input, process, and/or product evaluations.

____ Reach agreement with the client on the time frame, the evaluators, key evaluation questions, required reports, client and stakeholder responsibilities, and allowable cost for the evaluation.

____ Reach agreement with the client on the standards for use in guiding and judging the evaluation.

____ Advise the client to fund an independent metaevaluation.

____ Decide with the client whether to assist the client group to apply findings following completion and delivery of the final report.

Collecting Information

____ Consider collecting a wide range of information about the project, for example:

____ Context	____ Plans	____ Staff	____ Transportability
____ History	____ Schedule	____ Implementation	____ Judgments by stakeholders
____ Beneficiaries	____ Reputation	____ Main effects	____ Judgments by experts
____ Benefactors	____ Resources	____ Side effects	____ Contrast to similar projects
____ Goals	____ Costs	____ Sustainability	

(continued)

____ Choose the framework for collecting information (e.g., case study, sample survey, field experiment, or a multimethod study).

____ Determine the information sources: documents, files, databases, financial records, beneficiaries, staff, funders, experts, government officials, or community interest groups.

____ Determine the information collection instruments and methods, for example:

____ Interviews	____ Survey	____ Video records
____ Participant observers	____ Rating scales	____ Log diaries
____ Literature review	____ Knowledge tests	____ Goal-free study
____ Search of archives	____ Debates	____ Case study
____ Focus groups	____ Site visits	
____ Delphi	____ Photography	

____ Specify the sampling procedures for each source: purposive, probability, or convenience.

____ Seek to address each main question with multiple methods and data points.

____ Schedule information collection, denoting times when each information source and each method will be engaged.

____ Assign responsibilities for information collection.

____ Orient and train data collectors.

____ Give the client and other interested parties a rationale for the information collection plan.

____ Review the information collection plan's feasibility with the client, and consider making prudent reductions.

Organizing Information

____ Develop plans and assignments for coding, verifying, filing, controlling, and retrieving information.

____ Design a database for the obtained information, including appropriate software.

____ Specify the equipment, facilities, materials, and personnel required to process and control the evaluation's information.

Analyzing and Synthesizing Information

____ Identify bases for interpreting findings, such as beneficiaries' needs, objectives, standards, norms, the program's previous costs and performance, costs and performance of similar programs, and judgments by experts and program stakeholders.

____ Specify qualitative analysis procedures (e.g., thematic analysis, content analysis, summaries, scenarios, or contrasts of photographs).

____ Specify quantitative analysis procedures (e.g., descriptive statistics; trend analysis; cost analysis; significance tests for main effects, interactions, and simple effects; effect parameter analysis; meta-analysis; test item analysis; factor analysis; regression analysis; and charts, tables, and graphs).

____ Select appropriate computer programs to facilitate quantitative and qualitative analyses.

____ Plan to search for trends, patterns, and themes in the qualitative information.

____ Plan to contrast different subsets of qualitative and quantitative information to identify both corroborative and contradictory findings.

(continued)

____ Plan to address each evaluative question by referencing and citing the relevant qualitative and quantitative information.

____ Plan to use qualitative information to elaborate and explain quantitative findings.

____ Plan to state caveats as appropriate in consideration of any inconclusive or contradictory findings.

____ Plan to synthesize quantitative and qualitative information (e.g., by embedding quantitative information within a qualitative narrative or by embedding interview responses and other qualitative findings in the discussion of quantitative findings).

____ Anticipate that the client or other stakeholders may require recommendations to correct problems identified in the findings, and be prepared to explain that the same data that uncovered the problems are unlikely to provide valid direction for solving the problems.

____ Consider planning a follow-up evaluation to generate and validly assess alternative courses of action for solving identified problems; such procedures might include an input evaluation of available alternative solution strategies, creation and evaluation of new solution strategies, engagement of relevant experts, review of relevant literature, or a working conference to chart and assess possible courses of action.

Reporting Information

____ Clarify the audiences for evaluation reports (e.g., the program's client, staff, policy board, and beneficiaries).

____ Identify reports needed by different audiences, such as interim, final, or component-specific reports; context, input, process, and product evaluation reports; technical appendixes; executive summary; and an internal metaevaluation report.

____ For each report, determine the appropriate formats, such as printed, oral, electronic, multimedia, storytelling, or sociodrama.

____ Outline the contents of at least the main reports, showing how findings from different sources and methods will be synthesized to answer the main evaluation questions.

____ Consider dividing the final report into three subreports: Program Antecedents (for those who need background information), Program Implementation (for those who would replicate the program), and Program Results (for the entire audience).

____ In the technical appendix include information such as the following:

____ Resumés of evaluation staff and consultants	____ Log of data collection activities
____ Information collection instruments and protocols	____ List of interim reports
	____ The evaluation contract
____ Reports of findings for particular data collection procedures	____ Summary of evaluation costs
____ Data tables	____ Internal account of how well the evaluation met the evaluation profession's standards

____ Develop a plan and schedule for delivering reports to the right-to-know audiences.

____ As appropriate, obtain prerelease reviews of draft reports.

____ Conduct feedback workshops to assist the client group in reviewing and discussing draft evaluation reports.

(continued)

Administering the Evaluation

____ Delineate the evaluation schedule.

____ Define and plan to meet staff and resource requirements.

____ Ensure that the evaluation plan is sufficient to meet pertinent standards of the evaluation field.

____ Provide for at least internal formative and summative metaevaluations.

____ Delineate a budget for the evaluation.

____ Negotiate an evaluation contract, specifying audiences, evaluator responsibilities and protocols, and editorial and dissemination responsibility and authority, among other provisions.

____ Provide for reviewing and updating the evaluation plan, budget, and contract.

A. Focusing the Evaluation

____ A1. Conduct context evaluation to understand the social and political context and identify needs within the context.

____ A2. Conduct context evaluation to examine resources that can be used to meet the identified needs.

____ A3. Identify the evaluation audience; these may include project funder, project leaders, staff, project participants, and those who otherwise might be affected by the evaluation.

____ A4. Identify questions, information needs, and concerns of the audience, including those who might be adversely impacted by the evaluation.

____ A5. Conduct input evaluation to help clients design and refine a responsive project plan.

____ A6. Identify and address potential barriers and complicating factors that might hinder the evaluation.

____ A7. Advise the client to fund an independent metaevaluation.

____ A8. Reach agreement with the client regarding such matters as the time frame, evaluation personnel, required reports, client and stakeholder responsibilities, and allowable evaluation costs.

____ A9. Decide whether to proceed with the evaluation assignment.

B. Clarifying Values and Standards

____ B1. Examine the mission of the client organization to ensure that the evaluation is aligned with its values.

____ B2. Adopt a set of evaluation standards as the official standards for guiding and assessing the evaluation.

____ B3. Reach agreement with the client on standards for guiding and assessing the evaluation.

____ B4. Reach agreement with the client on evaluation model or approach to be applied.

____ B5. Develop an Evaluation Standards Attestation form.

C. Formulating Evaluation Questions

____ C1. Obtain and understand client and audience's information needs.

____ C2. Formulate process-focus questions.

____ C3. Formulate product-focus questions.

____ C4. Reach agreement with client on the list of questions to be answered.

(continued)

D. Determining the Technical Design

____ D1. Select research designs that will enhance the trustworthiness of the evaluation findings and can provide information for process and product evaluation purposes.

____ D2. Bear in mind that mixed designs might be needed and preferable.

____ D3. Reach agreement with client regarding the effectiveness and feasibility of the research designs.

E. Collecting Information

____ E1. Meet confidentiality requirement when collecting information.

____ E2. Consider using both quantitative and qualitative information collection methods.

____ E3. Consider collecting a wide range of information about the project.

____ E4. Consider addressing each main evaluation question with multiple methods and data.

____ E5. Decide on information to collect for process and product evaluation to assess project implementation and impact.

____ E6. Choose appropriate information collection methods and applicable instruments.

____ E7. Determine the information sources.

____ E8. Determine time line for each information collection instance.

____ E9. Assign responsibilities for each information collection instance.

____ E10. Review and reach agreement with the client regarding the information collection plan, and make needed adjustments.

F. Organizing Information

____ F1. Meet confidentiality requirement at all times.

____ F2. Keep data analysis needs in mind when developing the data organization plan.

____ F2. Establish a system to organize information that reflects the evaluation's structure.

____ F3. Develop a data management and organization plan, including data entry, data storage, data transfer, confidentiality assurance, data cleaning, and so on.

____ F4. Specify the equipment, facilities, materials, and personnel to process and control the evaluation information.

____ F5. Assign responsibilities for data organization.

____ F6. Develop database(s) for the information collected.

G. Analyzing Information

____ G1. Plan analyses to best answer evaluation questions and judge the project.

____ G2. Identify bases and criteria for judging and interpreting findings (e.g., beneficiaries' needs, project objectives, standards, norms, previous performance, expert judgment).

(continued)

____ G3. Select appropriate quantitative data analysis procedure for the quantitative data collected and determine appropriate computer program to facilitate it.

____ G4. Supplement the p-value with an effect size when applicable when conducting significance testing.

____ G5. Select appropriate qualitative data analysis procedure for the qualitative data collected and determine appropriate computer project to facilitate it.

____ G6. Seek to address each evaluation question by referencing the appropriate qualitative and/or quantitative analysis findings.

____ G7. Plan to state caveats in light of inconclusive or contradictory findings.

H. Reporting information

____ H1. Determine the full range of intended report recipients, their common evaluative information needs, and the specialized needs of different segments of the audience.

____ H2. Determine the types of report needed by different groups of audience. Some examples are: interim report, final report, component-specific report (context evaluation report, input evaluation report, process evaluation report, product evaluation report, sustainability evaluation report, transportability evaluation report), technical report, and an executive summary.

____ H3. Outline the contents of projected reports, including evaluation questions, needed information, and analysis and synthesis of findings.

____ H4. Schedule the completion and delivery of each report.

____ H5. Schedule production and review of draft reports and planning to obtain prerelease reviews of the drafts.

____ H6. Plan to meet regularly with the client throughout the evaluation to review and update the reporting plan as appropriate.

____ H7. Obtain and use audience's feedback on draft report to increase the clarity and correctness of the final report.

____ H8. Determine the appropriate format for each type of report. For example, electronic, printed, oral, storytelling, webinar.

____ H9. Consider dividing the final report into three subreports for ease of use by different audiences: project antecedents (project background information), project implementation, and project results.

____ H10. Include a technical appendix or a separate technical report to provide access to items of a technical nature—for example, the evaluator's résumé, data collection instruments, and detailed reports of findings from a particular set of data.

____ H11. Project ways to follow up delivery of reports by helping recipients to closely consider findings and determine how best to apply the findings.

____ H12. Protect the privacy rights of human subjects in all report types and delivery formats.

(continued)

I. Administering the Evaluation

____ I1. Ensure the designed evaluation has the potential to meet the pertinent evaluation standards.

____ I2. Include a schedule of evaluation activities in the evaluation design.

____ I3. Review the schedule of evaluation activities with the client and reach agreement on its feasibility.

____ I4. Consider using a photographic reprise or flowchart to depict key aspects of the evaluation components and process.

____ I5. Include staff assignments in the evaluation design.

____ I6. Reach agreement with the clients on the evaluation design.

____ I7. Assign evaluation responsibilities.

____ I8. Have a plan B for important, time-sensitive evaluation activities.

____ I9. Reach agreement with the client on the budget plan.

____ I10. Negotiate an evaluation contract with the client.

____ I11. Provide for internal formative and summative metaevaluations and advise the client to arrange for and fund an independent metaevaluation.

J. Promoting Evaluation Utilization

____ J1. Use random sampling when possible to enhance the evaluation finding's generalizability.

____ J2. Provide detailed project implementation report so that interested parties can study and replicate.

____ J3. Plan to form and regularly engage a stakeholder review panel to provide input throughout the evaluation process.

____ J4. Apprise the client of the need for follow-up evaluation use assistance.

____ J5. Include in the evaluation's budget and contract the advance provision and funding for providing evaluation use assistance to clients.

____ J6. Identify ways to engage other stakeholders.

____ J7. Provide evaluation information to help with the project's institutionalization.

____ J8. Present evaluation findings at conferences.

____ J9. Publish evaluation findings in journals and books.

CHAPTER 7

Budgeting Evaluations

"A sound evaluation budget is necessary to successfully execute an evaluation design."

A sound evaluation budget delineates the financial support needed to execute an evaluation design. This chapter identifies and explains six basics of evaluation budgeting; identifies main evaluation budget line items; explains ethical imperatives in evaluation budgeting; identifies, assesses, and provides guidelines for six major types of evaluation budget agreements; and explains the application of a generic evaluation budgeting checklist.

Overview

Over the years of reviewing many proposals for evaluation contracts, Stufflebeam would initially turn to the proposal's back pages to examine the evaluation's budget. All too frequently, he encountered an unexplained total cost figure, a grossly imprecise budget, or, incredibly, no budget at all. In proposals that lacked reasoned and sufficient cost projections, Stufflebeam often skipped the step of examining the evaluation design and, instead, immediately recommended against funding the evaluation proposal. In such cases, he decided that summarily panning a poorly budgeted evaluation proposal would serve the funder's interest because, otherwise, he or she might finance an evaluation plan that could not be executed successfully or that might

be grossly overpriced. Also, he averred that placing a stop recommendation on an evaluation proposal with a poor budgetary plan would be in the evaluator's interest because this might spare the evaluator the professional embarrassment of launching a predictably unsuccessful evaluation due to its flawed budget. Regarding the need for sound, advance evaluation budgets, the funder should not buy a "pig in a poke," and the evaluator should not proceed to execute an evaluation design that is not supported by an appropriate budget. Fortunately, over the years we have seen improvements in evaluators' development of sound, advance evaluation budgets and funders' insistence on complete and justified up-front evaluation budgets.

In this chapter, we discuss the basics of evaluation budgeting and then guide the reader through the fundamentals of preparing an evaluation budget. In particular, we discuss six fundamental factors to consider in developing an evaluation budget; identify and explain an extensive list of potential line items in evaluation budgets and discuss how to reference them in determining evaluation staffing positions; advise evaluators how to keep evaluation budgeting on a high ethical plain; identify, assess, and give examples of applying six major types of evaluation budget agreements; and present and explain how to apply a generic evaluation budgeting checklist.

Budgeting evaluations based on the CIPP Model is no different than budgeting an evaluation based on any other evaluation model. In budgeting evaluations based on the CIPP Model, the evaluator must first produce a design that is keyed to the types of evaluation to be conducted, that is, context, input, process, or product evaluation, and then cost out the work to be done. Accordingly, this chapter is applicable not only to evaluations based on the CIPP Model but to any and all evaluations that are grounded in a sound evaluation design.

Six Factors to Consider in Developing Evaluation Budgets

In this section, we identify and discuss six main factors that evaluators should reference and invoke in developing sound evaluation budgets.

Address the Interdependence of Evaluation Designs and Evaluation Budgets

Fundamentally, the tasks of designing and budgeting evaluations need to go hand-in-hand when planning and contracting an evaluation. In designing the evaluation, the evaluator should keep budgeting needs in mind and make budget-related notes that will be helpful later in producing the evaluation budget. After drafting the evaluation design, the evaluator should prepare a realistic budget for supporting all the designed tasks. A good budget plan should provide the best estimate of all the funds required to successfully carry out the evaluation. In developing the evaluation budget, the evaluator should aim to assure that qualified persons can successfully carry out the full range of evaluation activities for the duration of the projected evaluation. Systematically working through the budget planning process will help the evaluator think through real-life

implementation of the designed evaluation and make necessary adjustments in the design before negotiating an evaluation contract.

Adhere to Institutional Requirements for Sound Evaluation Budgets

The structure and specificity of an initial evaluation budget should be grounded in the evaluation funder's particular budgeting and reporting requirements and the evaluation organization's budgeting, accounting, and billing protocols. In developing a functional evaluation budget, the evaluator must assiduously take both of these grounding factors into consideration. Early in the budgeting process, the evaluator definitely should consult with the budget and human resources offices within her or his organization to verify and understand their particular budget process, rules, and stipulations. The evaluator should also make sure he or she understands and adheres to the funder's financial protocols.

As Feasible, Communicate with the Funder in the Process of Building the Evaluation Budget

When a request for an evaluation proposal allows exchange between the evaluator and the funder, the evaluator should communicate with the funder toward reaching agreement on a sound evaluation budget plan. Good communication between the evaluator and funder is of value to both parties. In such exchanges, the evaluator should make clear to the funder the intent to request all, but no more than the funds needed to conduct an effective evaluation. Their discussions should seek mutual understanding on the following:

- The link between the evaluation's design and its need for funds.
- The acceptability of providing funds for unpredictable contingencies.
- Any funding limit for the evaluation budget.
- The level of budget detail required by the funder.
- The protocols and schedule for submitting the evaluation's bills.
- The schedule of payments to the evaluator's organization.

Some but not all of these topics may be covered in the boiler plate of the funder's request for the evaluation. The main points here are that the evaluator needs to clarify such matters early in the process of making an evaluation budget and that communication with the funder toward reaching accord on budget agreements is highly desirable.

Provide for Periodic Budget Reviews and Updates

Even though a detailed evaluation design provides an essential basis for budgetary discussion and initial budgeting decisions, the funder may nevertheless have difficulty in fully projecting the extent of information requirements that might be added or dropped during the evaluation. Any new requirements during the evaluation likely will require added funds. Moreover, the discontinuation of certain evaluation tasks, along the way, could justify reducing the evaluation budget. Accordingly, it is reasonable for the evaluator to request that the original evaluation budget be subject to periodic review and revision. Such an agreement can work in two directions: the evaluation budget may be appropriately reduced if certain tasks are dropped, or the budget may be increased if the funder expands the scope of evaluation work. In the budgeting process, the evaluator should discuss with the funder the possible need to renegotiate the evaluation budget if and when the client group finds it important to request additional evaluation services or asks that certain evaluation tasks be eliminated. In general, it is desirable that the initial evaluation budget provide for needed modifications in order to address unanticipated or new client information needs that may emerge during the evaluation or to reduce the budget if certain originally projected tasks are discontinued.

Take Account of the Budgetary Implications of Formative versus Summative Evaluations

The degree of flexibility for an evaluation budget can vary depending on the degree to which the evaluation is or is not interactive with the client group and continually responsive to unfolding client group needs. Budgets for relatively fixed, preordinate evaluations—especially field experiments—may remain relatively unchanged throughout the evaluation because designs for such studies are well specified in advance and, more or less, intended to be held constant. At the same time, designs and budgets for formative evaluations are general and intended to evolve in order to continually

address emerging client group needs. Advance budgeting for formative evaluations is problematic because the needed evaluation procedures will be determined throughout the evaluation in response to the client group's evolving questions and information requirements. Two provisions relevant to funding formative evaluations are including a sizable **contingency fund** in the budget and agreeing with the funder that the evaluation budget will be subject to periodic review and updating. In the case of formative evaluation, it is important for the evaluator and client to reach accord on provisions for meeting the evaluation's evolving budgetary requirements.

Tailor Budgets in Consideration of the Particular Type of Evaluation Agreement

The level and type of detail needed for an evaluation budget can vary depending on the type of evaluation agreement. Such types of agreement may be a grant, a fixed-price contract, a cost-reimbursable contract, or a shared-cost cooperative agreement, among other possibilities. We discuss evaluation agreements in detail in Chapter 8. For our purposes here, we stress that the evaluator will need to budget in accordance with the type of agreement to be negotiated and simultaneously meet her or his organization's budgeting and fiscal accountability requirements.

Two examples illustrate the evaluator's need to tailor budgets in consideration of the type of evaluation agreement. Under a grant for an evaluation, the funder may pay a fixed amount for the evaluation and require only enough budget detail to justify the fixed amount. In such agreements, the funder would likely pay the evaluator's organization a lump sum or a series of scheduled payments. The evaluator would meet the funder's accountability requirements by delivering the promised evaluation products but would not be required to account for exactly how the granted funds were allocated to the different evaluation tasks. Under a grant, the funder's main concern is to ensure that the evaluator delivers high-quality evaluation products, irrespective of how funds were expended, as long as they were utilized to achieve the grant's goals.

In contrast to an evaluation grant, under an evaluation contract the funder is likely to require a fully detailed budget and scrutinize the breakouts of the different projected costs. Under these circumstances, the evaluator typically must provide as much budgetary detail as the evaluation design permits. As mentioned earlier, relatively fixed, preordinate evaluation designs will require relatively complete, up-front, detailed budgets. However, as also noted above, a contract for a formative evaluation design necessarily will lack the detail seen in the budget for a relatively fixed summative evaluation design. This is so because the formative evaluator's response to the client group's evolving evaluation needs cannot be precisely predicted. While all evaluation budgets should provide for financing unanticipated, emergent needs for funds, this is especially the case in formative evaluations. In general, we recommend that all budgets for contracted evaluations include a contingency funds section to cover unanticipated evaluation feedback requirements and also include an agreement with the funder that the evaluation design and budget will be subject to periodic reviews and updates.

Irrespective of the funder's requirement for only a general or a detailed budget, the evaluator's organization often has its own need for a high level of detail for internal accounting and auditing purposes. We recommend that the evaluator meet her or his organization's budgeting requirements by developing as much budgetary detail as the evaluation design allows and also provide the funding organization with the level of budget detail it requires. Whether or not the funder wants to see a fully specified budget, evaluators and their organizations will find detailed, up-front budgets to be valuable for purposes of both evaluation management and evaluation accountability.

Evaluation Budget Line Items

Although many items need to be included in an evaluation budget plan, most of them fall under certain line-item cost categories. The seven **common line items** in evaluation budgets are personnel, travel, consultants, equipment, supplies, services, and indirect costs (depicted in Figure 7.1).

Personnel

Evaluation often requires a team effort. Evaluators need to assemble a highly qualified team of individuals who can effectively implement the evaluation design. The principal evaluator will provide conceptual leadership, regularly interact with the client, supervise the other evaluation team members, lead in delivering re-

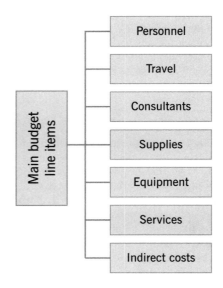

FIGURE 7.1. Main evaluation budget line items.

ports to the client group, and maintain the evaluation's accountability.

There are no set rules for constituting an evaluation team. In setting up such a team, the principal evaluator should identify the needed evaluation roles and figure out how best to staff them. The following are evaluation roles to consider in determining how best to staff an evaluation:

- Conceptual leadership
- Evaluation design and redesign
- Day-to-day evaluation management
- Regular interaction with the client
- Field-level data collection
- Program content expertise
- Instrument selection and construction
- Data entry
- Quantitative data analysis
- Qualitative analysis
- Information technology support
- Information management
- Report writing
- Report editing

- Report delivery
- Clerical support
- Fiscal management
- Evaluation accountability
- Metaevaluation

Evaluation roles and staff positions are not the same. In a small, one-person evaluation, the evaluator needs to fulfill all of the roles that the evaluation design requires. In a large, complex evaluation, the evaluator needs to set up an evaluation team to implement most, if not all, of the roles listed above. In that case, certain evaluation team members would likely play more than one role in the evaluation. Therefore, the lead evaluator needs to be skilled in preparing evaluation job descriptions for evaluation team members—and sometimes other evaluation participants, such as advisors—that are both efficient and effective in assigning evaluation staff members and other participants to the evaluation tasks to be carried out.

Table 7.1 illustrates how a lead evaluator might plan to establish an evaluation team. The row headings are the roles listed above, while the column headings are the particular evaluation positions the evaluator might decide to staff. X's in the matrix's cells denote, hypothetically, the roles to be assigned to each evaluation participant in a certain evaluation. After determining the row and column headings of such a matrix, the evaluator can use it to define the responsibilities of each evaluation participant.

In this matrix, note that key evaluation positions not often included in evaluation staffing plans are the evaluation review panel and an external evaluation subcontractor. The evaluation review panel can be especially useful in engaging a representative group of stakeholders in reviewing draft evaluation plans and reports, facilitating data collection, and helping disseminate findings. The subcontractor role can be useful for conducting a range of evaluation tasks, including performing substudies and issuing formative and summative metaevaluations of the evaluation project.

The size and composition of the evaluation team will vary according to the size and complexity of the evaluation and the available resources. For example, in the self-housing evaluation project described in Chapter 3, the evaluation team was quite large and included a wide range of evaluation roles. However, in the service-learning evaluation project illustrated in Chapter 5, the evaluation team was only composed of two university faculty members (as evaluators), a graduate student, and a support staff member.

When considering what types of personnel to involve, the evaluator must determine the types of staff that will be needed to implement the evaluation design. The evaluator may want to select staff from her or his organization and from outside organizations. Once the evaluator has determined how to staff the evaluation, he or she will have to estimate the cost of the evaluation of the projected evaluation team. Determining the costs of evaluation personnel often is more complex than simply setting pay rates, multiplying them by the number of projected hours of work for each staff position, and summing up the total cost. In reaching a reliable estimate of the total evaluation personnel cost, the lead evaluator especially will need to take into account the costs of recruitment and staff benefits, the varying staff benefits for different categories of personnel, and the fact that consultants will not be entitled to fringe benefits.

Travel

Travel costs typically include:

- Airfare
- Trip insurance
- Rental car
- Tolls
- Baggage
- Taxi
- Internet service
- Telephone
- Lodging
- Parking
- Meals
- Snacks and beverages for meetings
- Conference registration
- Gratuities

Evaluation staff may travel for different purposes related to the evaluation. The evaluation budget should provide for funding all the projected travel expenses. Evaluation team members might make trips to meet

TABLE 7.1. A Matrix for Defining Evaluation Staff Positions

Evaluation Roles	Evaluation Director	Traveling Observer	Technical Support Specialist	Secretary	Consultant	Evaluation Review Panel	Evaluation Subcontractor
Conceptual leadership	X						
Evaluation design and redesign	X						
Review of draft evaluation plans			X			X	
Day-to-day management	X						
Interaction with client	X						
Development of Traveling Observer Handbook		X					
Help cut red tape related to data collection						X	
Field data collection		X					
Program content expertise					X		
Instrument construction		X	X				
Data entry				X			
Quantitative data analysis			X				
Qualitative analysis	X						
IT support				X			
Information management				X			
Report writing	X	X					
Review of draft reports						X	
Report editing				X			
Report delivery	X	X					
Follow-up support for use of findings	X					X	
Clerical support				X			
Fiscal management	X			X			
Evaluation accountability	X	X	X	X			
Metaevaluation							X

with the client, observe project staff meetings, make site visits to different project sites, conduct **town hall meetings** or focus group sessions with project stakeholders, coordinate feedback workshops for the project staff, deliver reports to different stakeholder groups, and/or report on the evaluation at relevant conventions to disseminate evaluation findings. In summary, depending on the size and scope of the evaluation project, the evaluator may need to consider the following in budget planning:

- Day-to-day travel related to data collection, especially for evaluations that involve a lot of qualitative approaches such as interviews, focus groups, and event observations.
- Travel expenses of team members who work remotely from various locations.
- Off-site training sessions to build the evaluation team's expertise.
- Visits to the funding organization.
- Off-site review panel meetings and related expenses.
- Travel expenses of external consultants or subcontractors.
- Travel related to conferences or workshops, as specified in the evaluation's communication plan.

Consultants and Subcontractors

Many evaluators hire expert consultants, either external or internal, to strengthen the evaluation work or to carry out certain evaluation activities. They might also subcontract with outside groups to conduct certain evaluation tasks, such as substudies or external metaevaluation. The consultants usually provide an expertise, such as specialized evaluation skills, content area knowledge, or technical expertise, that is not available within the main evaluation team; or they provide the ability to do the work more quickly and at less cost. The same can be said for subcontractors and the added advantage of their independent perspective that can be invaluable in obtaining external metaevaluation reports.

Utilizing consultants and subcontractors will incur a variety of costs. The majority of the costs will be fees for services, which can be an agreed-on amount or, especially in the case of consultants, an hourly/ daily rate. Another cost might be the combination costs for communications with the lead evaluator and other members of the evaluation team. Such communication costs could include discussions with the evaluator regarding the scope of work and schedule of deliverables, as well as postage for mailing documents. A major cost might be travel for the consultant or subcontractor to visit the evaluation sites or to meet the evaluator or the evaluation team members in person for face-to-face consultations, together with the associated costs for support services. To ensure that the evaluation consultant or subcontractor provides high-quality service, the evaluator should consider establishing a contract that includes a phased payment schedule tied to observable milestones or completion of specific tasks.

Supplies

Evaluations require a large variety of materials and supplies, including:

- Stationery and other clerical supplies
- Copy paper
- Ink cartridge
- Coffee, food, and bottled water for meetings and other events
- Certificates or other recognition items for engaged stakeholders, such as review panel members
- Research scales/instruments
- Postage, envelopes, and other mailing supplies

While it can be hard to predict the changing needs and costs for even the best-developed evaluation design, there are some useful strategies to consider when estimating and ordering evaluation supplies. One way to think about materials and supply costs is to estimate them for each projected event or activity. Because evaluators develop budgets for evaluations that typically have predictable start and end points and intermediate deadlines for deliverables, the evaluator can find it useful to estimate supply costs for each deliverable. Another useful practice is to employ a cost-reimbursable provision for billing for materials actually used in the evaluation.

Equipment

Sometimes it is not easy to distinguish between supplies and equipment. A good rule of thumb is that equipment costs typically include items that need to be purchased for the evaluation but can be used for other projects at a later date. These items might include:

- Computers
- Router
- Computer software
- Printer
- Cell phones
- Desk phones
- Fax machine
- Projectors
- Tape recorders
- Video recorders
- Cameras
- Transcribing equipment
- Desks, chairs, and other office furniture
- Filing cabinets
- Manuscript binders and three-hole punch devices
- Staplers, scissors, tape dispensers, and other desk equipment

The evaluator should consult her or his organization's grants and contracts office about the policies regarding expenditures for equipment. In some cases, the funder will require that the evaluator's organization supply the equipment. In other cases, the funder may agree to pay for the equipment and provide ownership of it to the evaluator's organization. Often, evaluation shops may already have and be able to use much of the needed equipment, without charging anything to the funder or charging only a small amount for maintenance, and, possibly, depreciation.

Services

An evaluator needs to closely examine the evaluation design to estimate service costs. If the research involves a large survey that will need to be mailed out to the potential respondents, then substantial costs for mailing services, such as those for UPS or Federal Express, should be calculated into the budget. If a lengthy telephone interview is part of the evaluation design, then costs for sizable phone bills might need to be included in the evaluation budget. Other typical service costs include photocopying, poster making, computerized graphic arts, printing and binding costs for the various reports, and video making for oral reports.

Indirect Costs

Most evaluation project cost estimates are broken down into direct costs and indirect costs. Direct costs are costs that can be identified specifically with the evaluation project and therefore are included in the direct costs portion of the evaluation budget. The evaluator should project these costs in the budget, record associated expenditures as they occur, and bill for them in accordance with advance contractual agreements. In contrast to direct costs, indirect costs refer to those costs that have been incurred to address needs that span projects, programs, and other operations in the evaluator's parent organization and that cannot be readily and specifically partitioned to determine associated direct costs for a particular project. Indirect costs include such items as institutional governance and administration, project oversight and accounting by the parent organization's business office, proposal processing, personnel/human resources services, affirmative action oversight, institutional human subjects reviews, parking, heat and light, custodial services, security, office furniture and equipment, and other costs not directly and exclusively tied to the evaluation's explicit tasks.

Many organizations have an established indirect cost rate (ICR) that was negotiated with the federal government. For different types of organizations—such as universities or private companies—the negotiated indirect cost rates may vary widely (e.g., from 35% of the direct cost budget for a university to well over 100% of direct costs for a private research and development organization). In cases of federally supported evaluations, the evaluator should identify the negotiated rate and incorporate it into the evaluation budget.

In cases of other types of funders, such as foundations, the evaluator's organization may need to negotiate a special indirect cost rate with the funder. For example, when a foundation awards a grant, rather than a contract for an evaluation, the foundation may not allow charges for any indirect costs, or, if they do, only a much smaller rate than the government negotiated rate. In such cases, the evaluation budget may appropriately show the reduction in the parent organization's indirect cost rate as a local contribution to the evaluation.

Another variable is whether the evaluation work will be housed and operated from within the evaluator's parent organization or whether the work will be off-site. In the off-site case, the indirect cost rate may be considerably lower than the regular rate. Basically, the evaluator should consult with her or his organization's business office to determine the appropriate indirect cost rate to include in the evaluation budget. As an example of a university's charges for indirect costs, the East Carolina University's IGERT evaluation project charged a rate for "Research Off-Campus Remote," which was 26% of the direct costs.

Miscellaneous supplies purchased in bulk, such as pencils, pens, and paper, that are to be used for purposes beyond the evaluation project typically may be covered as indirect costs, whereas materials required for specific projects are charged as direct costs. In general, we suggest that the evaluator assiduously identify all costs that will be incurred directly for the evaluation project and include those costs in the direct cost part of the evaluation budget.

If the evaluator's institution does not have a current ICR, or if a funder does not accept the evaluator's institution's predetermined ICR, the evaluator's organization likely will need to negotiate an ICR with the funder. Some funders may require the evaluator or the evaluator's institution to recommend and justify an indirect cost rate for incorporation into the evaluation contract or grant. Ultimately, the evaluator's organization will need to reach an agreement with the funder on an appropriate indirect fund rate. In most organizations, the evaluator's business office can be very helpful in dealing with the indirect costs issue. We strongly advise evaluators to make effective use of such services and to do so early in the process of building an evaluation budget.

Ethical Imperatives in Budgeting Evaluations

Evaluators must construct their evaluation budgets on sound ethical grounds and maintain integrity, **transparency,** and accountability in all fiscal matters related to the evaluation. They should deal honestly with the funder in ensuring that the evaluation will have the necessary funds. The evaluation budget should be sufficient to enable the evaluator to implement the full range of the proposed tasks at a high level of quality and professionalism. In particular, a sound evaluation budget should meet the ethical requirements spelled out in the Joint Committee (2011) *Program Evaluation Standards.*

An Ethical Approach to Evaluation Budgeting

Evaluators should develop a budget professionally and prudently and should provide their best estimate of a full-cost evaluation budget. Ideally, an evaluation's proposed evaluation budget amounts should project just the right amount of funds needed to effectively carry out all the needed evaluation work. Because not all budgeting needs can be anticipated—especially in formative evaluations that evolve pursuant to ongoing interactions with the client group—such a full-cost budget should include a contingencies category of funds and should include a provision for periodically reviewing and updating the budget. In the interest of the evaluation budget's transparency, inclusion of a contingency funds category is preferable to the common and dubious practice of inflating most or all budget items in anticipation of unpredictable, emergent needs for added funds.

The goals of ethical evaluation budgeting are to implement the evaluation design and to meet requirements for fiscal integrity, transparency, and accountability. We strongly recommend that before proceeding with a planned evaluation the evaluator should take all necessary steps to assure that the evaluation will be supplied with the resources required to conduct a quality and professionally responsible evaluation. The evaluator can ensure the availability of the needed level of funds by reaching agreement with the funder on both the evaluation design and the funds required to carry it out. Because information needs may evolve during the evaluation, we again emphasize that the evaluator and the funder should reach agreement on both a budgeted amount for unpredictable contingencies and a provision for periodic reviews and updates of the evaluation budget.

We also stress that professionally responsible evaluators ground their evaluations in honest, competently prepared estimates of the funds needed for the projected evaluation. If an evaluation is fully designed in advance, the evaluator can easily provide a best estimate of the full-cost budget. If the evaluation is of the formative type and is expected to evolve over time, then the evaluator should provide a start-up budget aligned with what is known of the evaluation assignment and inclusive of a category of contingency funds.

In general, evaluators should budget only for the costs of activities required to fully implement the approved evaluation design. However, funding activities that are outside the evaluation design's requirements can be legitimate if the funder agrees, for example, to support evaluation staff members' attendance at professional meetings or if the funder agrees to a profit margin for an evaluation company.

The Special Case of Unanticipated Evaluation Costs

Understandably, all budget projections are estimates and inevitably include some inaccuracies. Therefore, evaluators should often request more funds than can be justified in the initial budget. Such contingency planning is in the best interests of both evaluator and funder. Thus, when unexpected costs arise, the evaluator will have money to cover them. If the evaluator worked under a fixed-price contract and ended the evaluation with a substantial budgetary surplus, we advise him or her to offer to return the remaining money to the funder or to recommend using the residual money to conduct additional work, such as assisting the client group to apply the evaluation's findings or providing training or related services to help build the organization's evaluation capacity. Based on our experience, some funders can take back the unused funds, but others may not have the authority to accept returned funds or added services. This is especially the case with federal government contracts. For example, Stufflebeam's fixed-price, large-scale evaluation for the U.S. Marine Corps ended with a $45,000 surplus. In that case, government policy prohibited the Corps from recovering the surplus funds or having the evaluation contractor apply them to deliver further evaluation service. Nevertheless, we believe evaluators exhibit professionalism when they make the funder aware of an evaluation's unused funds and suggest using the funds to benefit the funder's organization.

Ethical Challenges and Complications in Funding Evaluations

Two complications may threaten or thwart an evaluator's efforts to develop an ethically sound evaluation budget.

One such challenge commonly occurs when the funder insists on a certain scope of evaluation service, agrees on the needed evaluation operations, but commits to providing less than the needed level of funding. In such a case, the evaluator should not agree to carry out an evaluation that is doomed to fail due to inadequate funding. When such a dilemma arises, there are a number of ethical responses available to the evaluator:

reach agreement with the client to reduce the evaluation's scope of work; respectfully bow out of the potential assignment; agree to proceed on a partially pro bono basis; or convince the funder to provide the full level of needed funds.

A somewhat more complicated version of this challenge is the situation that arises when the funder refuses to increase the budget to the needed level or to reduce the evaluation's scope of work, but has the authority to insist that the evaluator proceed with the assignment anyway. Based on our experience, such problematic evaluation assignments occur all too frequently when the evaluator is an employee of the funder's organization. When such an evaluator cannot decline the problematic assignment, then he or she should issue a caveat in the final report. Such a statement should make clear that funding restrictions prohibited the evaluator from fully carrying out all of the necessary evaluation tasks; that the reliability and validity of the findings could not be assured; and that the client group should view the evaluation findings with a substantial level of circumspection.

Unethical Evaluation Budgeting Actions

Unfortunately, cases of unethical evaluation budgeting are not unknown. We strongly advise evaluators not to engage in either of the two unethical evaluation budgeting practices summarized next.

The first is a case in which the evaluator deceptively and purposely inflates the budget in order to make a large profit. This can occur more easily in sole-source evaluations with no competing evaluators—for example, when the funder chooses a particular evaluator without seeking competitive proposals. We judge the practice of deceptively and intentionally grossly overbidding an evaluation award to be opportunistic, unprofessional, and unethical. Such funder-gouging acts are contrary to professional evaluation service.

We also judge as unprofessional and unethical the budgeting practice of what is sometimes known as "**buying a contract.**" In such a case, the evaluator grossly underestimates a projected evaluation's cost in order to win a bidding competition and then, about midway in the evaluation, requests the additionally required funds. Our view is that such low-cost bidders know that down the road they will have to return to the bidder, with "hat in hand," apologize for underestimating the evaluation's costs, and state that successful completion of the evaluation will require additional funds. Such unethical behavior presents the funder with a dilemma. Although terminating the evaluation contract would be justified, the evaluation's client group would then not receive the needed interim and final evaluation reports. By terminating the evaluation contract midway in the evaluation process, the funder likely would consider most of the already expended funds to have been wasted. Faced with such bad choices, funders often give in to the evaluator's request for more money. However, the funder likely would never hire that evaluator again. Moreover, evaluators who engage in buying contracts with low bids injure their own reputations and also impair the credibility of the evaluation profession. Clearly, buying contracts with unjustifiable low bids is alien to the fundamental values of ethical budgeting and professional evaluation service.

Incompetent Evaluator Actions

Sometimes overbudgeting or underbudgeting is unintentional and not devious but the result of the evaluator's inexperience and limited competence. Unintentional overbidding or underbidding can happen when a novice evaluator requests either far more or far less than the needed funds. In the case of overbudgeting, sooner or later the funder will realize that the evaluator has greatly inflated the evaluation budget; consequently, the client and other stakeholders may lose confidence in the evaluator's reports. In the case of grossly underbudgeting, the evaluator may fail miserably to carry out the evaluation assignment or may have to face the embarrassment of admitting poor budgetary planning and asking the client for more money. We strongly advise novice evaluators to have their evaluation designs and budgets scrutinized by experienced evaluators and/or financial experts. Also, if the funder doubts the validity of the proposed evaluation budget, he or she should obtain an independent assessment of both the evaluation design and the evaluation budget.

Summary of Ethical Considerations in Budgeting

This section has projected a strong ethical position on evaluation budgeting. Evaluators should strive to budget, both up-front and throughout the evaluation, for what is required to produce a professionally responsible evaluation while exercising utmost fiscal integrity, transparency, and accountability. In general, we advise

evaluators to develop an up-front, full-cost budget, to include both a contingency funds section and an agreement for periodic review, and, as needed, update the evaluation budget. For **responsive evaluations,** in which information needs will continually evolve, we understand that the evaluator likely cannot develop an advance, full-cost budget. In such cases, we advise the evaluator to estimate those costs that are predictable; include a budgetary section to cover unanticipated contingencies; work out an agreement with the funder that cost estimates will periodically be revisited and updated; and adjust the evaluation budget as appropriate. Evaluators are advised to keep their budgeting transparent and are warned not to deceptively inflate budgets or engage in the practice of "buying contracts." We advise novice evaluators to obtain professional assistance in vetting their evaluation budgets and adjusting them as appropriate. Clearly, all evaluators should maintain highly ethical budgeting practices. Evaluation is a profession, and its practitioners should act ethically in all aspects of evaluation service, including budgeting.

Developing Different Types of Evaluation Budgets

Depending on the types of evaluation agreements, evaluation budgeting will vary. In this section, we discuss evaluation budgeting under six major types of evaluation budgets: fixed-price budgets, grants, cost-reimbursable budgets, cost-plus budgets, cooperative agreements, and **modular budgets**.

Fixed-Price Evaluation Budgets

The IGERT evaluation case described in Chapter 7 was budgeted under a fixed-price agreement. The funder stipulated that the evaluator would complete the evaluation work over the 5-year period and requested that the evaluator provide a budget that would allow the evaluator to complete the work effectively. The evaluator submitted the budget summarized in Table 7.2 to request $84,433 for the evaluation work.

The budget was submitted along with brief explanations for the different line-item costs. Under the fixed-price agreement, the funder found this level of specificity adequate because the contract required the evaluator to complete the stipulated work to the funder's satisfaction and bill no more for the evaluation work than the initially agreed-upon amount. In contrast to this chapter's preceding discussion of budgeting, this budget did not include a contingency funds line item, and, as it turned out, one was not needed.

Based on the evaluation design, this budget estimated that the evaluator's time in the evaluation would be equivalent to teaching four university courses. The evaluator determined her evaluation project salary needs by calculating the amount of money required to buy out one of the courses she had been teaching, based on her salary rate. She then calculated her total salary cost for the first year of the evaluation by multiplying the cost of the one course to be bought out times four. This calculation produced a total salary for the lead evaluator in the amount of $26,483. For each of the subsequent evaluation years, the evaluator determined her evaluation project salary by multiplying the previous year's salary by 1.05. Ironically, the three projected 5% increases turned out to be unneeded because— due to the U.S. financial recession that started in 2008 and lingered—her university did not approve any salary increases between 2008 and 2012. In spite of this real-world experience, we advise evaluators to budget appropriately for the evaluation staff's annual salary increases. Minimally, such increases should keep the staff members' salaries in line with the annual inflation rate.

The $5,273 for fringe benefits in Table 7.2 was determined by multiplying the university's 20% fringe benefit rate by the total salary amount ($26,483). After summing up the salaries and the fringe benefits, the total personnel costs came to $31,756.

The estimated $26,502 travel cost was budgeted to cover the evaluator's planned site visits and travel to give presentations at professional conferences. The consultant honorarium amount was determined by multiplying the number of consultant days (3) by a daily consultant rate of $1,000. This yielded the total consultant honorarium of $3,000. The $1,000 for consultant travel and support service was the sum of the estimated travel and lodging costs, plus support services for the consultant. Thus, the total consultant cost came to $4,000.

The equipment line-item estimate of $995 was for the cost of a video recorder and a tripod for videotaping focus group interviews plus a voice recorder for audiotaping individual interviews. The supplies line-item estimate of $2082 was included to cover commercial tests/instruments, books related to integrated education

TABLE 7.2. Budget for the IGERT Evaluation

Line Item	Cost	Total
A. Personnel		
1. Salaries	$26,483	
2. Fringe benefits	$5,273	
3. Total personnel		$31,756
B. Travel		$26,502
C. Consultants		
1. Honorarium	$3,000	
2. Travel and support service for consultants	$1,000	
3. Total consultants		$4,000
D. Equipment		$995
E. Supplies		$2,082
F. Services		$1,675
F. Total direct costs		$67,010
G. Total indirect costs		$17,423
H. Total project costs		$84,433

and IGERT, paper and related materials for producing the evaluation plan, materials for meetings, and materials for draft and final reports. The services line item of $1,675 was based on the evaluation's need for outside scoring of commercial tests, communication, postage, photocopying, and poster making.

The total project cost line item of $84,433 was the sum of the line items enumerated above plus the indirect cost figure of $17,423. This number was obtained by multiplying the evaluation's estimated direct cost of $67,010 by the university's indirect cost rate of 26% for its "Off Campus Research Remote" category. Adding the resulting indirect cost of $17,423 to the total direct cost yielded the bottom-line amount of $84,433.

Budgeting under Grants

The evaluation of the service-learning project that we discussed in Chapter 5 was funded under a grant agreement. An evaluation grant is a financial award to support a qualified evaluator (or evaluators) to conduct a study that is of interest to the evaluator(s), contains societal value, lies within the funder's mission, and is seen to be at a fundable level. In the service-learning evaluation example, Learning to Teach, Learning to Serve (LTLS) was a new project developed by the Student Coalition for Action in Literacy Education (SCALE). LTLS's goal was to develop a replicable model that could be used across the state of North Carolina, as well as in other states, to enhance teacher education through service learning and to change the face of teaching. LTLS is working with North Carolina institutions of higher education to infuse teacher education programs with service-learning instruction.

SCALE proposed a 3-year project to offer participating institutions the possibility of multiple-year funding, training, and networking opportunities. Each institution was expected to develop or enhance teacher education courses to include service learning, research, and reflection opportunities for preservice teachers. Each course would include a service-learning component that provides the preservice teachers with the opportunity to serve as literacy and/or ESOL tutors in the local community for at least 30 hours per semester. East Carolina University's College of Education formed a faculty LTLS taskforce and secured grant funds for implementing a service-learning project in its teacher education program. Two professors in research and evaluation developed and submitted an evaluation grant application to SCALE that included evaluation goals, an evaluation design, and an associated budget for evaluating the service-learning project. The budget for evaluating the project is shown in Table 7.3.

TABLE 7.3. Budget for the LTLS Service-Learning Project

Line Item	Cost	Total
A. Personnel		
1. Salaries	$7,029.08	
2. Fringe benefits	$1,524.56	
3. Total personnel		$8,553.64
B. Travel		$507.01
C. Consultants		$250.00
D. Equipment		$125.00
E. Supplies		$64.35
F. Total direct costs		$9,500.00
G. Total indirect costs		$500.00
H. Total project costs		$10,000.00

The personal costs for this project reflect the projected amount of work for the two evaluators identified in the evaluation design. Usually, a basic personnel cost is determined for each staff member by multiplying her or his daily rate by the number of days to be worked on the project. In the case of the LTLS project budget, however, because the personnel only included the two evaluators who were faculty members at East Carolina University (ECU), the lead evaluator first estimated the amount of time that each evaluator would work on the project based on the evaluation design, then estimated the corresponding percentages of a full-time equivalent (FTE) staff member for each one, and finally converted the FTE percentages to salary amounts. These amounts totaled $5,000 for evaluator A and $2,029.08 for evaluator B. With an approximately 22% fringe benefit rate, the corresponding cost of fringe benefits was $1,076.61 for evaluator A and $447.95 for evaluator B. The total estimated personnel cost thus came to $8,553.64. In the LTLS evaluation, ECU paid the graduate student's stipend. That contribution is not shown in Table 7.3, although it could have been listed as a university contribution.

Because many evaluators may be unfamiliar with how their organization calculates benefits for different categories of staff members, we advise such evaluators to ask their organization's financial personnel to help calculate personnel salary and fringe benefit costs.

Like the personnel costs, the LTLS's estimated travel costs were derived from the evaluation design. The travel costs included expenditures for mileage in traveling to and from the project site to conduct interviews and make observations. Costs for out-of-state travel to conferences were not included in this evaluation budget because the LTLS project director allocated project funds to cover those travel costs. Absent that contribution, the evaluators would have calculated and reached an estimate for the out-of-state travel. These costs may include conference registration, airfare, lodging, meals, taxi, and baggage handling.

The consultant honorarium was determined by adding up the number of consultant hours in the evaluation design (two) and multiplying them by the agreed-on hourly rate of $125. This yielded the total consultant fee of $250. The $125 cost for equipment was included to acquire a small portable projector for the evaluation team's use in presenting project findings. It is noted that certain institutions may put equipment items costing less than a certain value in the supplies category instead of the equipment category, even though the item can be used in other projects.

The supply line-item estimate of $64.35 covered such consumable items as books, paper, and related materials. These were used for such purposes as producing evaluation plans, survey instruments, materials for evaluation meetings, and interim and final reports. Some evaluation budgets include a "services" line item to cover the costs of items such as phone communication, photocopying, computer use, graphic design, and mailing services.

The total direct cost line item of $9,500 was the sum of the above described line items: total personnel, travel, consultants, equipment, and supplies. The indirect cost of $500 was roughly 5% of the total direct cost of $9,500. Notice that the indirect cost percentage was rather low. This was because the evaluation was funded under a grant rather than a contract. As mentioned previously, granting organizations typically provide funds for projects of interest to the proposing organization. Since the funded project is in the organization's interest, it is understandable that the granting organization expects the recipient organization to have some "skin in the game," often in the form of covering most or all of their own indirect cost expenses. The funding organization's rationale is that the grant award is a charitable contribution to support the recipient's goals and program and is not a particular service to the granting organization. Further, the proposed work is often central to the recipient's organization, and thus it should make some in-kind contributions. Adding the $500 indirect cost and the $9,500 direct cost yielded the bottom-line total amount for the evaluation of $10,000, which was the upper limit of annual evaluation funds that SCALEs offered.

Notes explaining each budget line item were appended to the evaluation grant proposal. SCALE deemed the proposed evaluation study as worthy, aligned with its mission, well planned and budgeted, and financially supportable. Consequently, the foundation awarded a $10,000 grant to fund the evaluation. SCALE expected the evaluators to use the funds wisely but not to return any unused funds.

Budgeting under Cost-Reimbursable Contracts

Under a cost-reimbursable evaluation contract, an evaluator's organization and a funder agree on a budget that is keyed to executing an approved evaluation design and to a schedule of payments based on bills for completed evaluation milestones. The funder pays the evaluator's institution for actual costs of evaluation activities up to the agreed-upon total evaluation cost. The funder may provide an initial amount of funds to support the launching of the evaluation. Thereafter the funder reimburses the evaluator's organization in response to bills for actual costs of completed evaluation activities. Such bills must include both documentation of work completed during the billing period and the documented cost of that work. Based on the evaluation agreement, such bills may be submitted on a quarterly basis or some other schedule. A key feature of this type of budgeting is that the evaluator's organization is paid, up to a total cost limit, for submission of deliverables and actual documented expenditures. In submitting the bills, the evaluator's organization must account for and report work performed plus actual evaluation expenditures. As long as the cumulative spending total does not exceed the contract's total funding amount and the evaluation has been performed satisfactorily, the funder will pay for the evaluation's full cost, but no more than that. If the evaluator needed less than the originally budgeted amount, the funder would keep the surplus funds. If the evaluator had expended more than the originally budgeted amount, his or her organization likely would have to bear those expenses.

Usually, a cost-reimbursable budget breaks out cost estimates more specifically than was seen in the service-learning evaluation project example discussed above. A cost-reimbursable contract usually requires quite specific budget notes that explain each budget item. Reporting on completed tasks and associated expenditures against the detailed line-item budget usually can serve as a sufficient basis for reimbursement. As with other types of evaluation agreements, a detailed work plan in the evaluation design will provide a foundation for detailing the budget's line items and writing the corresponding budget notes.

The cost-reimbursable budget is undoubtedly in the funder's best interest because it minimizes potential risks. The funder needs to pay for nothing but completion of the agreed-on tasks, reports, and possibly other named products, and the funder won't be paying for expenditures that exceed the agreed-on funding ceiling. Further, if the original budget is insufficient to complete the project, the funder has authority to decide for or against providing additional funds needed to complete the evaluation assignment.

Under the cost-reimbursable budget, the evaluator assumes a certain degree of risk. The main risk is that the evaluator would have to incur the additional cost for completing the evaluation work if he or she had agreed to an insufficient budget. The evaluator can avoid such a pitfall by agreeing with the client on a schedule for periodically reviewing and making appropriate adjustments in the budget and also including in the budget a category for funding unpredictable contingencies. As this discussion shows, in negotiating a cost-reimbursable agreement, the evaluator should meticulously project as much as possible the evaluation's full cost.

The evaluator's organization should also build safeguards into the evaluation contract to prevent or effectively address the possible occurrence of the funder either being slow in paying submitted bills or defaulting on their payment altogether. If there is any worry that such a circumstance might occur, we advise the evaluator to engage his or her organization's lawyer to make sure the evaluation contract includes legal safeguards and corrective actions for a case in which the funder fails to live up to the contractual agreement for paying the evaluation's justified and duly presented bills. Below we revisit a somewhat painful example, discussed previously in Chapter 2, to underscore the importance of reaching contractual agreements to assure prompt and just payments for work performed.

In one of Stufflebeam's evaluations, budgeted under a cost-reimbursable arrangement, the funder—the National Assessment Governing Board (NAGB)—refused to pay the evaluation's final bill. The evaluation was a follow-up evaluation to a previous formative evaluation that had found many flaws in the subject project. NAGB had paid for the formative evaluation in accordance with the contracted budget. Subsequently, NAGB returned to the evaluator and requested an immediate summative evaluation of the project. This follow-up evaluation was needed because NAGB's parent organization—the United States Congress—stipulated that its continued financial support to the funder would be conditioned on receiving a summative evaluation of the subject project. NAGB then informed the evaluator that it urgently needed a follow-up summative evaluation of the project. NAGB's leader also said the organization needed the evaluation report before a new contract could be processed through slow government channels. As a "do-gooder," Stufflebeam acquiesced and proceeded to conduct and report the needed summative evaluation. Again the evaluation found the subject project to be seriously flawed. Being outraged by this finding, NAGB refused to pay for the evaluation and got away with this decision because there was no completed contract for the work. When the Congress got hold of the summative evaluation report that NAGB had rejected, the House of Representatives decided to defund NAGB, but the U.S. Senate overturned the House's decision. The evaluator's organization bore the approximately $5,000 cost of the summative evaluation. In retrospect, in the absence of an iron-clad contract, the evaluator should have declined to conduct the summative evaluation.

Budgeting under Cost-Plus Agreements

A **cost-plus agreement** provides the evaluator the funds needed to conduct the evaluation, together with an additional amount of funds for purposes beyond those of the contracted evaluation. Depending on the intended use of the additional funds, this type of agreement can be further divided into three types: cost plus a fee, cost plus a grant, and cost plus a profit.

The **cost plus a fee** budget allows the evaluator to use the additional funds to help sustain the contracting organization's regular operations. Such operations might include administering the organization, meeting with an organizational advisory board, and writing funding proposals. In this type of budget, the evaluator would include an **institutional sustainability fee** line item in the budget and provide a note briefly explaining how the added money would be used.

The **cost plus a grant** budget allows the evaluator to use the additional funds to help support the organization's substantive mission, such as research, support of graduate students, or writing journal articles. In this budget type, the evaluator should provide a budget line item for the grant amount and provide a note summarizing the intended use of those funds.

The **cost plus a profit** type of budget is typically used by evaluation firms that offer their services with the explicit goal of realizing a financial gain. The evaluator should explicitly specify the proposed amount of profit as a line item in the budget. One way to determine the proposed profit amount is to calculate it as a percentage of the evaluation's direct cost, for example, 10%.

The risks associated with cost-plus budgets are minimal as long as the evaluator and funder agree on the funds for the main evaluation work and those for funding some other specified organizational purpose. Of course, the evaluator must clarify, for example, with a budget note, how the added funds will be used and subsequently be accountable for that use. The main part of the budget will fund the designed evaluation work, and the added amount will serve other organizational purposes.

Overall, we judge the cost-plus approach to be ethical and to provide relevant budgeting options for addressing the varying missions of different kinds of organizations. Moreover, we see cost-plus budgets to be helpful in furthering the professionalization of evaluation by supporting such activities as research on evaluation and evaluation training.

Budgeting under Cooperative Agreements

A **cooperative agreement** typically stipulates that the funder and the evaluator would collaborate in conducting the evaluation. This entails the evaluator and the funder sharing authority over and responsibility for completing the evaluation.

Evaluation under cooperative agreements can work satisfactorily if there is appropriate differentiation and clear specification of evaluator and funder roles. For example, the funder can help establish connections and rapport between the evaluator and the stakeholders; help assure effective stakeholder involvement and cooperation; and facilitate such evaluation activities as data collection, evaluation site access, and clerical support. Also, by cooperating in the conduct of the evaluation, the funder is likely to develop a sense of ownership of the evaluation and be prone to apply its findings and promote stakeholder's use of the findings as well. The funder may also appreciate being empowered to directly oversee and influence the evaluation work. This latter point is where a cooperative agreement can become dysfunctional and even send the evaluation "off the tracks."

Cooperative agreements, though providing many benefits, may be hazardous to the proper conduct of an evaluation. Problems may occur when funder and evaluator roles are not clearly differentiated or when the funder pulls rank to unduly influence or constrain data collection, preparation of reports, or dissemination of findings. The evaluation contractor should have authority to make decisions in these matters, and that authority should be clearly defined in the evaluation agreement.

Under a cooperative agreement, the funder has a potential conflict of interest that might or might not surface during the evaluation. Such funder conflicts of interest may include inappropriate funder interventions such as taking action to ensure that obtained findings are neither negative nor embarrassing; insisting on staffing the evaluation work with evaluators of the funder's choice; or preventing the dissemination of negative findings. In our experience, conducting evaluations under cooperative agreements at a minimum puts the evaluation work under a continuing cloud of possible inappropriateness and may actually impair the evaluation's integrity, viability, validity, credibility, or utility.

A case in point occurred when Stufflebeam conducted a large-scale evaluation under a cooperative agreement with a federal government agency. Soon after the evaluation began, the evaluation's federal "co-director" insisted that the evaluation's staff positions be filled with women. She also began asserting her authority regarding selection of evaluation tools and procedures and preparation of reports. Stufflebeam deemed all of her actions to be violations of the cooperative agreement, in addition to being inappropriate and counterproductive. He tried but failed to get the federal evaluation "co-director" to curtail her inappropriate interventions and instead concentrate on her defined role in the evaluation design. When the evaluation contractor's constructive efforts in this regard failed, he went to Washington to see his federal counterpart's superior. He reported chapter and verse to the federal official why the cooperative agreement wasn't working as it should. He emphasized that if the co-director's inappropriate intervention continued, the evaluation would fail, and he offered to have the evaluation agreement terminated. Subsequently, the federal agency replaced their representative; the new evaluation co-director effectively carried out the role defined for him in the cooperative agreement, and the evaluation proceeded to a successful conclusion.

The fact that the evaluation ultimately succeeded is testimony to the possibility that evaluations under cooperative agreements can work as intended. However, the case just described also shows that evaluations conducted under cooperative agreements can sometimes be problematic. The central issue is that evaluating under a cooperative agreement can easily erode the evaluator's independence. In such an agreement, the funder clearly has a potential conflict of interest, especially if the evaluation findings tend in the negative direction. In any evaluation, the evaluation contractor needs authority to take the necessary actions to produce and report valid findings. Evaluators should not put themselves in a position where they have the responsibility but not the authority to do what is needed to produce a successful evaluation. Under a cooperative agreement, the funder can wield undue influence and might inappropriately or incompetently influence the evaluator's decisions and actions, thereby seriously impairing the evaluation's quality and integrity. Moreover, if the funder heavily impacts the evaluation's conclusions and findings, or stops the evaluator from releasing certain embarrassing findings, then the evaluator's credibility and integrity can be seriously damaged. When an evaluation fails, the funder will suffer loss of the funds as well as the value and usefulness of the evaluation. We think an evaluation is more likely to fail under a cooperative agreement because of the funder's built-in conflict of interest.

We consider a cooperative agreement to be the weakest and most problematic type of evaluation arrangement. If evaluators have to enter into such an arrangement, it is critical for them to negotiate a contract that clearly stipulates that the evaluator will have appropriate authority over expenditures, staffing, procedures, and reporting of findings. Additionally, it is wise to request and secure an agreement that the evaluation will be subjected to a standards-based independent metaevaluation.

Modular Budgets

In a modular evaluation budget, the evaluator breaks out funding for main budget modules: line-item costs, costs of each evaluation task, and/or costs for each project year or other time period. The evaluator then develops different budget charts to display combinations of the different budget breakouts.

Modularizing an evaluation budget is helpful to both funder and evaluator. The funder can reference modularized budgetary breakouts in prioritizing projected evaluation tasks and deciding how much support to provide for each one. The funder can also reference the breakouts to decide how much money to allocate to cover the evaluation's financial needs in each projected evaluation year or other time period. The evaluator can use a modularized breakout of the budget to divide up the evaluation's budget between the lead evaluation organization and one or more subcontractors; this would be the case especially in large-scale evaluations. Also, the evaluator might be able to define costs specifically for the initial evaluation work but provide only general estimates for later-scheduled work. Modular presentations of an evaluation budget can be usefully applied with all of the other budget types: **fixed-price contract**, grant, **cost-reimbursable contract**, cost-plus agreement, and cooperative agreement. In general, evaluators serve both themselves and the evaluation's funder by breaking out costs by line item, task, and year (or other performance period) and appending the breakouts to the evaluation proposal.

The first step in the process of modular budgeting is to develop a master budget for carrying out the main evaluation tasks in each evaluation year (or other performance period). Such a master budget estimates the full cost of each line item and breaks it out by year (or other performance period) and by main evaluation tasks. This provides the building block for developing summary budget charts that divide the amount for each line item by either main tasks or years (or other performance periods). In general, the first essential step in developing budget breakouts is to build a master budget that shows—for each evaluation year or other period—the line-item cost of each main evaluation task. To aggregate costs into summary charts showing costs for line items and years (or other performance periods) or for line items and tasks, the evaluator must first delineate the line-item costs projected for each task during each evaluation year.

Table 7.4 contains a made-up example framework designed to help readers see how to construct a foundational, master budget for use in developing summary budget charts. This example framework is simpler than those that would accompany complex evaluations. Detailed foundational budgets for such more complex evaluations might include a longer list of line items, more than 2 years (or other performance periods), and/or more than three main tasks. The simple framework in Table 7.4 is easy to display and can be expanded, as much as needed, to accommodate the budgeting requirements of different evaluations.

Often an evaluator will find it useful to break down a master budget chart, such as the one above, into a separate chart for each year or other performance period. The separate chart would include the row line items, the evaluation task columns, and a total costs column to the right of the task columns. Including the line-item totals for each performance year or other period would ease the evaluator's charge to aggregate costs by line items, tasks, and performance periods into the summary charts presented next.

TABLE 7.4. Example Framework for Delineating Each Evaluation Period's Line-Item Costs for Each Main Task

Line Item	Year (or Period) 1			Year (or Period) 2			Totals			
	Task 1 Data Collection	Task 2 Data Analysis	Task 3 Reporting	Task 1 Data Collection	Task 2 Data Analysis	Task 3 Reporting	Task 1 Data Collection	Task 2 Data Analysis	Task 3 Reporting	Totals
Evaluator	$1,300	$900	$600	$1,400	$900	$700	$900	$1,100	$3,000	$10,800
Secretary	400	300	300	400	300	300	300	200	500	3,000
Fringe benefits (40%)	680	480	360	720	480	400	480	520	1,400	5,520
Research assistant	400	300	300	400	300	300	250	350	400	3,000
Consultant	100	150	50	50	200	50	100	175	25	900
Travel	250		50	250		50	250		50	900
Materials	50		50	50		50	50		50	300
Services	20		30	20		30	20		30	150
Indirect (30%)	960	639	522	987	654	564	705	702	1,637	7,370
Totals	4,160	2,769	2,262	4,277	2,834	2,444	3,055	3,047	7,092	31,940

Below we present two example frameworks for breaking out and effectively communicating an evaluation's projected costs. These frameworks are based on the budget for an actual 5-year budget request. The frameworks are: line items by tasks (Table 7.5) and line items by years (Table 7.6). These tables illustrate how an evaluator can inform the potential funder of the plan for spending the full cost budget to carry out each main evaluation task and what level of funding will be needed in each projected evaluation year (or other time period). Table 7.5 shows line item and task cost totals across all 5 evaluation years and also shows the projected evaluation's total cost. Table 7.6 also shows line-item cost totals across all 5 years but also shows the total projected cost for each project year, as well as the projected evaluation's total cost.

The charts in this section are intended mainly to help the evaluator communicate an evaluation's budget in terms that are both of interest and clear to the funder and other interested parties.

Summary of Major Budget Types

In Table 7.7, we summarize the six major budget types described in this chapter. We denote each type's key characteristics and relative benefits for and risks to the evaluator and the funder. Evaluators sometimes cannot choose the type of budget to utilize because the funder may stipulate the type of budget to be submitted. When the evaluator can propose the type of budget to be used, we advise that he or she consider the type of evaluation budget that would be most compatible with the particular evaluation and her or his organization's accounting operations.

Overall, we advise against using cooperative agreements because they can put the evaluation's integrity and quality at risk by taking away or compromising the evaluation's independence. If a cooperative agreement must be used, it should be used with caution and effective safeguards. Clearly, differentiating the roles, authorities, and responsibilities of the funder and

TABLE 7.5. A Generic Modular Evaluation Budget Showing Line Items by Task

Line Item	Task A Planning, initial pilot study, instrument development, background study, and stakeholder engagement	Task B Data Collection and regular meetings with a stakeholder review panel	Task C Data Analysis, reporting, and follow-up assistance	Task D Evaluation Training and other evaluation capacity building services	Total
A. Personnel					
A1. Lead evaluator	$15,647	$17,574	$18,396	$19,474	$71,091
A2. Evaluation manager	22,174	22,909	22,815	23,756	91,654
A3. Editor/support staff	2,995	3,190	3,230	3,326	12,741
A4. Fringe benefits (40%)	16,326	17,469	17,776	18,622	70,193
A5. Graduate research assistant	5,628	5,628	5,629	5,630	22,515
A6. Consultant	10,150	10,250	10,375	10,400	41,175
A7. Total personnel	72,920	77,020	78,221	81,208	309,369
B. Travel	18,800	21,065	23,108	24,185	87,158
C. Materials, equipment, and services	4,550	4,750	5,041	5,400	19,741
F. Total direct costs	96,270	102,835	106,370	110,793	416,268
G. Indirect costs	33,695	35,992	37,230	38,778	145,695
H. Total evaluation costs	$129,965	$138,827	$143,600	$149,571	$561,963

TABLE 7.6. A Generic Modular Evaluation Budget Showing Line Items by Year

Line Item	Year 1	Year 2	Year 3	Year 4	Year 5	Total
A. Personnel						
A1. Lead evaluator	$13,390	$13,792	$14,206	$14,632	$15,071	$71,091
A2. Evaluation manager	17,264	17,781	18,315	18,864	19,430	91,654
A3. Editor/support staff	2,400	2,472	2,546	2,622	2,701	12,741
A4. Fringe benefits (40% of salaries)	13,222	13,618	14,027	14,447	14,880	70,194
A5. Graduate research assistant	4,241	4,368	4,499	4,634	4,773	22,515
A6. Consultant	11,280	5,544	8,821	9,112	6,418	41,175
A7. Total personnel	61,797	57,575	62,414	64,311	63,273	309,370
B. Travel	15,773	16,562	17,390	18,260	19,173	87,158
C. Materials, equipment, and services	3,572	3,751	3,939	4,136	4,343	1,9741
D. Total direct costs	81,142	77,888	83,743	86,707	86,789	416,269
G. Indirect costs	28,400	27,260	29,310	30,347	30,376	142,632
H. Total evaluation costs	$109,542	$105,148	$113,053	$117,054	$117,165	$561,962

evaluator will help the evaluator maintain his or her independence and appropriate level of authority and thus protect the evaluation's prospects for success. We think the five other budget types are potentially useful to evaluators and funders and relatively free of the problems seen in cooperative agreements. The choice of one of these five over the others is largely a function of the scope and type of evaluation to be conducted as well as preferences of both the evaluator and the funder.

Checklist for Developing Evaluation Budgets

To provide readers with practical assistance, we discuss the generic checklist for budgeting evaluation displayed in Checklist 7.1 (at the end of this chapter). This checklist is a 2015 update of Stufflebeam's checklist that appeared in Stufflebeam and Coryn (2014). It includes directions for both developing and reviewing evaluation budgets and financial agreements. The checklist lists and delineates ten tasks needed to develop a sound evaluation budget. Importantly, it is intended for reference in developing the initial budget and in reviewing and updating the budget during the course of the evaluation.

1. Ensure That the Evaluation Design Has the Needed Details

A good evaluation design serves as the basis for developing a complete, functional, and defensible evaluation budget. At the beginning of the budget development process, the evaluator needs to examine the evaluation design to ensure that it includes enough details for building the needed budget. Task 1 of the checklist specifies the essential design components: personnel, consultants, tasks, activities, nonpersonnel resources, funding period, funding schedule, subcontracts, metaevaluation, and provisions for reviewing and updating the budget.

These components should be clearly defined in the evaluation design. If certain essential design elements are missing or are not sufficiently clear, then the evaluator should improve the design. In the case of a formative evaluation where not all design and budget details can be specified in advance, the evaluator should confirm with the funder that the evaluation budget will be periodically reviewed and updated as needed.

2. Determine the Type of Budget Agreement

Different types of budget agreements require different costing approaches and levels of detail. Often it is the

TABLE 7.7. Summary of Different Types of Evaluation Budgets

Key Characteristics	Benefits for the Evaluator	Benefit for the Funder	Risks to the Evaluator	Risks to the Funder
Fixed-price contract				
A fixed amount is paid to the evaluator to complete the agreed-upon scope of work.	The evaluator might make a profit if the needed funds were overestimated.	The funder is likely to receive the needed service at agreed-upon price.	The evaluator might incur a financial loss if the fixed price was insufficient.	The funder might pay much more than the evaluation's actual cost.
Grant				
The grant is awarded to support the evaluator's proposed study with minimal funder oversight and control and often without paying for indirect costs.	The evaluator enjoys the freedom to pursue a study of interest and to apply the granted funds as needed.	The funder can support projects well linked to its mission with minimal oversight required.	Risks are nonexistent if the evaluator receives sufficient external and internal resources to complete the study.	Risks are minimal if the evaluator is competent and responsible in completing the proposed study and achieving its objectives.
Cost-reimbursable contract				
Actual expenditures are reimbursed by the funder, up to a given limit.	The evaluator receives sufficient funding for executing an agreed-upon evaluation design.	The funder invests only the amount of funds that are actually expended in completing the evaluation and that do not exceed the agreed-upon funding limit.	The evaluation may fail if the evaluator underbid the job and did not reach agreement for periodic review and update of the budget.	The funder has minimal financial risks but may risk receiving all the needed evaluation reports and services if the funding limit was set too low.
Cost-plus agreement				
Funds cover execution of the evaluation design plus other purposes of interest to the evaluator.	The evaluator receives funds to conduct the evaluation plus additional funds for other purposes (profit, organizational sustainability, research, training, publishing, etc.).	The funder obtains the needed evaluation and makes an agreed-upon, worthy supplemental contribution to the evaluator's organization.	Risks to the evaluator are minimal as long as he or she accurately estimated funding needs for the evaluation and the other agreed-upon purposes.	Risks are minimal as the funds will support the desired evaluation and cover an additionally agreed-upon award to the evaluator.
Cooperative agreement				
Evaluator and funder share authority and responsibility for conducting the evaluation.	The funder might help with a variety of evaluation tasks related to stakeholder cooperation, data collection, report dissemination, and so on.	The funder can exercise close oversight and participation in the evaluation to ensure that the funder's interests and needs are fully addressed and to facilitate the work.	Risks are substantial because the evaluator can lose independence and the funder can impose inappropriate influence on the evaluation.	There might be conflicts between funder and evaluator regarding conduct of the evaluation, and consequently the evaluation's integrity and quality may be compromised.
Modular budget				
The budget is broken out by line items, evaluation years, and evaluation tasks.	The evaluator can allocate funds to line items, tasks, and time periods and use the breakouts to properly inform the funder of how the funds will be applied.	The funder can decide what tasks to fund and can project funding needs for the evaluation's succession of years or other time periods.	The breakout might tempt the funder to drop certain parts of the evaluation, even important parts.	The funder may receive an evaluation of lesser quality if the funder dropped some important parts of the evaluation.

funder who dictates the type of budget to be employed. When given the choice, the evaluator and her or his organization should choose the budget type that will best meet the evaluation's needs and be compatible with the organization's financial accounting system.

3. Determine the Needed Level of Budget Detail

The evaluator should determine how much budget detail to provide based on the funder's requirements, those of her or his organization, and the complexity of the evaluation assignment. Typically, a grant or a fixed-price contract requires only a general representation of estimated costs. The other types of evaluation agreements usually require substantially more detail. Task 3 lists eight possible ways to break out and explicate an evaluation's projected costs. At a minimum, all types of budgets should break out costs by line items. As explained previously in this chapter, the budgets for complex, multiyear evaluations often should be broken out by line items, tasks, and years, and, as appropriate, also by funder and local contributions. In a full implementation of the CIPP Model, the evaluation's project costs may usefully be broken out by the main tasks of context evaluation, input evaluation, process evaluation, and product evaluation. Generally, it is good practice to prepare and use budget breakouts as planning and management tools, even if the funder issued no requirements for breaking out the evaluation's projected costs into summary charts, such as those that were illustrated in this chapter's section on modular budgets. For all types of budgets, it is good practice to append notes that explain key budget items.

4. Determine Pertinent Cost Factors

The checklist presents an extensive list of potential cost factors under Task 4. The evaluator should consider these factors in the process of determining which ones will be needed to flesh out the evaluation's specific costs. We advise evaluators to inquire whether the funder has a budget ceiling for the projected evaluation. The evaluator would find the funder's answer to this question important in determining the scope of evaluation work that can be conducted or in deciding on the projected evaluation's feasibility under the known funding limit. If the evaluation is to go forward, the evaluator will find advance information about the evaluation assignment's funding limit to be useful for keeping evaluation activities and expenditures within the set funding limit. Moreover, knowing the evaluation's budget ceiling can help evaluators and their institutions determine whether to contribute local funds to the evaluation. For example, the evaluator's organization might agree to reduce its indirect cost rate so that the evaluator can use a larger portion of the evaluation's funds to carry out the evaluation work.

Not all factors listed under Task 4 need to be incorporated into an evaluation budget. For example, to calculate personnel costs, the evaluator should use either daily rates or hourly rates, not both. Some evaluations may not involve consultants or travel. As another example, the evaluator would consider projecting increased costs to cover inflation and salary increments only in the case of multiyear evaluations.

Personnel costs are a major category in many evaluations. When the evaluation design identifies specific staff and consultants, the evaluator likely can stipulate their pay rates. When such staff and consultants are still undetermined, the evaluator should provide cost estimates and note that those rates may have to be adjusted up or down once actual staff members and consultants have been selected. Form 7.1 (at the end of this chapter) is a worksheet for figuring personnel costs by category. The daily rates provided in the form are only examples, as these can vary depending on many factors—for example, the evaluation organization's salary policies, union contracts, geographic region, and supply and demand of appropriately qualified consultants. Notice that separate estimates are given for core evaluation staff, on the one hand, and graduate students and consultants on the other. This practice reflects the fact that universities do not give fringe benefits to graduate students and consultants. Under contracts with federal funders, we advise evaluators to designate consultants as independent contractors. This avoids complications regarding the evaluation organization's decision not to pay unemployment compensation taxes in behalf of these evaluation participants and emphasizes the independent perspectives of these outsiders.

When working with evaluations that span multiple years, evaluators can complete a separate worksheet for each project year. The evaluators should project and provide for annual increments, 5% for example, related to inflation and salary increase.

5. Determine Line Items

Task 5 calls for the evaluator to determine all line items to be included in the evaluation budget. Under Task 5 we listed items that commonly appear in evaluation budgets. The evaluator should checkmark all items in the list that are germane to carrying out the evaluation design. The purpose of this process is to help evaluators assure that they will not under-budget the needed scope of work.

6. Group Line Items into Budget Categories

The evaluator should complete Task 6 by grouping the line items identified in Task 5 into functional budget categories. Typically, these include personnel, travel, equipment, supplies, consultants, services, and indirect costs. Two other important groups of costs can be subcontracts and metaevaluation. The purpose of grouping the list of detailed line items is to provide the funder with an organized, efficient presentation of the evaluation's projected costs. The categories identified above are examples and may be replaced with some other set of advance organizers, depending on the preferences of the funder and/or the evaluator's organization.

7. Determine Local Contribution

Task 7 is included in the checklist in case the evaluator's organization agrees to contribute in some way to covering the evaluation's costs. Such local contributions are common under grant agreements, especially those that mainly serve the evaluation organization's mission. In some cases, the funder, such as a charitable foundation, will require some type of local contribution, such as reducing or eliminating indirect cost charges. In other cases, the evaluator's organization may strongly desire to conduct a certain evaluation and agree upon a local contribution because, otherwise, the evaluation's funding limit would be too low to conduct a quality evaluation. As seen in Task 7's checkpoints, the evaluator's organization might agree to reduce or eliminate indirect cost charges, contribute part or all of the lead evaluator's involved time, pay for the involvement of graduate assistants, directly fund certain evaluation tasks, and so on. A caveat is that under a federal funding agreement, the evaluator should determine the legality of reducing her or his organization's federally audited indirect cost rate. Often such a reduction would be illegal. Also, in a competitive bidding situation, certain local contributions to lower the proposed budget could be contrary to stipulations in the request for proposal and thus be considered unethical. Accordingly, evaluators should be careful to ensure that any local contribution will be legal and ethical. As appropriate, evaluators should report any local contribution in the budget by including a "Local Contribution" budget category.

8. Compute Evaluation's Costs and Charges

Having completed Tasks 1 through 7, the evaluator can quite accurately compute the evaluation's projected costs and charges. The budget display format will depend on the evaluation design, the funder's requirement, the requirement of the evaluator's institution, and the evaluator's preference. A good practice is to develop the budget in its most detailed level and then aggregate as appropriate, especially as seen in this chapter's section on modular budgeting. For instance, for a multiyear evaluation involving multitasks, the evaluator could first develop a line-item budget, broken out by tasks for each year. At this stage, the evaluator should confirm her or his previous decision to include or not include a line item for unpredictable contingencies. Such a provision in the budget could prove essential to ensuring that unpredictable costs can be covered as needed as the evaluation unfolds. This is especially so for formative evaluations. Each year's budget display should be supplemented with a set of explanatory budget notes. Next, evaluators should consider aggregating the master set of figures in various ways to meet the needs of different audiences. It is often a good idea to append a detailed set of budget notes to the evaluation proposal.

9. Document Fiscal Accountability Provisions

In the evaluation proposal, we advise evaluators to provide the funder with documentation of how the evaluation's finances will be monitored, controlled, audited, and reported effectively to assure the utmost fiscal accountability. In proposals for small, single-evaluator evaluations, the evaluator should explain how he or she will keep track of expenditures and maintain an internal accounting record. In large-scale evaluations based in organizations, the evaluation proposal should be submitted through the organization's financial office. The proposal should identify the organizational agent that will submit bills and answer any financial related questions the funder may have. The proposal should also explain how the organization's financial office will oversee, control, and audit the evaluation's expenditures and bill for evaluation payments. Many funders will require such information, but, whether or not this is so, the evaluator should address these matters in the evaluation proposal and thereby forestall any confusion and disputes that might otherwise arise.

10. Clarify Requirements for Payment

The final budget preparation task is for the evaluator to reach an agreement with the funder on funder and contractor responsibilities regarding payment for the evaluation. We advise evaluators to consider the following:

- Identify the office and person(s) in charge of making the payment on behalf of the funder.
- Clarify the funder's requirement in regard to financial reports, including their schedule.
- Clarify the amounts and schedule of payments to be received from the funder.
- In the case of large or longitudinal evaluation, seek legal advice before a contract is finalized.

Summary

Effective evaluation budgets provide sound financial bases for evaluators to carry out successful evaluations. In opening the chapter's discussion, we posited that an evaluation proposal should not be approved if it doesn't include a sound budget to support effective execution of the evaluation design. Developing an evaluation budget can be a complex and tedious process, especially when the evaluation is large and complex. However, evaluators can follow a systematic, step-by-step process to create the needed budget.

This chapter has presented practical advice on key topics pertinent to developing evaluation budgets. We grounded the chapter in six basic factors of sound evaluation budgeting: addressing the interdependence of evaluation designs and budgets; adhering to institutional budgeting requirements; communicating with the funder during the budgeting process; providing for periodic budget reviews and updates; differentiating budgeting needs for formative and summative evaluations; and tailoring budgets to accommodate different types of evaluation agreements. Subsequently, we discussed major line-item budget categories including personnel, travel, consultants, supplies, equipment, services, and indirect costs, and sometimes a category of local contribution.

We then stressed and discussed the imperative that evaluators must be totally ethical in budgeting evaluation efforts, and we offered relevant practical advice. Particularly in our discussion of budgeting ethics, we proposed a general approach to ethical budgeting; discussed the special case of budgeting for unpredictable evaluation costs; identified common ethical challenges and complications in evaluation budgeting; gave our views of appropriate responses to such challenges and complications; identified what we consider to be unethical evaluation budgeting practices; and also discussed ethical breaches in evaluation budgeting that arise from incompetence.

Next we discussed the different types of evaluation budgets, including fixed-price, grant, cost-reimbursable, cost-plus, cooperative agreements, and modular budgets. We identified conflict-of-interest hazards in cooperative agreements and generally warned against entering into such agreements. Regarding the different evaluation budget types, we provided detailed discussion of the utility of breaking out evaluation costs by line items, years or other performance periods, and tasks. We also discussed the key characteristics, risks, and benefits of each of the six identified budget types.

Finally, we presented and explained a checklist for working through ten steps in the evaluation budgeting process: determining the evaluation design's completeness, the needed type of evaluation agreement, the needed level of budget detail, the pertinent cost factors, appropriate line items, functional grouping of line items, any local contributions, ways to compute evaluation costs, provisions for fiscal accountability, and provisions for billing and payments.

REVIEW QUESTIONS • • • • • • • • •

1. Summarize how you would explain this chapter's six basics of evaluation budgeting to a colleague.

2. What is this chapter's rationale for stating that an evaluator can more easily work out the details of a preordinate evaluation than those of a responsive evaluation?

3. Identify and briefly define the line-item budget categories identified in this chapter.

4. Summarize the key points in this chapter's recommended general ethical approach to evaluation budgeting.

5. Identify and define at least two common ethical challenges and complications in evaluation budgeting and give your views of how evaluators should respond to each one.

6. Identify and define at least two unethical evaluation budgeting practices that evaluators should avoid.

7. Summarize difficulties that evaluators often encounter relating to budgeting for unpredictable evaluation costs and give your view concerning how evaluators should address such difficulties.

8. Identify the risks and benefits involved in budgeting under a cooperative evaluation agreement and summarize the advice you would give to an evaluator who has to budget and expend evaluation funds under such an agreement.

9. Briefly identify and summarize five key decisions that an evaluator needs to make in the course of developing an evaluation budget.

10. Identify and summarize the three types of cost-plus budgets. Then summarize in a matrix the risks and benefits of each cost-plus budget type to the evaluator and to the funder.

11. Describe the steps you would follow to calculate an evaluation's total personnel costs.

12. Identify at least three reasons why a funder might prefer a cost-reimbursable evaluation budget.

13. Define what is meant by modular evaluation budgets. Then give your view of when a modular budget would be useful and of the potential utility of the different types of modular budgets presented in this chapter.

14. Use the figures in Table 7.4 to construct a budget chart that summarizes projected evaluation costs by line items and tasks.

15. Find a completed evaluation work plan; summarize the plan; then apply the evaluation checklist in Form 7.1 to draft a budget for carrying out the work plan.

SUGGESTIONS FOR FURTHER READING

Horn, J. (2001). *A checklist for developing and evaluating evaluation budgets.* Kalamazoo: Western Michigan University, The Evaluation Center. Retrieved from *www.wmich.edu/evalctr/archive_checklists/evaluationbudgets.pdf.*

Shenson, H. L. (1990). *The contract and fee-setting guide for consultants and professionals.* Hoboken, NJ: Wiley.

Stufflebeam, D. L., & Coryn, C. L. S. (2014). *Evaluation theory, models, and applications* (2nd ed.). San Francisco: Jossey-Bass.

1. **Examine the evaluation design to ensure that it includes the needed details for developing a sound evaluation budget. (Check those that are included in the present design.)**

   ____ 1.a. Personnel

   ____ 1.b. Consultant

   ____ 1.c. Tasks

   ____ 1.d. Activities

   ____ 1.e. Nonpersonnel resources

   ____ 1.f. Funding period

   ____ 1.g. Funding schedule

   ____ 1.h. Subcontracts

   ____ 1.i. Provisions for updating the budget as appropriate

   ____ 1.j. Metaevaluation

2. **Determine the type(s) of evaluation budget agreement. (Check all that apply.)**

   ____ 2.a. Fixed-price contract

   ____ 2.b. Grant

   ____ 2.c. Cost-reimbursable contract

   ____ 2.d. Cost-plus-a-fee agreement

   ____ 2.e. Cost-plus-a-grant agreement

   ____ 2.f. Cost-plus-a-profit agreement

   ____ 2.g. Cooperative agreement

   ____ 2.h. Modular budget

3. **Determine the appropriate level of budget detail. (Check all that apply.)**

   ____ 3.a. Line-item budget

   ____ 3.b. Line items by task and year (or other evaluation period)

   ____ 3.c. Line items by tasks

   ____ 3.d. Line items by year (or other evaluation period)

   ____ 3.e. Years by tasks

   ____ 3.f. Total budget amount with a narrative explanation

   ____ 3.g. Breakout of the local contribution

   ____ 3.h. Budget notes

(continued)

---

4. Determine pertinent cost factors. (Check all that apply.)

____ 4.a. Budget ceiling

____ 4.b. Allowance for pre-award costs

____ 4.c. Hiring costs

____ 4.d. Name and/or job title and **hourly** salary rate for each staff member

____ 4.e. Name and/or job title and **daily** salary rate for each staff member

____ 4.f. Fringe benefit rate for each category of staff

____ 4.g. Number of workdays for each staff member

____ 4.h. Number of work hours for each staff member

____ 4.i. Daily per diem rate for staff

____ 4.j. Projected number of staff trips

____ 4.k. Estimated average travel cost per staff trip

____ 4.l. Name and/or job title and **daily** rate for each consultant

____ 4.m. Number of workdays for each consultant

____ 4.n. Name and/or job title and **hourly** rate for each consultant

____ 4.o. Number of work hours for each consultant

____ 4.p. Projected number of consultant trips

____ 4.q. Projected total travel days for each consultant

____ 4.r. Daily per diem rate for consultants

____ 4.s. Projected average travel cost per consultant trip

____ 4.t. Indirect cost rate

____ 4.u. Factor for annual staff salary increments

____ 4.v. Factor for annual level of inflation

____ 4.w. Institutional sustainability fee factor (in cost-plus-a-fee or cost-plus-a-grant awards)

____ 4.x. Profit factor (in cost-plus-a-profit)

____ 4.y. Other

5. Determine line items. (Check all that apply.)

____ 5.a. Personnel salaries

____ 5.b. Personnel fringe benefits

____ 5.c. Total personnel

____ 5.d. Travel

____ 5.e. Consultant honoraria

____ 5.f. Consultant travel

____ 5.g. Consultant materials and other support costs

(continued)

____ 5.h. Total consultant costs

____ 5.i. Equipment

____ 5.j. Supplies

____ 5.k. Telephone

____ 5.l. Photocopying and printing

____ 5.m. Binding

____ 5.n. Video making

____ 5.o. Poster making

____ 5.p. Computer use

____ 5.q. Postage

____ 5.r. Total services

____ 5.s. Unpredictable contingencies

____ 5.t. Total direct costs

____ 5.u. Total indirect costs

____ 5.v. Institutional sustainability fee

____ 5.w. Supplemental grant

____ 5.x. Contractor profit

____ 5.y. Subcontracts

____ 5.z. Metaevaluation

____ 5.aa. Other costs

6. **Group line items into budget categories. (Check all that apply.)**

____ 6.a. Personnel

____ 6.b. Travel

____ 6.c. Consultants

____ 6.d. Equipment

____ 6.e. Supplies

____ 6.f. Services

____ 6.g. Subcontracts

____ 6.h. Total direct costs

____ 6.i. Indirect costs

____ 6.j. Total project costs

____ 6.k. Budget notes

____ 6.l. Metaevaluation

(continued)

7. Determine local contribution(s), if any. (Check all that apply.)

____   7.a.   Reduction or elimination of the indirect cost charges

____   7.b.   Contributed time of staff members

____   7.c.   Institutional funding of certain expenses

____   7.d.   Other

8. Compute cost and charges. (Check all that apply.)

____   8.a.   Charges by year (or other work period)

____   8.b.   Charges by project task

____   8.c.   Charges by subcontract

____   8.d.   Overall charges

____   8.e.   Local contribution

____   8.f.   Budget notes to be added

____   8.g.   Independent budget review to be obtained

____   8.h.   Metaevaluation

9. Document fiscal accountability provisions (Check all that apply.)

____   9.a.   Responsibility for internal accounting

____   9.b.   Responsibility for financial reporting

____   9.c.   Responsibility for internal auditing of project finances

10. Clarify requirements for payment. (Check all that apply.)

____   10.a.   Funding source and contact persons

____   10.b.   Financial reporting requirements

____   10.c.   Schedule of financial reports

____   10.d.   Amounts and schedule of payments

Personnel Categories	Task 1		Task 2		Task 3		Total	
	Days	Cost	Days	Cost	Days	Cost	Days	Cost
Core evaluation staff								
Principal investigator: $800/day								
High-level methodologists: $700/day								
Field researcher: $400/day								
Technical support staff: $300/day								
Clerical staff: $150/day								
Total core staff without fringe								
Fringe benefit rate (e.g., 30%)								
Total core staff with fringe loaded								
Graduate students								
Advanced students: $175/day								
Entry-level students: $125/day								
Total graduate students								
Consultants								
High-level consultants: $800/day								
Midlevel consultants: $600/day								
Total consultants								
Total personnel								

Note: Rates presented in the form are only examples.

From *The CIPP Evaluation Model: How to Evaluate for Improvement and Accountability* by Daniel L. Stufflebeam and Guili Zhang. Copyright © 2017 The Guilford Press. Permission to photocopy this material is granted to purchasers of this book for personal use or use with individual clients (see copyright page for details). Purchasers can download enlarged versions of this material (see the box at the end of the table of contents).

CHAPTER 8

Contracting Evaluations

"Negotiating an evaluation contract is vital to safeguarding an evaluation's success."

This chapter is intended to assist evaluators and their clients to develop, adopt, and implement clear, enforceable contracts or memorandums of agreement for funding and successfully executing an agreed-upon evaluation design. We define terms associated with advance evaluation agreements, explain the role and importance of such agreements, discuss the essential features of an evaluation agreement, discuss who should be involved in the contracting process, describe the process of negotiating agreements, and present a checklist for developing and judging an evaluation agreement.

Overview

This chapter is about **evaluation contracts** and **evaluation memorandums of agreement**. The first term refers to formal, legally enforceable agreements, while the second term refers to agreements that are less formal and not necessarily formalized to be legally binding. For efficiency of presentation, throughout the chapter we mainly use the term *contracting* to cover both forms of an evaluation agreement.

Evaluation contracting is dependent on prior steps of designing and budgeting evaluations. We covered these two topics separately in Chapters 6 and 7 because they represent two initial steps in the process of establishing the foundation for a successful evaluation. The

third such step is to negotiate with the client a written agreement stipulating how the evaluation will be carried out and funded. Evaluation design, budgeting, and contracting are interrelated, with an evaluation budget being dependent on the existence of an approved evaluation design, and the evaluation contract being dependent on the previous development of an evaluation design and the associated budget. Once the evaluator and client have agreed on an evaluation design and the evaluation budget, the natural next step is to explicate and commit their agreements to writing. Basically, the evaluator and client should prepare, agree on, and sign a contract for funding and conducting the evaluation work. In the remainder of this chapter, we address the following questions:

- What are the definitions of evaluation contracts and evaluation memorandums of agreement?
- What are the most important reasons for negotiating evaluation contracts?
- What are essential features of a sound evaluation contract?
- Who should be involved in developing evaluation contracts?
- What is involved in negotiating an evaluation agreement?
- What is a comprehensive set of checkpoints for developing and finalizing an evaluation contract?

What Are Definitions of Evaluation Contracts and Memorandums of Agreement?

As stated earlier, an evaluation agreement can be one of two types: a formal contract or a less formal memorandum of agreement. In external evaluations, the formal contract is typically more applicable and, therefore, preferable; memorandums of agreement are typical and can serve usefully in internal evaluations. In this section, we define and discuss the two types of agreement.

Regardless of its type, the evaluation agreement should provide a framework of mutual understanding for proceeding with the evaluation work. Both types of agreement pertain to an evaluator and a client, or sponsor, reaching and signing an advance written agreement for each party's responsibilities for implementing an evaluation.

Although a solely oral evaluation contract could be legally binding, such agreements are built on soft ground, hard to remember, and difficult to enforce. These agreements include only weak bases for addressing disputes about what might or might not have been agreed to previously. Written agreements provide a concrete record of what was agreed to. They help forestall possibilities for disputes that might emerge due to either party's misunderstanding or misremembering what was previously agreed to. For practical reasons, and to avoid unnecessary complications, we advise evaluators and their clients to document their agreements in writing.

Evaluation Contracts

An evaluation contract is a legally enforceable, written agreement between an evaluator and a client, or sponsor, concerning an evaluation's specifications and funding, and both parties' associated responsibilities.

The evaluation contract should:

- Be built on the previously agreed-upon evaluation design and evaluation budget.
- Be detailed and explicit in addressing the full range of issues that are vital to the evaluation's success.
- Either append or reference the separate evaluation design and budget documents as part of the evaluation agreement.
- Define, at least in general terms, what would constitute a breach of contract by either party and what actions could appropriately be taken to address such breaches.
- Be consistent with federal and state laws and statutes, as well as policies of the involved organizations.
- Define bases and procedures for contract reviews and revisions or even cancelation.
- As applicable, include a sign-off by the legal office in the evaluator's parent organization.

Evaluation contracts are between two parties. Frequently, the parties include a client who needs an evaluation of his or her program and an evaluator selected by the client to conduct the evaluation. In other cases, the contracting parties include an evaluator and a sponsor who will fund the evaluation, so that a designated client group will receive and use the evaluation's findings. Even though evaluation contracts often understandably reflect inputs from a wide range of stakeholders, none of them should become an independent third-party signer of the evaluation contract. An evaluation contract among more than two parties would create confusion and chaos on important issues such as the appropriate allocations of authority, responsibility, and accountability. Clearly, an evaluator should never enter into a three-or-more party contract.

Evaluation Memorandums of Agreement

An evaluation memorandum of agreement is similar to an evaluation contract, except that it is less formal. It is an evaluator's write-up of the agreements reached and documented between the evaluator and a client for proceeding with an evaluation. An evaluation memorandum of agreement should specify what is to be done, by whom, how, where, when, and what funds and resources will support this effort. A memorandum of agreement could be based on the minutes of evaluation planning meetings or various communications with the client. Ultimately, it should be signed and dated by both the evaluator and the client.

Once an evaluator drafts the memorandum of agreement, he or she should submit it to the client, who often would be an official or a project director in the evaluator's organization. Following the client's review of the drafted memorandum the two parties should meet to finalize and sign the agreement. An evaluation memorandum of agreement suits internal evaluations well where a formal written contract would seem atypical, awkward, and unnecessary.

An example of an evaluation memorandum of agreement occurred when the Principal Investigator (PI) of a college of education's grant-funded project invited a professor in the college to evaluate the project. After thoroughly discussing the project's need for evaluation with the PI, the evaluator prepared an evaluation design and associated budget and, based on these documents, drafted a memorandum of agreement for the PI's consideration. After talking through the drafted design, budget, and memorandum of agreement, the evaluator and PI agreed on some changes. The evaluator then revised the three documents and submitted the amended memorandum of agreement with appended copies of the evaluation design and budget to the PI. The PI accepted the revised agreement with its appendices, both parties signed and dated the agreement, and the evaluator proceeded to carry out the evaluation.

What Are the Most Important Reasons for Negotiating Evaluation Contracts?

It is imperative for evaluators to secure advance written evaluation contracts before setting out to work on the evaluation assignments. Evaluation agreements can ensure the evaluation's utility, feasibility, propriety, accuracy, and accountability, as well as the evaluation's technical feasibility and fiscal viability; provide safeguards to forestall disputes; and serve as a basis for settling disputes if they occur. Evaluation agreements also give evaluators an opportunity to deal up-front with potential political complications and protect the evaluation's integrity. Having or lacking an advance evaluation contract can literally mean the difference between succeeding in an evaluation or failing.

Clarifying the Evaluation's Basics

The evaluation contract should give assurance that the evaluation will be properly focused to meet the information needs of the client and other members of the evaluation's audience. Specifically, the contract should identify the program or project to be evaluated; the intended users and uses of findings; the evaluation model to be employed; the types of evaluation to be conducted; the evaluation standards to be met; the main questions to be answered; the evaluation's time frame; the nature and timing of main interim and final reports; and provisions for supporting use of the findings. Although most or all of these basics will be included in the evaluation design, the client should add any of them to the contract language that are not clearly present in the evaluation design.

Assuring the Evaluation's Adherence to the Standards of the Evaluation Profession

The process of effectively negotiating an evaluation contract requires the evaluator to carefully design the evaluation to meet the standards for sound evaluations (e.g., utility, feasibility, propriety, accuracy, and accountability). This process also engages the client in examining the evaluation design closely to ensure its quality, feasibility, and potential utility. In carrying out the evaluation, the evaluation contract provides a tangible basis for guiding and supporting its effective execution, settling any disputes that may arise during the course of the evaluation, and ultimately defending the soundness of the final report. Also, as circumstances warrant, the client or evaluator can reference the evaluation contract to assure the evaluation's audience that the evaluation was conducted in accordance with documented, advance agreements. By referencing and sharing the evaluation contract, the client or evaluator can strengthen the audience's confidence and trust in the evaluation's findings.

Assuring the Evaluation's Feasibility

Evaluations typically involve many operational details that require cooperation by many persons in the evaluation's environment, and an advance evaluation contract is important to assure the evaluation's feasibility. Such details include protocols for entering program facilities, contacting program participants, collecting information, keeping collected information secure, editing reports, and disseminating evaluation findings. Although the evaluator should have woven the full range of important implementation tasks into the evaluation design, he or she should also reference or spell out such implementation items in the contract so that the evaluator can efficiently and effectively carry out the work with the cooperation and support of the client and other stakeholders. The evaluator should also make the evaluation's technical design a part of the contract by either appending it to the contract or referencing it as an integral part of the agreement.

Assuring the Evaluation's Fiscal Viability

The evaluator should make sure that the evaluation contract provides for adequate funding of the evaluation. Fiscal viability of any program evaluation is dependent on a sound evaluation budget, the associated funds, and a functional schedule for remitting payments for completed evaluation tasks. The evaluation contract should include the budget, as either an appendix or a statement that the separate budget is part of the evaluation agreement. Key cost items to be referenced include evaluation personnel, consultants, equipment, materials, facilities, travel, communication, incentives, and indirect costs (see Chapter 7).

Forestalling and Settling Disputes

The evaluator and client should reach explicit agreements within a contract to forestall, as much as possible, disputes that may emerge during the evaluation. When written in explicit terms, the contract provides documentation of concrete use in avoiding disputes that otherwise could arise due to a lapse of memory by either party to the contract or, as sometimes happens, a client wanting to suppress or whitewash unwelcome, though valid evaluation findings. For example, in some of Stufflebeam's contracted evaluations the client, upon seeing a draft of the final report, volunteered to edit the report, even though the evaluation contract explicitly assigned editorial authority over reports to the evaluator. In those cases, the client's usurping of the evaluator's authority to edit reports would have violated the terms of the evaluation agreement and impaired the evaluation's independence and integrity. However, Stufflebeam referenced the evaluation contract and maintained his authority to edit the final evaluation report. Here we see that it is highly important that evaluation contracts be specific and clear regarding all key

matters in the evaluation. To the extent an evaluation contract is vague and open to opposing interpretations, the evaluation is susceptible to a variety of issues, including disagreements about such matters as proper procedures, access to information, cooperation by program personnel, editing of reports, dissemination of findings, and paying for the evaluation work.

Although an evaluation contract is an important safeguard against misunderstandings, flawed memories of what was agreed to, and disputes during an evaluation, the contract may not address all areas of needed agreement that may arise during the evaluation. For example, changes in the program plan may raise new questions for the evaluation, or dynamics in the program's environment may require side investigations that were not provided for in the evaluation's design, budget, and contract. Accordingly, a sound evaluation contract should provide for renegotiating and updating the contract as needed.

Dealing Effectively with Potential Political Complications

An important reason for negotiating evaluation agreements concerns the politics of evaluation. Evaluations can be intensely political. Political influences can hinder an evaluation, cause it to fail, or make it a pawn to certain parties who might seek to misrepresent or misuse evaluation findings. An evaluator's failure to uncover and mitigate potential mischief on the part of evaluation users can result in seriously unjust impacts on certain stakeholders. After completing one of his evaluations, Stufflebeam learned that the client, who headed the subject project's parent organization, initially had no interest in obtaining information regarding the project's value or its strengths and weaknesses. The client's real reason for contracting the evaluation was to use the evaluation report as a pretext for firing the project's director, who had a personality conflict with the client. Even though the evaluation report was unmistakably positive, the client referenced the few indications of project weaknesses as the basis for firing the director. This unfortunate case teaches us that before entering into an evaluation contract the evaluator should obtain candid inputs from stakeholders who might be harmed by the evaluation and take steps to protect the evaluation from corrupt use or even reject the evaluation assignment altogether.

A main source of political threats is interest groups wanting to repress or alter an evaluation's findings or even preclude the final evaluation report from being released to the rightful audiences. Sometimes, a client might seek an evaluation just to use the findings as a means to attack an opponent or to gain an advantage over certain stakeholders. Evaluators should be cautious lest they become the client's hired gun in her or his contest with political rivals. Whenever feasible, evaluators need to examine the politics surrounding a request for an evaluation before signing on to do the work. Evaluators should make a thorough search for the political forces that could have a negative influence on a projected evaluation. We emphasize again that before accepting an evaluation assignment, and especially before finalizing an evaluation contract, the evaluator should search out and get input from a range of representative stakeholders.

Stakeholders who are vulnerable and/or in a position to be harmed by an evaluation often can alert a potential evaluator to possible illicit political influences. Therefore, to gain a fuller and deeper understanding of the possible illicit political forces, evaluators are advised to communicate with people who might be negatively affected by the evaluation and give them the opportunity to freely express any concerns they might have about the projected evaluation.

This kind of groundwork is highly valuable in helping evaluators decide what to include in an evaluation agreement, especially whether it is necessary to install appropriate safeguards in the agreement to circumvent undue political influences. Evaluators should adopt all feasible and effective measures to prevent any parties from interfering with or corrupting the evaluation. One safeguard that is effective in militating against political interference is to engage and meet regularly with an evaluation review panel that is broadly representative of all the different evaluation stakeholder groups. If the client and evaluator cannot agree to and institute apparently needed safeguards, then the evaluator would be wise to decline the evaluation assignment.

However, it is often not easy for evaluators who are being approached to conduct studies in their own organization to reject an evaluation assignment. In such a case, the evaluator will need to seriously engage in appropriate background work before finalizing an evaluation agreement. In writing the agreement, the evaluator should key it to professional evaluation principles and standards and identify relevant safeguards for assuring the evaluation's integrity and credibility. As mentioned earlier, one such powerful safeguard is to appoint and meet regularly throughout the evaluation with a rep-

resentative stakeholder review panel. It is also a good idea to advise the client to contract for an independent metaevaluation or to provide funds for the evaluator to engage a metaevaluator. If the evaluator encountered problems during the evaluation that compromised the evaluation's findings, he or she should state appropriate caveats in the final evaluation report.

Protecting the Evaluation's Integrity

As we have noted, negotiating an evaluation agreement that is sound and explicit can safeguard an evaluation's integrity by providing protection against improper client and evaluator actions. One such protection is the assurance that the client is not exerting any undue or unethical influence on the evaluator. An agreement should also accord the evaluator independence and the authority to report the findings in a fair, objective, and uncensored manner. Establishing evaluation agreement guidelines in advance helps ensure that evaluation sources and the data collected are trustworthy and credible, while certifying the reliability and validity of the reported findings.

What Are the Essential Features of Evaluation Contracts and Memorandums of Agreement?

In the Joint Committee on Standards for Educational Evaluation (2011), the "formal agreements" standard states that "evaluation agreements should be negotiated to make obligations explicit and take into account the needs, expectations, and cultural contexts of clients and other stakeholders" (p. 87). Evaluators should write evaluation agreements that contain mutual understandings of the specified expectations and responsibilities of both the client and the evaluator. An evaluation agreement should be keyed to the evaluation's assignment, design, and budget, and to professional standards for sound evaluations. The agreement should define and differentiate the evaluator's and client's areas of authority and responsibility. The agreement should be stated clearly, recorded in writing, and signed by both the evaluator and client and, as appropriate, by officials of the evaluator's and client's organizations. Generally, it is prudent to include the evaluation design, the budget, and selected professional evaluation standards as an essential part of the agreement—either in the contract's body or by reference. Also, the contract should provide for needed reviews and revisions of the contract during the evaluation, as well as include clear terms and a process for terminating the contract, if necessary. Beyond the above general requirements for a sound evaluation contract, the evaluator and client should address a number of additional matters, as follows.

Assuring Consistency with Organizational Contracting Requirements

Evaluators should adhere to their own organization's grant-making and contracting practices as well as those of the evaluation's client organization and funder (if these are different). In the process of developing an evaluation contract the evaluator often should consult her or his organization's attorney. Attorneys can be particularly helpful in protecting the evaluation organization's interests and those of program participants and other stakeholders, especially in regard to deliverables, editing, dissemination, liability, and payments.

Identifying and Addressing Specific Issues That Could Cause the Evaluation to Fail

An evaluation agreement or contract should be negotiated and completed prior to starting an evaluation study. It should cover the full range of issues that might hinder the evaluation or cause it to fail. Many of these issues are usually not included in the evaluation design, yet too often evaluators mistakenly consider the evaluation design to be a complete written agreement. Evaluators should consider addressing such issues as the following in the agreement:

- Standards for judging the evaluation
- Evaluation's objectives and scope of work
- Design
- Access to needed information
- Evaluation participants' protection
- Protocols for collecting information
- Individual and joint responsibilities for conducting the evaluation
- Evaluation information security
- Stakeholder cooperation agreement
- Evaluation reports and their due dates
- Other evaluation deliverables and their due dates
- Protocols for reporting information
- Reporting schedule

- Right-to-know audiences
- Safeguards against possible threats to the evaluation's integrity
- Provisions for keeping and reporting financial information
- Terms of work compensation
- Editorial responsibility and authority
- Dissemination of reports
- Utilization of findings
- Evaluation use for educational purposes
- Presentation of evaluation features and results
- Publication of evaluation features and results

Adhering to the Contractual Agreements

The Joint Committee (2011) *Program Evaluation Standards* requires that "having entered into an agreement, both parties have an obligation to carry it out in a forthright manner or to renegotiate it" (p. 87). Neither the client nor the evaluator should act unilaterally in any matter for which the evaluation agreement requires joint decision making, including materially changing the evaluation's scope, design, time line, or budget without agreeing with the other party to amend the contract. Instead, they should negotiate terms that both parties accept. In short, both parties should candidly communicate with each other and reach written agreements regarding all matters related to the evaluation's procedures, implementation, funding, and reporting, together with any other key evaluation matters not included in the initial contract.

Overall, evaluation contracts should:

- Be built on background discussions with representatives of the full range of evaluation stakeholders.
- Define and address pertinent conflicts of interest.
- Define, identify, and effectively address potential biases, both perceived and real.
- Be keyed to the standards of the evaluation profession.
- Make the agreed-upon evaluation design and budget a party to the contract.
- Be clear about the terms and schedule of payments for evaluation work.
- Determine the criteria for proper spending by the evaluator.

- Provide criteria and procedures for reviewing and updating the contract as appropriate.
- As feasible, provide for an independent metaevaluation.
- Make clear the consequences of violating any of the terms of the agreement, with the ultimate goal of protecting the integrity of the program evaluation.

Who Should Be Involved in Developing Evaluation Contracts?

Key parties to be involved in contracting include stakeholders who can help identify issues to be addressed, the evaluators and clients as the contract's signatories, officials in the evaluator's and client's organizations who may countersign the agreement, and attorneys who can help ensure the agreement's legal viability.

Stakeholders should be consulted in the process of reaching the needed agreements. It is important to consult with stakeholders prior to finalizing an evaluation agreement. This will not always be easy or even feasible, especially in national competitions for awards to conduct large-scale evaluations funded by such organizations as federal agencies, charitable foundations, or corporations. However, when feasible, evaluators should consult with stakeholders, or at least take their interests into account prior to finalizing an evaluation agreement.

In addition to negotiating with the client, the evaluator should strive to consult people who, though not party to the written agreement, will be involved in, affected by, or interested in the evaluation. It would be risky to expect that people will automatically participate in the evaluation without preagreement. Evaluators should not put the evaluation at risk by leaving stakeholder participation in the evaluation to chance, but should instead take the necessary steps to obtain their agreements to cooperate. For example, to ensure success in data collection, respondents' cooperation should be obtained in advance. When this is not feasible, evaluators should explicitly include in the evaluation design and contract provisions for consulting stakeholders and obtaining their inputs and agreement to participate in the evaluation.

Among stakeholders who should be contacted are those whose work will be assessed, those who will contribute information, administrators and staff members with whom the evaluation will be conducted, members of the media, leaders of pertinent community organizations, as well as interested community members. We repeat that evaluators should reach out to those who might be harmed by an evaluation and give them the opportunity to share their thoughts and air their concerns. Ideally, all of the stakeholder consultation work should take place before an evaluation agreement is signed.

We stress, however, that the only contractual signatories are the evaluator or evaluation organization and the client or client's organization. Although evaluations will involve stakeholders other than the organization and/or evaluator, these stakeholders have no authoritative powers in the contracting process. Giving others power to make decisions or to influence the evaluation process can create chaos; thus, the evaluator (or his or her organization) and the client (or his or her organization) should hold all formal decision-making power in the contracting process.

What Is Involved in Negotiating an Evaluation Agreement?

In initiating the contracting process, the evaluator should seek to develop a foundation of effective communication, trust, confidence, and cooperation. The evaluator should be receptive to hearing the client's concerns, taking account of other stakeholders' inputs, and making clear, substantive responses to any and all stated concerns. The evaluator should stress to the client and others the importance of grounding the contract in the standards of the evaluation field and the evaluation's design and budget that were previously developed. Securing mutual understanding of what the evaluation should accomplish and how the different participants should work together to accomplish the evaluation's aims are important prerequisites to successfully addressing sensitive negotiating matters. The process of negotiating and executing a sound evaluation contract sets the stage for efficient and effective execution of the evaluation design based on a constructive relationship between the evaluator and client. Importantly, the process of negotiating an evaluation agreement engages the client and evaluator in a productive process of closely examining and possibly strengthening the evaluation design and budget; informing and obtaining feedback from stakeholders regarding draft agreements; and clarifying and agreeing on evaluator and client expectations, responsibilities, and rights in the evaluation.

The evaluation contracting process generally involves the following 11 steps.

1. Meet with the client to hear and thoroughly explore the request for an evaluation.

2. Meet with representatives of the full range of stakeholders to hear their ideas and concerns regarding the projected evaluation. Make sure to seek out and hear from persons who might be harmed by the evaluation.

3. Draft an evaluation design and associated budget.

4. Finalize the evaluation design and budget based on substantive exchange with the client.

5. Draft the evaluation contract, including referencing or appending the agreed-upon evaluation design and budget.

6. Review the draft contract with a relevant attorney and others as appropriate, and modify it as needed.

7. Review the draft budget with the client and modify it as appropriate.

8. Receive the finalized, signed contract from the client.

9. Secure any needed approvals of the contract from the evaluator's parent organization.

10. Recycle the contracting process if necessary.

11. Finalize the agreement with the client and evaluator parties, affixing signatures and dating the contract.

This process can be seen more clearly in Figure 8.1.

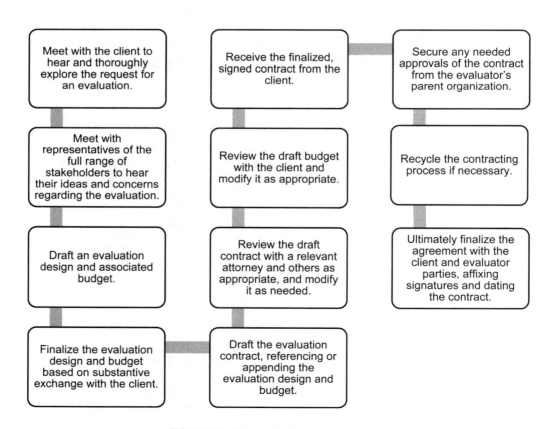

FIGURE 8.1. The evaluation contract process.

What Is a Comprehensive Set of Checkpoints for Developing and Finalizing an Evaluation Contract?

In Checklist 8.1 (at the end of this chapter), we provide an evaluation contracting checklist to help evaluators and clients identify key contractual issues and reach and record their agreements for carrying out an evaluation. Even though not all items included in the checklist will apply in all evaluation agreements, it is prudent to consider all of the checkpoints both when starting a negotiation and when reviewing a draft set of agreements. Then, the contracting parties can select those items that should be incorporated into the agreement or revise the draft as needed.

We suggest that the evaluator code applicable items that are important with a checkmark (✓), code those that are not applicable as "NA", and leave those without agreement blank. Those left blank may still be viewed as important and can be revisited and recoded accordingly. The checklist serves as a tool for evaluators to use in detailing and negotiating evaluation agreements; they can also sign, date, and retain the completed checklist as a convenient summary of what they intend to cover in the official evaluation agreement.

Summary

This chapter has addressed the fundamentally important evaluation task of negotiating written evaluation agreements. Such an agreement can be a formal, legally enforceable contract or a less formal memorandum of agreement. The formal contract applies especially to external evaluations, while the less formal often is sufficient and more appropriate for internal evaluations. Evaluators should negotiate advance agreements with their clients as a means of assuring the evaluation's integrity, viability, credibility, and effectiveness; and especially of forestalling or providing the means for addressing possible disputes during the evaluation.

Both evaluation contracts and memorandums of agreement should be written clearly in enforceable language; grounded in professional standards for sound evaluations; keyed to the evaluation design and budget; reflective of inputs from stakeholders; clear concerning evaluator and client authority and responsibility; oriented to ensuring the evaluation's feasibility, efficiency, fiscal viability, and effectiveness; open to later amendment or termination; and negotiated and signed by the evaluator and the client prior to starting the evaluation. The chapter concludes with an evaluation contracting checklist that presents the full range of issues to consider and, as appropriate, address when developing or assessing an evaluation agreement. Sound evaluation contracting provides a systematic approach to making an evaluation as fail-safe as possible.

REVIEW QUESTIONS • • • • • • • • • • •

1. What are the similarities and differences between evaluation contracts and evaluation memorandums of agreement?

2. Formulate and explain an example to illustrate how an evaluation client might use an advance contract to avoid an evaluator's potential future misunderstanding and unauthorized action concerning dissemination of the evaluation's findings.

3. From the evaluator's perspective, list at least five undesirable possible consequences of conducting an evaluation without an advance written evaluation contract.

4. From the client's perspective list at least five undesirable possible consequences of commissioning an evaluation without an advance written evaluation contract.

5. List what you see as five of the most important features of a sound evaluation contract.

6. Who should sign an evaluation contract? Please explain.

7. Identify and justify your choices of at least six important contractual issues that an evaluator should identify, examine, and resolve before finalizing an evaluation contract.

8. List the process steps you would follow in negotiating an evaluation contract.

9. Identify an evaluation project with which you are familiar; list at least three possible threats to that evaluation's success; then draft a contractual statement to help prevent each of the threats.

10. List at least ten reasons for negotiating advance evaluation agreements.

11. Reference this chapter's evaluation contracting checklist to list what you see as at least five im-

portant contractual safeguards to assure proper dissemination of evaluation findings.

SUGGESTIONS FOR FURTHER READING

American Evaluation Association Task Force on Guiding Principles for Evaluators. (2013). Guiding principles for evaluators. *American Journal of Evaluation, 34,* 145–146.

Joint Committee on Standards for Educational Evaluation. (2011). *The program evaluation standards: A guide for evaluators and evaluation users* (3rd ed.). Thousand Oaks, CA: Sage.

Patton, M. Q. (2008). *Utilization-focused evaluation* (4th ed.). Thousand Oaks, CA: Sage.

Stufflebeam, D. L., & Coryn, C. L. S. (2014). *Evaluation theory, models, and applications* (2nd ed.). San Francisco: Jossey-Bass.

Basic Considerations

___ a. Object of the evaluation (e.g., a named program)

___ b. Purpose of the evaluation (i.e., how the findings will be used)

___ c. Client (including the client's organization)

___ d. Other right-to-know audiences

___ e. Authorized evaluator(s)

___ f. Guiding values and criteria

___ g. Standards for guiding and judging the evaluation

___ h. Contractual questions

Information

___ a. Required information

___ b. Information sources

___ c. Respondents selection criteria and process

___ d. Information collection procedures

___ e. Information collection tools

___ f. Provisions to obtain needed permissions to collect data

___ g. Follow-up procedures to ensure adequate information

___ h. Provisions for ensuring the quality of obtained information

___ i. Provisions for storing and maintaining security of obtained information

Analysis

___ a. Procedures for analyzing quantitative information

___ b. Procedures for analyzing qualitative information

Synthesis

___ a. Participants in the process of reaching conclusions

___ b. Procedures and guidelines for synthesizing findings and reaching conclusions

___ c. Decisions on whether evaluation reports should include recommendations

Reports

___ a. Deliverables and due dates

___ b. Interim reports format, content, length, audiences, and delivery methods

___ c. Final report format, content, length, audiences, and delivery methods

___ d. Permissions and restrictions related to publishing information from or based on the evaluation

(continued)

Reporting Safeguards

____ a. Anonymity, confidentiality

____ b. Prerelease review of reports

____ c. Conditions for participating in prerelease reviews

____ d. Rebuttal by evaluees

____ e. Editorial authority

____ f. Authorized recipients of reports

____ g. Final authority to release reports

Communication Protocol

____ a. Contact persons

____ b. Rules for contacting program personnel

____ c. Communication channels and assistance

Evaluation Management

____ a. Assignment of evaluation responsibilities

____ b. Time line for evaluation work by the client and evaluators

Client Authority and Responsibilities

____ a. Access to information

____ b. Services (e.g., clerical, office equipment, telephone)

____ c. Personnel

____ d. Information

____ e. Facilities

____ f. Equipment

____ g. Materials

____ h. Transportation

____ i. Work space

Evaluation Budget

____ a. Budget type (fixed-price, cost-reimbursable, or cost-plus agreement)

____ b. Payment amounts and dates

____ c. Conditions for payment, including delivery of requested reports

____ d. Budget limits or restrictions

____ e. Agreed-on indirect cost and overhead rates

____ f. Contracts for budgetary matters

Review and Control of Evaluation

____ a. Provisions for contract amendment and cancellation

____ b. Provisions for periodic review, modification, and renegotiation of the design as needed

____ c. Provision for evaluating the evaluation against professional standards of sound evaluations

Preparer: _____ Date: _____

CHAPTER 9

Collecting Evaluative Information

"Sound evaluative conclusions must be based on a sufficient range of valid information."

This chapter is a guide to information collection in the context of the CIPP Model. The chapter makes the case for collecting sound and useful information; discusses main types of evaluative questions and potentially relevant information; reviews a range of useful quantitative and qualitative procedures; stresses the importance of employing multiple sources, evaluators, and procedures; and discusses the utility of the Joint Committee's professional standards for developing and judging information collection plans. Examples of data collection plans and procedures in evaluations that employed the CIPP Model are interjected throughout the chapter.

Overview

This chapter focuses on the information collection component of the CIPP Evaluation Model. Basically, the chapter is a practical guide for evaluators to follow in planning and implementing a sound process of information collection. Throughout the chapter, we reference and provide examples of information collection as it was employed in a wide range of evaluations that employed the CIPP Model.

We begin the chapter by stressing the importance of collecting information that is **objective,** reliable, and valid. We then enumerate the types of questions that evaluations typically address and present a wide array of the types of potentially relevant evaluative information. In consideration of these questions and types of information, we discuss and illustrate the application of many quantitative and qualitative information collection methods and comment on the mutually reinforcing qualities of these two types of methods. Next, we emphasize the importance of employing an information collection approach that uses multiple sources of information and multiple procedures. Subsequently, we reference the Joint Committee's professional standards on information collection and point up their relevance for developing and judging information collection plans. Finally, we discuss the procedures involved in organizing information for analysis.

The Rationale for Sound Data Collection in Evaluation Studies

An evaluation's central goal is to judge the merit and value of a program or other entity. Rendering sound judgments requires relevant, valid information. Information collection is the process of systematically gathering and validating information on variables that are relevant to answering stated evaluation questions and fully judging a program's value. Although information collection methods may need to vary by the discipline of the evaluation's targeted program, all evaluations require sound information collection processes. Sound information will ensure that the evaluation's users are not misled by faulty data and erroneous conclusions. Without a foundation of sound information, any evaluation is doomed to fail. But with a supply of cogent, reliable, and valid information an evaluator may confidently answer a client group's questions and render a defensible judgment of the subject program.

Overarching Questions to Ask When Planning Data Collection

Planning a sound information collection process requires that the evaluator ask a series of overarching questions, such as:

- What is the evaluation's purpose?
- Who will use the information and how?
- What do the intended users want to learn about the subject program?
- What are the most important evaluation questions?
- What information should be collected, both to answer the client group's questions and to assess the program's merit and worth?
- Where will the information be collected?
- What information collection methods will be most appropriate?
- When and how often will the information be collected?
- Who will collect the information?
- What orientation and training should the information collectors receive?

Questions such as these are important because they help assure that the obtained information will be relevant and sufficient to answer the client group's evaluation questions and to judge the program's quality and value.

Information Needs and Relevant Procedures for Context, Input, Process, and Product Evaluations

The four types of evaluation (context, input, process, and product) serve distinct purposes and address different sets of generic evaluation questions. In correct applications of the CIPP Model, evaluators should reference such questions in deciding what information to collect.

Context Evaluation Questions and Information Needs

As discussed in Chapter 2, the purpose of context evaluation is to define the relevant context; identify the targeted beneficiaries and assess their needs; identify and assess assets and opportunities for addressing the needs; diagnose problems underlying the needs; and judge whether program goals and priorities are sufficiently and appropriately responsive to the assessed needs.

In its formative role, context evaluation asks:

- What are the highest-priority needs in the program area of interest?
- What beneficiary group should be served?
- What is an appropriate breakout of the target group's needs?
- What potential goals would be reflective of the assessed needs?
- What potential problems and barriers to the program's success need to be addressed and overcome?
- What assets and potentially available opportunities are available to assist in meeting beneficiaries' assessed needs and achieving the drafted goals?

Summatively, context evaluation might ask questions such as:

- To what extent did this intervention address high-priority needs?
- To what extent did the program's goals reflect beneficiaries' targeted needs?

• To what extent did the goals take account of and target ways to overcome barriers to the program's success?

• To what extent did the goals incorporate use of available assets and opportunities to enhance prospects for success?

The evaluator needs to compile and assess background information on the intended beneficiaries' needs and relevant assets and opportunities from such sources as health records, school grades and test scores, funding proposals, previous evaluation reports, funding programs, and newspaper archives; engage a data collection specialist to monitor and record data on the program's environment, including related programs, area resources, area needs and problems, and political dynamics; interview program leaders and staff to review and discuss their perspectives on beneficiaries' needs and to identify any problems the program will need to solve; and interview other stakeholders to gain further insight into the needs of intended beneficiaries, relevant assets or opportunities, and potential problems for the program.

The information needed to answer these questions would include the program's history, intended beneficiaries, beneficiaries' assessed needs, program goals, program/area assets, potential funding opportunities, benefactors, and any obstacles to program success. Depending on relevance and availability, the information collection plan might also include any proposal or mandate that led to the program's establishment; personnel records germane to the targeted beneficiaries, (e.g., health records, diagnostic test results, educational level, and employment); students' achievement test scores, attendance records, school grades, and participation in a free and reduced cost school lunch program; the program's database, website, listserv, and/or newsletter; previous evaluations of the program or similar programs; relevant research literature, such as results of surveys, rating scale studies, public hearings, and **epidemiological studies**; relevant funding programs; and public records, including newspaper archives relevant to the program's economic, cultural, and political environment.

Evaluators should use such data collection procedures as document retrieval and review, interviews, site visits, literature reviews, case studies, surveys, focus groups, hearings, diagnostic tests, **system analysis, demographic analysis**, **secondary data analysis**, epidemiological studies, historical analysis, and the **Delphi technique**.

Input Evaluation Questions and Information Needs

The purpose of input evaluation is to identify and assess system capabilities, alternative program strategies, and (as appropriate) alternative external contractors; assess the chosen strategy's procedural design, budget, schedule, staffing, and stakeholder involvement plans; and help assure that the selected inputs are responsive to targeted program goals and beneficiaries' needs.

In its formative role, input evaluation asks:

• What are the most promising potential approaches to meeting the targeted needs and achieving the stated goals?

• How do these alternatives rate on past uses, potential for success, costs, political viability, feasibility, and so on?

• How can the needed intervention be most effectively designed, staffed, funded, and implemented (e.g., through merging the best features of the assessed alternative approaches)?

• Is the produced action plan sound and workable?

• What are predictable barriers to effective implementation?

In its summative role, input evaluation asks:

• What program approaches were considered?

• What approach was chosen and, compared with other viable strategies, why?

• How well was the chosen strategy converted to a sound, feasible work plan?

Evaluators need to identify existing program approaches that could serve as models for the contemplated program; reach agreement with the client on criteria for evaluating competing program approaches; and collect required information on the identified program approaches and compare them on agreed-upon criteria.

The information needed to answer the input evaluation questions includes such categories as program assessment criteria, alternative program approaches, selected program approach, operational plans (schedule, staff, consultants, facilities, equipment, materials, internal evaluation, external evaluation), budget, and contract. Information is also needed for arrangements for accounting, administrative oversight, and area support.

In identifying and assessing alternative program approaches, evaluators can employ evaluation techniques such as literature searches, document analysis, interviews, background checks, visits to exemplary programs, advocate teams studies, and pilot trials. In evaluating the program staff's action plan for carrying out the chosen program approach, the evaluator can employ expert reviews, cost analysis, and instruments to assess program staff members' relevant knowledge and attitudes.

Process Evaluation Questions and Information Needs

The purpose of process evaluation is to identify or predict defects in the procedural design or its implementation, provide information for preprogrammed implementation decisions, affirm activities that are working well, and record and judge procedural events and activities.

In its formative role, process evaluation asks:

- To what extent is the program proceeding on time, within budget, and effectively?
- What, if any, impediments to successful implementation need to be addressed?
- If necessary, how should the design be improved?
- If indicated, how should program implementation be strengthened?

In its summative role, process evaluation asks:

- To what extent was the program carried out as planned or modified with an improved plan?
- How effectively did staff identify and overcome problems of implementation?
- How well was the program executed?

The information needed to answer the process evaluation questions might include minutes of staff meetings, field notes, program progress reports, expenditure reports, field observer reports, photographic records, beneficiary feedback, staff interviews, oversight personnel interviews, media releases, program website, program listserv, program newsletter, videotapes or audiotapes of program events, or focus group feedback. Such information should be keyed to such uses in the subject program as identifying potential procedural barriers, assisting program implementation decisions, and documenting the actual program process and costs.

Evaluators often appropriately engage **resident observers** or **visiting investigators** to monitor and document the program's implementation. In order to study and document the program's ongoing operations, the observer or visiting investigator may choose from a wide array of information collection techniques. These techniques include both structured and unstructured observation, formal and informal interviews, rating scales, questionnaires, **records analysis**, periodic photographing of program events and environment, case studies of program beneficiaries, town hall meetings, and focus groups.

Product Evaluation Questions and Information Needs

The purposes of product evaluation are to identify intended and unintended outcomes; relate them to goals and assessed needs and to context, input, and process information; and judge accomplishments in terms such as **quality**, worth, probity, equity, cost, **safety**, and significance.

In its formative role, product evaluation asks:

- To what extent is the program effectively addressing the targeted needs?
- To what extent is the program reaching all the intended beneficiaries?
- To what extent is the program achieving its goals?
- What, if any, unexpected accomplishments are emerging?
- What, if any, negative effects are emerging?
- Is there a need to modify program plans to increase success or eliminate bad outcomes?

In its summative role, product evaluation asks:

- To what extent did this program successfully address the originally assessed needs and stated goals?
- To what extent did the program reach all the intended beneficiaries?
- What, if any, were the unanticipated positive outcomes?

- What, if any, were the unexpected negative outcomes?
- What conclusions can be reached in terms of the program's quality, impacts, cost-effectiveness, sustainability, and broad applicability?
- To what extent has the program been replicated elsewhere, and, if so, with what results?

The information needed to answer the product evaluation questions might include milestone reports; measures of **main effects** and **side effects**; results of wide searches for the full range of program effects; beneficiaries' assessments of the services they received; staff reports on perceived program outcomes; documentation of results from various specific data collection techniques; expert judgments of program outcomes; periodic photographs of the program's environment and impacts; contrasts of the program's outcomes with those of similar programs; plans for sustaining the program; and any evidence of program replication.

To obtain product evaluation information such as those enumerated above, the evaluator should identify and utilize relevant program records. These may be in the form of the program's website, database, minutes of meetings, newsletters, achievement or diagnostic test results, reports to the program's funder, financial records, minutes of program meetings, and so forth. Beyond examining extant program information, the product evaluator typically will gather additional information using a variety of information collection procedures.

These procedures may include rating scales, checklists of expected outcomes, achievement tests, interviews, surveys, a photographic record, cost-effectiveness analysis, goal-free evaluation (a search for program impacts that may or may not be associated with program goals), study of program effects on experimental and comparison groups, study of the trend in program outcome measures taken during the course of the program, and surveys. Other product evaluation techniques include focus groups (involving a cross-section of stakeholders) to discuss the desirability and practical possibilities of sustaining the program, program hearings, epidemiological studies, and a search for and assessment of similar programs that might be plausible alternatives to the program being evaluated.

The evaluator should engage the program's director to supply information on the program's cost of implementation and outcomes. Relevant documentation includes program plans, staff assignments, budgets, expenditure records, records and reports of program accomplishments, assessments by the program's funder, and any plans for long-term implementation of the program.

Typically, the evaluator should interview a wide range of respondents to determine and assess program outcomes. These respondents include the program's leaders, staff, beneficiaries, and others possessing in-depth information about the program. These respondents should be asked to give their views on whether the program reached the right beneficiaries, what was achieved, and what program features should be sustained. Usually, the evaluator should also interview area stakeholders as well as experts in the substance of the program. These individuals may include community leaders, employers, school and social program personnel, clergy, city officials, police, judges, home owners, administrators of similar programs, and researchers in the program's disciplinary area. Such informants may be sufficiently informed about the program to provide informed perspectives on its quality, best and worst features, and effects on the community. As appropriate and feasible, the evaluator might also conduct in-depth case studies of the program experiences of selected beneficiaries.

An Overview of the Information Collection Task and Some Examples

When put together, the information collection plan should be sufficient to fully assess the subject program but should also be parsimonious in avoiding the collection of unneeded information. At the outset of the information collection process, the evaluator should consider a broad range of potentially relevant information, then narrow the set of information to those categories that are most germane to the current evaluation assignment. The CIPP Evaluation Model is a source of a wide range of potentially useful information categories to consider, as seen in Table 9.1. In choosing categories of information for an evaluation, the evaluator should seek to address each main evaluation question with multiple types of information.

In an evaluation study of a patient safety initiative, Farley and Battles (2009) conducted a comprehensive examination of varying types of activities within the patient safety initiative operated by the **Agency for Healthcare Research and Quality (AHRQ)**:

For the *context evaluation,* the evaluation documented historical events leading up to the start of the patient safety initiative and identified external expectations and challenges for the initiative both at the project's inception and throughout its implementation. Information for this analysis was obtained from written documents, websites, and other factual sources. In addition, individual interviews were conducted with key national stakeholders, including AHRQ staff, to understand their views on the history of patient safety and related issues, AHRQ's initiative, and progress in improving patient safety. Data from the interviews were organized and summarized by topic area and analyzed to identify key themes and differences in viewpoints among stakeholders. Interview results also were considered within the context of factual information obtained from other sources. Similar data collection and analysis methods, including interviews and analysis of written or electronic documents, were used for the input evaluation, which described and assessed the goals and strategies that AHRQ established for the patient safety initiative.

The *process evaluation* drew upon a variety of data collection methods, since so many different kinds of activities were involved. It relied extensively on individual or group interviews with stakeholders, including leads of funded projects, representatives of organizations involved in patient safety, and AHRQ staff. Data also were coded from the project proposals, which allowed us to profile projects by type of patient safety issue addressed, practices tested, health care settings, contribution to scientific evidence, and other factors.

As described above, the *product evaluation* consisted mainly of exploratory analyses of existing measures and data, which therefore did not involve primary data

TABLE 9.1. Potentially Useful Sources of Evaluative Information

Context Evaluation	Input Evaluation	Process Evaluation	Product Evaluation
• Program's economic, cultural, and political environment	• Program assessment criteria	• Staff meetings	• Milestone reports
• Program's history	• Alternative program strategies	• Progress reports	• Main effects
• Intended beneficiaries	• Selected program strategy	• Expenditure reports	• Side effects
• Beneficiaries' assessed needs	• Operational plan	• Implementation evaluation reports	• Goal-free evaluation reports
• Program goals	• Schedule	• Activity records	• Beneficiaries' judgments
• Program/area assets	• Staff	• Minutes of meetings	• Staff self-assessments
• Benefactors	• Consultants	• Photographic records	• Expert judgments
• Obstacles to program success	• Facilities	• Beneficiaries' feedback	• External evaluation reports
• Similar programs in the area	• Equipment	• Staff interviews	• Observer reports
• Relevant literature	• Materials	• Oversight personnel interviews	• Photographic records
• Program website	• Internal evaluation	• Media releases	• Contrast to similar projects
• Program listserv	• External evaluation	• Program website	• Sustainability potential
• Program newsletter	• Budget	• Program listserv	• Transportability potential
• Program hearings	• Contract	• Program newsletter	• Accomplishment reports
• Health records	• Accounting	• Videotapes of program events	• Program website
• School grades	• Administrative oversight	• Audiotapes	• Program listserv
• Diagnostic test results	• Reputation and area support	• Field notes	• Program newsletter
• Funding proposals	• Program website		• Focus groups
• Previous evaluation reports	• Program listserv		• Program hearings
• Funding programs	• Program newsletter		• Diagnostic test results
• Newspaper archives			• Epidemiological results
• Epidemiological results			• Survey results
• Survey results			• Rating scale results
• Rating scale results			• Achievement test results
• Achievement test results			• Personnel records
• Personnel records			• Organizational database
• Organizational database			• Videotapes of realized benefits for intended beneficiaries (e.g., new or rehabbed houses)

collection. The Evaluation Center researched written materials to identify existing measures that might be used to assess outcomes using administrative data, assessed the technical basis for the outcome measures, and estimated baseline trends for some of them. Standard methods for working with administrative data were applied, including construction of variables for measures being tested, case mix adjustments, and statistical inference. (p. 639)

The above examples illustrate that collection of a sufficiently broad range of pertinent and defensible information armed the evaluators, in both cases, to answer evaluation questions confidently, present defensible conclusions, and confidently advise the client group to embrace and apply the evaluation's findings.

Types of Information Collection Methods

Information collection methods for evaluations may be seen as varying along a continuum, with quantitative methods at one end and qualitative methods at the other.

Quantitative Data Collection Methods

Quantitative data collection methods employ structured data collection instruments that fit diverse experiences into predetermined response categories. They produce results that are easy to summarize, compare, analyze, and generalize. Quantitative data-gathering methods that may be applied in a diverse set of fields include:

- Standardized achievement tests
- Rating scales
- Cost accounting
- Q-sorts
- Pre-scaled questionnaires
- Scaled opinion survey instruments
- Recording, in preset categories, certain occurrences (e.g., the number of students absent from school on a particular day)
- Extraction of data from census records
- Health indicators, such as blood pressure, body temperature, and ferritin iron level
- Checklists
- Relevant data from management information systems
- Recording of measures of ambient temperature over defined time periods
- Recording of numbers of different types of crimes in a time period for a given locale
- Procedures for scoring different sports events

Qualitative Data Collection Methods

Qualitative data collection methods play an important role in evaluation by providing information useful to understand the processes behind observed quantitative results. Qualitative methods can be used to support quantitative surveys by providing direction for generating evaluation hypotheses, strengthening the design of survey questionnaires, and, ultimately, interpreting quantitative evaluation findings. In reporting quantitative information, it can be useful to readers to interject quotations and other information from interviews and other qualitative methods that enhance the meaning of the quantitative results.

Qualitative information collection methods all tend to be open-ended and have less structured protocols (i.e., evaluators may change the information collection strategy by adding, refining, or dropping techniques or informants); rely more heavily on interactive interviews (i.e., respondents may be interviewed several

BOX 9.2.–Quantitative Outcome Measures Example

Gavidia-Payne et al. (2003) conducted an outcome evaluation of a statewide child inpatient mental health unit and utilized a range of standardized quantitative outcome measures:

- *Strengths and Difficulties Questionnaire (SDQ).* The SDQ is a 25-item measure used to assess change in child behavior and functioning. It contains five subscales: hyperactivity, emotional symptoms, conduct problems, peer problems, and prosocial behavior. With the exception of the latter subscale, lower scores on the SDQ subscales indicate better behavior and functioning.

- *Health of the Nation Outcome Scales for Children and Adolescents (HoNOSCA).* The HoNOSCA is a brief, clinician-rated consumer outcome questionnaire, which is designed to measure consumer health status and treatment outcomes in child and adolescent mental health, over several aspects of health functioning. Higher scores on the HoNOSCA are indicative of more unhealthy child functioning.

- *Piers–Harris Children's Self-Concept Scale (P-H).* The P-H is an 80-item self-report measure completed by children (with the assistance of a researcher, if necessary), designed to measure children's self-concept across six domains: behavior, intellectual and school status, physical appearance and attributes, anxiety, popularity, and happiness and satisfaction. In addition, the P-H includes a response bias and consistency index that can be used to filter invalid responses. Higher scores on the P-H indicate higher self-esteem than low scores.

- *Parenting Scale (PS).* The PS is a 30-item self-report measure completed by parents, designed to facilitate the early detection of dysfunctional discipline and assist in the prevention and early treatment of behavior problems. The PS has three subscales: laxness, overreactivity, and verbosity. Lower scores indicate more functional parenting practices.

- *Parenting Sense of Competence Scale (PSOC).* The PSOC is a 16-item self-report measure designed to assess parenting self-esteem. The scale reflects the degree to which the parent feels comfortable with various aspects of his or her role as a parent. It includes two subscales: satisfaction and efficacy. Higher scores indicate greater parenting efficacy and satisfaction.

- *Center for Epidemiological Studies Depression Scale (CES-D).* The CES-D is a 20-item self-report measure designed to assess depressive symptomatology in adults. The measure has no subscales; lower scores indicate fewer depressive symptoms. The CES-D is not a clinical tool and therefore is used only as an indicator of depressive symptomatology.

- *McMaster Family Assessment Device (FAD).* The FAD is a 60-item self-report instrument that assesses family functioning on several dimensions and distinguishes between healthy and unhealthy families. The FAD has six subscales: problem solving, communication, roles, affective responsiveness, affective involvement, and behavior control, plus one global functioning scale. Lower scores indicate "healthier" family functioning.

times to follow up on a particular issue, clarify concepts or check the reliability of data); and use triangulation to increase the credibility of their findings (i.e., evaluators utilize multiple data-collection methods to check the authenticity of their results). In addition their findings are usually not generalizable to any specific population, but rather use of each qualitative method produces a single piece of evidence that can provide in-depth information in response to a particular evaluation question.

Qualitative information collection usually requires more time to obtain feedback from a range of respon-dents than does typical quantitative data-collection procedures such as surveys. For example, the evaluator needs to record the information obtained thoroughly, accurately, and systematically, using field notes, sketches, audiotapes, photographs, and other suitable means. As in the collection of quantitative information, qualitative information collection must meet the standards of utility, feasibility, propriety, and accuracy, which, for qualitative information collection, can be especially challenging in relationship to such standards as human rights and respect, transparency and disclosure, cost-effectiveness, and reliability. Common qualitative information collection procedures include open-ended questionnaires, individual and group interviews, observation methods, and document reviews. The method that employs some or all of these types of methods is the in-depth case study, which may be a study of an active program or a historical analysis of a past program.

A case study involves an up-close, in-depth, and detailed examination of a subject (the case), as well as its related contextual conditions. The "case" being studied may be an individual, organization, event, or action, existing in a specific time and place. Thomas (2011) defines case study this way: "Case studies are analyses of persons, events, decisions, periods, projects, policies, institutions, or other systems that are studied holistically by one or more methods. The case that is the subject of the inquiry will be an instance of a class of phenomena that provides an analytical frame—an object—within which the study is conducted and which the case illuminates and explicates" (p. 513).

Case study research can mean single and multiple case studies, can include quantitative evidence, relies on multiple sources of evidence, and benefits from the prior development of theoretical propositions (Yin, 2014). As such, case study research should not be confused with qualitative research, for case studies can be based on any mix of quantitative and qualitative information.

Multiple Information Sources, Evaluators, and Methods

When contemplating the collection of information for an evaluation, the evaluator should remember that sound information collection typically requires the use of multiple methods. Evaluators should consider collecting a wide range of information about the program—from multiple sources, through the engagement of multiple evaluators, and by applying multiple procedures. Such a multifaceted investigative approach is necessary for triangulating both quantitative and qualitative findings to form a full understanding of a program and to increase the credibility, trustworthiness, and utility of conclusions. In general, for each evaluation question, multiple types of information should work together to reach as much consensus as is warranted. Clearly, conclusions based on multiple pieces of information, gathered from different sources, and collected by multiple evaluators can enhance an evaluation's trustworthiness.

When a research scale is needed for information collection, if possible, the evaluator is advised to use an existing research scale with reported, known psychometric properties. This suggestion mainly reflects the reality that program evaluations rarely afford the evaluator the time and resources required to develop and validate new evaluation instruments. That is because the instrument development and **validation** process is usually long, tedious, and costly. However, the evaluator also should not use instruments just because they are readily available. Making the wrong move to use easily available instruments that lack validity to address an evaluation's questions is tantamount to dooming the evaluation to failure. Such unprofessional evaluation behavior will open the door to inappropriate uses of the evaluation's findings and ultimately discredit the evaluator.

In general, evaluators should keep the process and product evaluation purposes in mind, and determine the appropriate time line for each information collection task. They should also make clear the information source(s) from which the information should be collected, and assign responsibilities for each information collection instance so that they can be carried out on time and accurately.

Professional Standards for Information Collection

Although evaluation is a relatively young discipline, this field has established a set of clear standards, an extensive literature base, and strong procedures for collecting evaluation information. The Joint Committee on Standards for Educational Evaluation (2011) stipulates that evaluation information collection should meet the following standards:

- Relevant Information
- Human Rights and Respect
- Explicit Program and Context Descriptions
- Reliable Information
- Valid Information
- Information Management

Evaluators need to gain a solid understanding of the professional standards for collecting sound evaluation information and follow them carefully and systemati-

BOX 9.3. Information Collection Methods Used in the IGERT Project

The evaluator in the QSE[3] IGERT project example employed multiple quantitative and qualitative data collection methods to collect a full range of information from a variety of sources at the appropriate time points to provide rich and thorough information for the evaluation:

- Conducted content analysis of publications describing other IGERT projects prior to the project.
- Administered the California Critical Thinking Skills Test (CCTST) to detect growth in the IGERT fellows' critical thinking skills before the project implementation, at the end of each year during the project implementation, and after the project implementation.
- Administered the Interpersonal Reactivity Index to detect growth in the IGERT fellows' interpersonal reactivity before the project implementation, at the end of each year during the project implementation, and after the project implementation.
- Administered the Problem Solving Inventory to detect growth in the IGERT fellows' problem solving before the project implementation, at the end of each year during the project implementation, and after the project implementation.
- Administered the Self-Efficacy Scale to detect growth in the IGERT fellows' self-efficacy before the project implementation, at the end of each year during the project implementation, and after the project implementation.
- Interviewed IGERT faculty council members prior to the project and annually during the project implementation to obtain their feedback on the QSE[3] project and impacts on IGERT-participating faculty and IGERT fellows.
- Conducted focus group interview of IGERT fellows annually during the project implementation to obtain their feedback on the QSE[3] project activities and impacts on the IGERT fellows.
- Applied a survey annually during the project implementation to obtain IGERT fellows' opinion regarding the QSE[3] project and its effectiveness.
- Observed weekly colloquia throughout the project implementation process to evaluate project implementation and effectiveness.
- Observed annual symposia throughout the project implementation process to evaluate project implementation and effectiveness.
- Conducted content analysis of IGERT fellows' work for course assignment throughout the project implementation process and at the end.
- Conducted content analysis of IGERT fellows' conference presentations and research publications throughout the project implementation process and at the end.

cally to meet these standards. In Table 9.2, we list the important standards related to information collection, quote the associated statements in the Joint Committee's standards (1994, 2011), and provide suggestions on how to meet these standards. In the following sections, we discuss these standards and recommendations. For more details, readers are advised to read the full text of each standard in the Standards (1994, 2011). Note that six of the seven standards included in Table 9.2 are found in the 2011 edition of the Joint Committee Standards and that one (Defensible Information Sources) appears in the 1994 edition. We included Defensible Information Sources in the table because, in our judg-

ment, it is more instructive to evaluators than what the 2011 edition contains on that topic.

Meeting the Relevant Information Standard

This Joint Committee standard states, "Evaluation should serve the identified and emergent needs of stakeholders" (2011, p. 45). To optimize evaluation utility, information must be relevant. To ensure that information is relevant, evaluators need to collect information that is connected to the purposes of the evaluation and the needs of the stakeholders, of high value, from trustworthy information sources, and enough for evaluation credibility.

TABLE 9.2. Professional Standards on Information Collection and How to Meet Them

Information Collection Standards	How to Meet the Standards
Relevant Information standard: "Evaluation information should serve the identified and emergent needs of intended users" (Joint Committee, 2011, p. 45).	— Communicate with stakeholders to understand their information needs and views concerning what constitutes relevant, credible, acceptable information. — Collect information that is connected to the purposes of the evaluation and address the needs of the stakeholders. — Collect information from trustworthy sources. — Collect information that is valuable and important. — Ensure adequate scope for assessing the evaluand's value. — Ensure that the information will address the evaluation's key questions. — Allocate time, resources, and personnel to information collection. — Allow flexibility for revising the information collection plan when needed.
Human Rights and Respect standard: "Evaluation should be designed and conducted to protect human and legal rights and maintain the dignity of participants and other stakeholders" (Joint Committee, 2011, p. 125).	— Understand stakeholders' cultural and social backgrounds, local traditions, and institutional protocols. — Adhere to federal, state, local, and tribal regulations and requirements. — Inform the client and stakeholders of the evaluation's provisions for adhering to ethical principles and codes of professional conduct. — Establish rules and procedures to ensure that the evaluation team members develop and maintain rapport with stakeholders and protect their rights. — Inform stakeholders of their rights to participate, withdraw from the study, or challenge decisions during the evaluation process. — Ensure that the interactions and communications between evaluation team members and the stakeholders are functional and respectful.
Explicit Program and Context Descriptions standard: "Evaluations should document programs and their contexts with appropriate detail and scope for the evaluation purposes" (Joint Committee, 2011, p. 185).	— Describe all important aspects of the program and how they evolve over time (e.g., design, recipients, staff, resources, procedures, activities). — Identify model/theory used to structure or carry out the program. — Describe how people experienced and perceived the program. — Describe contextual factors that appeared to greatly influence the program. — Identify other programs/projects or factors in the context that may have affected the evaluated program. — Report how the program's context compares to other contexts in which the program might be adopted.
Defensible Information Sources standard: "The sources of information used in a program evaluation should be described in enough detail, so that the adequacy of the information can be assessed" (Joint Committee, 1994, p. 141).	— Obtain information from multiple, defensible sources. — Use pertinent, previously collected information once validated. — Consider employing both qualitative and quantitative collection methods. — If feasible, obtain information from the population instead of samples. — Employ sampling procedures that enhance representativeness. — Document and report sampling designs and procedures. — Document and report any potential biasing features in the information. — Include sampling procedures and data collection instruments in the evaluation report's technical appendix or in a separate technical report.

(continued)

TABLE 9.2. *(continued)*

Information Collection Standards	How to Meet the Standards
Valid Information standard: "Evaluation information should serve the intended purposes and support valid interpretations" (Joint Committee, 2011, p. 171).	— Carefully plan, monitor, and document the information collection process. — Follow a sound instrument development procedure to create an instrument that will yield high validity. — Select existing instruments that have evidenced high validity, and validate them again in the current evaluation use. — Employ multiple information collection methods to provide cross-checks and balance on possible weak measures. — Ensure that the combination of data-collection methods collectively and effectively addresses all of the study's questions. — Report validity claims and evidence for each data-collection procedure in the evaluation report's methods section or technical appendix.
Reliable Information standard: "Evaluation procedures should yield sufficiently dependable and consistent information for the intended uses" (Joint Committee, 2011, p. 179).	— Secure the expertise needed to investigate information reliability. — Determine, justify, and report the type(s) of reliability of choice and the acceptable levels of reliability. — Select instruments with acceptable reliability for answering questions similar to those in the target evaluation. — Assess and report reliability of the chosen extant instruments when used in the target evaluation. — When constructing new instruments, carefully develop and follow a blueprint. Engage stakeholders to review draft instruments for feedback. Pilot-test and refine new instruments to achieve acceptable reliability. — If possible, engage multiple data collectors and examine their findings for consistency. — Train data collectors and those who code, score, and analyze information to improve consistency of scoring and findings. — Examine and report consistency of scoring and coding among different scorers or coders. — Document procedure used to ensure reliability in the method section of an evaluation report or in a separate technical report.
Information Management standard: The standard specifies that "evaluations should employ systematic information collection, review, verification, and storage methods" (Joint Committee, 2011, p. 193).	— Use information sources and information collection procedures that will enhance the information's usefulness, accuracy, and trustworthiness. — Establish and implement information collection protocols to ensure that the collection of information is systematic and error-free. — Establish and implement quality control protocols to ensure the quality of the collection, processing, validation, storage, retrieval, and preparation of evaluation information. — Carefully document and securely retain the original, processed, and analyzed information. — Competently prepare information for analyses.

The *relevant information standard* stresses two main requirements on information: scope and selectivity. The scope requirement emphasizes that evaluations should collect information that has sufficient breadth to address an evaluation audience's important information needs and provide sufficient basis to support a judgment of the evaluand's merit and worth. Evaluators should collect information on all the important variables about the evaluand, among which are:

* Participant needs
* Program goals and assumptions
* Program design
* Program implementation
* Program costs
* Program outcomes
* Program's positive and negative side effects

To serve evaluation's purpose of assessing merit and worth, evaluators should collect information that will collectively answer all the essential evaluation questions, regardless of whether the client and stakeholders specifically requested the information. The Joint Committee (1994) version of the standard also states: "Evaluators should determine what the client considers significant but should also suggest significant areas the client may have overlooked, including areas identified by other stakeholders" (p. 37).

The selectivity requirement advises evaluators to be selective in deciding what information to collect. Sometimes it's infeasible or unwise to satisfy all the information interests of all stakeholders, and the evaluators will need to collect less information than the client requests. Evaluators should identify the potential body of relevant information, including what is requested by the client and stakeholders and what is needed to render a judgment of an evaluand's merit and worth. The evaluators should subsequently work with the client and stakeholders to distinguish the most important pieces of information from those that are unnecessary or of minor importance. Ultimately, the evaluators should decide on a list of information to be collected, in consideration of necessity, importance, and practicality. Here we see an example of the trade-off decisions that an evaluator often has to make when a conflict arises between, for example, meeting the requirement of information scope and that of such feasibility concerns as cost.

Shams, Golshiri, Zamani, and Pourabdian (2008) reported a CIPP evaluation of mothers' participation in improving the growth and nutrition of their children. They used a wide range of relevant information in the five stages of the evaluation work. In the first stage (contractual agreements), all stakeholders and beneficiaries were identified, including mothers and their children, their neighbors, relatives and acquaintances, local health workers, related experts in the District Health Center, and some professors in the Medical and Health Faculty. The goals and objectives of the project were clarified. Also, after receiving the stakeholder's viewpoints about the processes of planning and implementing the project evaluation, the details of the plan were clarified.

In the second stage (context evaluation), background information was collected with the help of the stakeholders: the percentage of children under care of the local health center and those under special care, together with information concerning resources, possibilities, problems, district needs, and the like.

In the third stage (input evaluation), a wide range of project inputs were identified; some of them were as follows: international experiences and models that have been used for increasing the levels of community participation; the program's proposed strategy to assess needs and feasibility; sufficiency of the program's budget to fund the needed work; sufficient, feasible, and political support for the program's work plan; and instructions for training some of the stakeholders to carry out the plan.

In the fourth stage (processes evaluation), the beneficiaries were gathered in a seminar and were given explanations for the generalities, goals, and potential positive effects of the project. At the end of the seminar, volunteers came forward and formed a project **steering committee**, which included local health workers, program leaders, and the previously mentioned volunteers. The committee made decisions concerning how to implement the plan and address potential problems. The model's educational contents consisted of the three subjects of growth monitoring, complementary nutrition, and stages of a child's nutritional development (homeostasis, attachment, separation, and individuation). Pursuant to the process evaluation feedback, the project team produced essential program materials, including the instructional plan and suitable pamphlets. The ensuing 10 months of intervention included two educational sessions for mothers every week. The team of instructors comprised three persons (one pediatrician and two specialists in community medicine). Before and after the instruction, the participating mothers' knowledge and practice were assessed through a three-part, 45-item questionnaire keyed to the mothers' instructional program. The instrument's content validity was assessed via reviews by experts and examination in consideration of relevant literature. The questionnaire's reliability was determined to be 72.53 by applying a **test–retest** method, then calculating the Cronbach alpha statistic.

In the fifth stage (product evaluation), the project was assessed for its impacts, effectiveness, sustainability, and transportability. Identified outcomes included:

- Effects on persons associated with the targeted beneficiaries, including spouses of beneficiaries, relatives, acquaintances, and their neighbors.
- Effects on the self-confidence of participating beneficiaries as evidenced in a standard Kopper–Smith questionnaire before and after intervention.
- Effects on meeting important community needs, especially the needs to improve children's growth and nutrition.
- Long-term sustainability effects of the project, such as continuation of the activities via a nongovernmental organization.
- Transportability effects of the project (in other regions and for development of other health services).

The data collected from the project questionnaire were analyzed using the SPSS software program and suitable statistical tests, including Wilcoxon, paired t-test, and McNamar (Shams et al., 2008, p. 26).

Meeting the Human Rights and Respect Standard

This standard states, "Evaluations should be designed and conducted to protect human and legal rights and maintain the dignity of participants and other stakeholders" (Joint Committee, 2011, p. 125). Many program evaluations require the evaluator to gather information from people associated with the program or other evaluands. Without due process and care, it's very easy for evaluators to inadvertently violate these people's rights or harm them in some way. These violations can have serious consequences: harm the affected persons, evoke legal prosecution, bring about profes-

sional sanctions, stir up dissension, discredit the evaluation, and so on. Evaluators should systematically and meticulously identify and make provisions for adhering to all applicable rights of those involved in or affected by the evaluation. Some rights are based in law, and others derive from ethics and common courtesy. Evaluators should honor the rights of evaluation participants not only to decide on how much and for how long they would be involved in information collection, but also to decline to participate. Additionally, evaluators must respect the cultural and societal values of all evaluation participants (Morris, 2003).

Evaluators should strictly follow the Human Rights and Respect standard (Joint Committee, 2011). An added layer of safeguard is to have an appropriate human subjects Institutional Review Board (IRB) examine the evaluation design and associated information collection tools. In fact, it is almost always mandatory for evaluators to go through the IRB process before they start the information collection process. Irrespective of such a requirement, evaluators should share with human subjects the procedure they and the clients will follow in the information collection process and how the information will be used. Evaluators should not access individual-level records without securing written permission from duly authorized parties. When evaluators want to tape-record or video-record interviews or other activities, they should obtain prior permission from the respondents, participants, and client. When confidentiality or **anonymity** is infeasible, the evaluators should be up-front with the human subjects about this limitation rather than making or inferring unrealistic promises. When minors are involved in program evaluation, as often occurs with school-based educational studies, both parental consent and the minors' agreement are needed before the evaluators can proceed to data collection.

Meeting the Explicit Program and Context Descriptions Standard

This standard states, "Evaluations should document programs and their contexts with appropriate detail and scope for the evaluation purposes" (Joint Committee, 2011, p. 185). To ensure the usefulness of an evaluation, the *explicit program description* standard obligates evaluators to make it clear to the audience what was evaluated. Sufficient details are needed to describe how the program was designed and how it was actually implemented, for these can differ greatly.

Further, many readers need details beyond a general characterization of the program. For example, readers interested in replicating the program need all of the particulars concerning such matters as administration, staffing, procedures, facilities, equipment, and costs, for such purposes as contrasting the program with alternative approaches and replicating the program with great fidelity. In failed programs, in order to diagnose the causes for failure, funders and administrators need specific information regarding any deviations between actual operations and plans. Researchers who want to understand a program's effects also need detailed information about the program's actual operations so that they can link specific parts of the program to the observed outcomes.

To fully describe the planned version and the implemented version of the program, the evaluator typically needs to collect information on:

- How the program was structured, governed, staffed, financed, and carried out
- Where the program was conducted
- What facilities were used
- What orientation and training the participants received
- How the relevant community was involved
- How program funds were budgeted and spent

Explicit context description helps readers identify possible influencers of the program. A program's context can heavily influence how the program is designed and operated and what it achieves. It has been established, for example, that Georgia's Vidalia onions and peaches can taste differently when planted in growing environments other than Georgia. Analogously, because of their respective environmental circumstances, programs with the same design can differ considerably in implementation and outcome. Proactive context evaluations can help the evaluator's client group understand local circumstances, identify and address problems and needs, and develop goals. Similarly, evaluation audiences need retrospective context evaluations to help them understand why a program succeeded or failed. Audiences considering replicating a successful program need to know what influential contextual dynamics would have to be present in the new setting. Audiences may consider replicating an unsuccessful program in a very different setting if the program's failure

was decidedly due to its particular and idiosyncratic environment.

Clearly, evaluators need to collect considerable contextual information to help readers understand how a program acquired certain characteristics and why it succeeded or failed. Important contextual variables might include:

- Program's geographical location
- Relevant political and social milieu
- Economics of the community
- Pertinent needs and issues in the area
- Pertinent legislation
- Availability of special funds for work in the program area
- Highly influential persons
- Highly influential environmental events
- Program's rationale
- Program's means
- Program's organizational home
- Program's timing
- Program's potential contributions to the locale
- Program participants and their program-related needs
- Competing programs in the area
- Pertinent state and national influences

Evaluators should draw information from multiple sources to fully describe a program's context. Examples of environmental circumstances include media records, newspaper accounts, area demographic statistics, area economics data, and pertinent legislation. Evaluators should also keep a log of unusual circumstances, both positive and negative, that might have an impact on the program. The evaluator should use existing sources of information about the program, which might include program descriptions, funding proposals, minutes of board and staff meetings, expense reports, progress reports, and final reports. The evaluator might collect additional information from photographic records, interviews, focus groups, and observations. It is wise to obtain holistic descriptions, detailed descriptions of individual program components, and, as applicable, time-specific descriptions for use in documenting and contrasting program changes and trends.

Meeting the Defensible Information Sources Standard

This standard states, "The sources of information used in a program evaluation should be described in enough detail, so that the adequacy of the information can be assessed" (Joint Committee, 1994, p. 141). Accessing defensible sources of information and utilizing sound **sampling** methods are critical in the process of producing sound evaluation reports. To render a full judgment of the program, evaluators should collect information from multiple sources using a variety of appropriate techniques. Information sources may include program participants and beneficiaries, program staff, administrators and policy board members, program informants, advisory board members, newspaper and public records, program proposals and reports, program records, and persons who might be affected by the program's spillover effects.

If appropriate, evaluators should employ both qualitative and quantitative information collection techniques and take advantage of the strengths of each, to best tap the information sources. Involved persons may be surveyed, interviewed, tested, asked to complete rating scales, and engaged in focus groups or hearings. Documents may be reviewed and coded for content analysis. Program activities can be observed, photographed, and recorded. Rich information obtained from multiple sources using a variety of techniques helps overcome limitations of individual sources and methods, and enables evaluators to cross-check the findings and render more trustworthy answers to each major evaluation question.

In large evaluation studies, it is often infeasible for evaluators to collect all relevant information from each information source. For instance, an evaluator cannot observe, test, and interview every participant every day. In reality, evaluators often collect information only from a sample of each data source. For example, they typically choose to collect information from selected participants (e.g., 50 out of 1,000) during selected time periods, or they only examine a sample of records and documents out of all records and documents. Such selectivity is called sampling, which is the process of selecting a number of individuals from a population, preferably in a way that the individuals are representative of the larger group from which they were selected.

Sampling may eventuate in both biased and missing information. If the information obtained from the sample is not representative of information that might have been obtained from all members of the population, the evaluator's inferences to characteristics of that population will be erroneous and misleading. The Joint Committee (1994) advised evaluators to "document, justify, and report their sources of information, the criteria and methods used to collect them, the means used to obtain information from them, and any unique and biasing features of the obtained information" (p. 141). The Committee pointed out that "poor documentation and description of information sources can reduce an evaluation's credibility" (p. 142). Thus, evaluators need to create safeguards to improve information sufficiency, representativeness, and transparency in their findings. We advise evaluators to document information sources, information selection processes, and instruments used to collect the information in an evaluation's technical appendix or separate technical report.

Evaluators can draw samples from a defined population using a sampling technique that may be selected from methods of probability sampling or nonprobability sampling. The difference between nonprobability and probability sampling is that **nonprobability sampling** does not involve random selection and probability sampling does. The purpose of probability sampling is to make inferences about a population from information obtained from a sample selected from that population. Such inferences are usually in the form of an estimate of a population parameter (e.g., mean, standard deviation) with a bound on the error of estimation. Each observation from a population provides a certain amount of information about the population parameter.

Random Sampling

Random sampling, unlike nonrandom sampling, ensures that every member of the population has an equal chance of being selected. Nonrandom sampling cannot ensure the sample's representativeness whereas random sampling strongly enhances the probability that the sample is representative of the population. Generally, evaluators should try to obtain a sample that is representative of the population, which means they should use random sampling if possible.

Within the evaluation field, however, important caveats are in order regarding sampling. It is often very important to give all interested stakeholders an opportunity to provide their inputs regarding the program's functioning and accomplishments. Such participation can greatly motivate the involved stakeholders to respect and utilize the evaluation's findings. Also, quite often in evaluation studies, it is not feasible to collect random samples, and even if one could, the available inference is limited to the time at which the sample was drawn. In the dynamic enterprise of program evaluation, the nature and composition of the served population may change significantly over time. As with information collection, where the collection of multiple measures is required, use of multiple modes of sampling and sampling times is often to be recommended; this practice provides opportunities to contrast the information obtained by application of the different sampling procedures and, as applicable, to the different times when the samples were drawn.

The three most common ways of obtaining random samples are simple random sampling, stratified random sampling, and cluster random sampling.

Simple random sampling is a sampling process in which every member of the population has an equal and independent chance of being selected. An everyday example is randomly drawing names from a hat. A formal way of drawing a random sample can be done by using what is known as a table of random numbers (Fraenkel, Wallen, & Hyun, 2015). Such a list can be found in the back of most statistics books. The advantage of simple random sampling is that, if large enough, it is very likely to produce a representative sample. Although there is no guarantee of complete representativeness, the likelihood of it is greater with large random samples than with any other method. Any differences between the sample and the population should be small and nonsystematic; that is, they are the result of random chance rather than systematic bias.

However, when evaluators want to ensure that certain subgroups are present in the sample in the same proportion as they are in the population, evaluators should utilize **stratified random sampling**. A stratified random sample is obtained by separating the population into discrete, nonoverlapping groups called strata (e.g., males and females) and then selecting a simple random sample from each stratum. The advantage of stratified random sampling is that it increases the likelihood that the members in each stratum will be proportionally represented in the overall sample. Aggregating sampled results from all subgroups, which may or may not be of interest in the particular evaluation, ensures that the units in each stratum will fairly represent their population proportionality in the summary statistics reported for the total sample.

Frequently, evaluators cannot select a random sample of individuals because of administrative or other restrictions. This is especially true in schools, where evaluators often have to obtain measures from all students in the classrooms involved rather than sampling only some students in individual classrooms. In **cluster random sampling**, the evaluator divides the population of interest into clusters (or identifies clusters that already exist, such as school classrooms) and then randomly selects a sample of clusters of the desired size. Just as simple random sampling is especially applicable and useful to the evaluator when findings must be generalized to a population containing many individuals, cluster random sampling is similarly applicable and useful when the evaluator must generalize to a population with very many clusters. Cluster random sampling has a number of advantages: it can be used when it is difficult or impossible to select a random sample of individuals; sometimes it is the only feasible way to collect the needed information from the population (e.g., students in schools); and it consumes less time and complications of data collection than is involved in sampling and obtaining measures from individuals. The serious downside of cluster random sampling is it poses a much bigger probability of obtaining a sample that is not representative of the population than simple random sampling.

Nonrandom Sampling

Three types of nonrandom sampling methods often used in evaluation studies are *systematic, convenience,* and *purposive.*

A **systematic sample** is obtained by selecting every *n*th name in a population until a predetermined sample size is obtained. This approach may be an acceptable, though less precise, alternative to drawing a random sample. When this method is employed, the evaluator needs to justify in the evaluation report or backup technical documentation why the sample was drawn systematically rather than randomly. Moreover, the evaluator should carefully examine the population list to decide whether a cyclical pattern exists. If it does, steps should be taken to achieve representativeness by randomly selecting individuals from each of the cyclical segments.

A **convenience sample** is any group of individuals who are conveniently available to be studied. Such a sample may include persons who strongly desire to have their inputs considered in the evaluation. A convenience sample almost certainly is not representative of the population of interest, but when coupled with a demonstrably representative sample, it can add an important dimension to the evaluation. It can increase the evaluation's depth of information, for example, by obtaining and reporting testimony from interested parties that helps illuminate the information obtained from the random sample. Input from persons in the convenience sample may raise new, important evaluation questions for study. Also, engaging stakeholders through convenience sampling can lead them to pay attention to and act on the evaluation's findings. This benefit shows that convenience sampling is a powerful means of helping secure utilization of evaluation findings. Nevertheless, evaluators should not employ a convenience sample solely to reach conclusions about population parameters.

A **purposive sample** is a sample selected because the evaluator needs to develop findings pertaining to a certain subgroup of individuals. Examples could be a school district's top three administrators, the most recent dropouts from families in a self-help housing project, those secretaries who, over the past 5 years, won their organization's outstanding secretary award, or a basketball team's seniors. In all of these cases, the evaluator purposely selects and studies a certain subgroup from a population to address a particular evaluation question pertaining directly to the sampled individuals. In cases of purposive sampling, the evaluator is looking not to infer to a larger population but to present findings about some aspects of interest that apply only to the particular subgroup. Such uses of purposive sampling are akin to collecting information from all members of a population, when there is no need or issue regarding inference or generalization.

Estimating and Addressing Error in Random Samples

Drawing conclusions about a population after studying results from a random sample will not be completely satisfactory for one important reason: the sample will entail an element of sampling error. If the random sample is of sufficient size, however, the error is likely to be sufficiently small to warrant confidence in the resulting inference. Regardless of the sample's size, the evaluator should calculate and report the amount of likely error. On the matter of sufficient sample size, a rule-of-thumb answer is that a sample should be as large as the evaluator can obtain with a reasonable expenditure of time and energy. In general, evaluators should obtain as large a sample as they reasonably can.

Some conventional guidelines have been established with regard to the minimum number of subjects needed (Fraenkel, Wallen, & Hyun, 2015). For descriptive statistics, a sample with a minimum of 100 is essential. For correlational studies, a sample of at least 50 is deemed necessary to establish the existence of a relationship. Finally, for experimental and causal–comparative studies, a minimum of 30 individuals per group is required, although sometimes experimental studies with only 15 individuals in each group can be defendable if they are tightly controlled; studies with only 15 subjects per group probably should be replicated before too much is made of any findings. In qualitative studies, the number of participants in a sample is usually between 1 and 20.

Nonresponse is one of the most pervasive problems affecting a sample's representativeness. **Nonresponse error** occurs when the characteristics of actual participants differ from those of sampled members who failed to participate as requested. Dillman, Smyth, and Christian's social exchange theory approach (2009) provides valuable guidance for addressing and reducing nonresponse problems.

Alternatives to Sampling

Not all evaluations have to employ sampling of respondents. In some, often smaller evaluation studies, the evaluator can collect information from all of a program's participants and each staff member (i.e., taking a census instead of selecting a sample). When information is gathered from all members of a population, the results can be reported directly. In such cases, there is no need to make inferences about the population based on a sample because evaluators have drawn information from the entire population. Doing so considerably simplifies the evaluators' tasks of analyzing and reporting findings. In planning data-collection activities, it is often appropriate to consider the feasibility and desirability of taking measures from all members of a population of interest. If so, the evaluator should take population measures, thereby relieving themselves from sampling and making inferences. Otherwise, the evaluator should select and apply appropriate sampling procedures.

Evaluators should report the information source selection experience forthrightly regardless of whether they employ sampling or a population census approach. They should describe the sources of information, document the techniques and processes by which information was collected from each source, and document any changes and noteworthy experiences that took place in the process. For information that was collected according to a prespecified plan, evaluators should report the original plan, any deviations from the plan, and reasons for the deviations to aid interpretation of evaluation findings. Finally, we reemphasize that evaluators should document and report both strengths and deficiencies in their information sources and, as appropriate, caution the audience not to place undue confidence in the obtained information.

Meeting the Valid Information Standard

The valid information standard states, "Evaluation Information should serve the intended purposes and support valid interpretations" (Joint Committee, 2011, p. 171). A commonly used definition of a valid instrument is that it measures what it is supposed to measure. A more theoretically sound definition of validity revolves around the defensibility of the inferences made from the information collected through the use of an instrument. Evaluators use information gathered with instruments to make inferences about the subject program's outcomes and other characteristics. For the evaluation to be accurate, these inferences must be correct . Therefore, evaluators need instruments that yield data that are fully defensible for reaching valid conclusions about the assessed program.

Validity is the most important property to consider when creating or selecting an instrument for information collection because the instrument must measure what it is intended to measure. Drawing correct conclusions based on data obtained from the administration of a particular instrument is what validity is all about. If the instrument does not accurately measure the intended variable, then the obtained results may lead to invalid inferences. In recent years, validity has been defined as referring to the *appropriateness, correctness, meaningfulness,* and *usefulness* of the specific *inferences* researchers (or evaluators) make based on the data they collect (Fraenkel, Wallen, & Hyun, 2015).

Validity is not an all-or-none proposition; it is rather one of degree. Validity refers to the degree to which evidence supports any inferences one makes based on the data he or she collects using a particular instrument. It is the inference derived from applying the instrument that is validated, not the instrument itself. Such infer-

ences should be appropriate, meaningful, correct, and relevant to the evaluation questions of interest.

Five classes of validity are applicable in evaluations: internal validity, external validity, construct validity, statistical conclusion validity, and content validity. Their applicability can vary depending on the nature and needs of different evaluations. For example, content validity is highly applicable to evaluations of standardized subject matter achievement tests but not so much to typical project evaluations.

Internal validity and external validity are largely functions of an evaluation study's design. **Internal validity** refers to the truthfulness or correctness of inferences about whether the relationship between two or more variables is causal. Inferences are said to possess internal validity if a causal relationship between two variables is accurately demonstrated. A causal inference may be based on a calculated relationship when three criteria are satisfied: the "cause" precedes the "effect" in time (temporal precedence); the "cause" and the "effect" are related (covariation); and there are no plausible alternative explanations for the observed covariation (nonspuriousness). Internal validity is especially applicable in validating the results of randomized, controlled experimental studies.

External validity, also known as generalizability, refers to the extent to which a study's results can be generalized (applied) beyond the study's environment or possibly some different time period. External validity is mainly a function of the extent to which the study's environment and special circumstances are representative of other settings of interest. Usually, the best an evaluator can do in this regard is to fully describe the evaluation's environment and its characteristics of design and operation—such as governance, beneficiaries, staffing, funding, and facilities—so that interested parties can consider how much the circumstances of the evaluated program match those of their situation.

Construct validity is mainly a function of a measurement's theoretical underpinnings. It refers to the degree to which an instrument measures an intended hypothetical psychological construct or nonobservable trait. How well does a measure of a construct (e.g., mathematical reasoning) explain differences in the behavior of an individual or an individual's performance on tasks believed to be related to the construct (e.g., math achievement scores)? More straightforwardly, for example, does the mathematical reasoning instrument truly measure mathematical reasoning? With a self-designed instrument, an evaluator must perform a series of studies to gather a variety of evidence to demonstrate that the scores from the instrument can be used to draw conclusions about the variable measured by the instrument. An example of a piece of evidence is the following: Students who received high scores on the mathematical reasoning instrument also made high scores on mathematical tests that required mathematical reasoning. When possible, evaluators are advised to use existing instruments with well-documented construct validity evidence.

Statistical conclusion validity is largely a function of analysis. It concerns the correctness of inferences regarding the covariation between two or more variables. In program evaluation, this especially concerns the validity of statistical inferences about the cause-and-effect relationship between the implementation of a program plan and the observed program outcomes, as well as the strength of the relationship between the two sets of observations. This type of validity is the bedrock construct in controlled, **variable manipulating,** randomized experiments.

Kline (2008) has provided an accessible introduction to the four concepts of validity discussed earlier in the chapter and how each can be addressed in a study. Although these four concepts are the main ones treated in the research and evaluation literature, we add a fifth one, which the field of standardized achievement testing labels content validity.

Content validity refers to the validation of conclusions that are drawn from scores by examinees on a test. A familiar example is the General Educational Development (GED) test battery. This battery of four subject matter tests—mathematical reasoning, science, social studies, and reasoning through language arts—is administered to adults who have not received a high school diploma but want to demonstrate their achievement of the equivalent of a high school education. The GED tests are aligned with current high school standards employed across the nation, as well as associated content in widely used textbooks and other instructional materials. The pass–fail decisions that GED authorities make from the examinees' test scores are based on cut scores they set on the test results based on their examination of GED test scores by a national sample of high school graduates. Such cut scores are arbitrary in that they are based on the judgments of experts. Validation of the GED tests involves studies to assess the contents of the four tests against the framework of current high

school standards and associated subject matter content taught in high schools throughout the United States, plus evaluation of the rationale and evidence underlying the cut scores.

Simpler instances of content validity apply to classroom achievement tests. Consider, for example, a sixth-grade classroom teacher who develops a test to examine his students' mastery of the geography lessons he taught during the first semester. To assure the test's content validity, the teacher should develop a test plan that is keyed to the semester's objectives and breakdown of geography topics taught. Often such a test plan is in the form of a matrix whose rows are learning objectives, whose columns are content topics, and whose cell entries are percentages of items to be included in the test. To assure the test's content validity, the teacher would next develop items to match the test plan's specifications. Ideally, the teacher would develop from two to four times the number of items needed for the test; pilot test and analyze difficulty levels and discriminative power of the pilot-tested items; select the best performing items for inclusion in the test in accordance with the test plan; thoughtfully set cut scores for use in grading test results; administer the test; and assess its reliability. Although such a comprehensive validation process is desirable, unfortunately the totality of such a process is not feasible in most teachers' classroom situations. Evaluations of the content validity of a classroom subject matter test, such as that described above, basically involves scrutinizing the teacher's test plan to obtain reasonable assurance that it matches what students were taught; examination of the conformance of the test's items to the test plan; examination of any pilot testing of the test's items; calculation of the test's reliability; and assessment of the teacher's rationale for assigning grades based on the test scores.

Clearly, validation is necessary to ensure the appropriateness and correctness of obtained information for answering an evaluation's questions. According to the Joint Committee (1994), "Validation is the process of compiling evidence that supports the interpretations and uses of the data and information collected using one or more . . . instruments and procedures" (p. 145). Figure 9.1 shows the series of tasks in a sound process to validate the interpretation and use of information collected using an instrument or a procedure.

It is incorrect to generally state that an instrument or procedure is valid or invalid. Rather, an evaluator should judge the extent to which the inferences or conclusions generated from particular use of an instrument or procedure are valid. The key determinant of validity is how fully and dependably the information answers the evaluation's questions. Evaluators should avoid the common mistake of assuming that their use of a particular instrument or procedure is justified because an investigator reported high validity in another study. Rather, they need to validate *their own* inferences or conclusions pursuant to their evaluation's particular questions and based on assessments of the study's procedures, instruments, and obtained information.

When choosing an existing instrument, the evaluator should pay attention to the validity information provided by the test publishers. Test publishers typically make it clear what an instrument is intended to measure and provide relevant evidence. Because of feasibil-

ity constraints, evaluators often have to adopt existing instruments or procedures whose uses in the particular study may not yield optimal validity. To overcome this potential weakness, we advise evaluators to employ multiple information collection methods to provide cross-checks and balance on possible weak measures, and to ensure that the combination of methods effectively addresses all of the study's questions. The evaluators should validate each set of inferences made based on the corresponding information collected separately and carefully, and then examine the collections of inferences and conclusions to ensure that they are coherent, consistent, sufficient, and defensible. They should also report any limitations in the evaluation information and accordingly provide appropriate warnings and guidance to the evaluation's intended users.

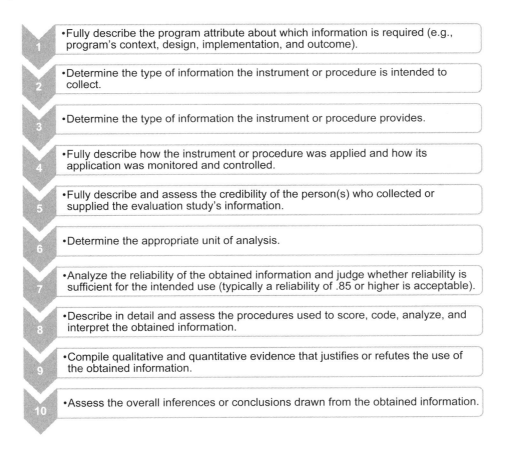

1. •Fully describe the program attribute about which information is required (e.g., program's context, design, implementation, and outcome).

2. •Determine the type of information the instrument or procedure is intended to collect.

3. •Determine the type of information the instrument or procedure provides.

4. •Fully describe how the instrument or procedure was applied and how its application was monitored and controlled.

5. •Fully describe and assess the credibility of the person(s) who collected or supplied the evaluation study's information.

6. •Determine the appropriate unit of analysis.

7. •Analyze the reliability of the obtained information and judge whether reliability is sufficient for the intended use (typically a reliability of .85 or higher is acceptable).

8. •Describe in detail and assess the procedures used to score, code, analyze, and interpret the obtained information.

9. •Compile qualitative and quantitative evidence that justifies or refutes the use of the obtained information.

10. •Assess the overall inferences or conclusions drawn from the obtained information.

FIGURE 9.1. Tasks in a sound process to validate the interpretation and use of information.

Meeting the Reliable Information Standard

This standard states, "Evaluation procedures should yield sufficiently dependable and consistent information for the intended uses" (Joint Committee, 2011, p. 179). In psychometrics, reliability is the consistency of the scores obtained—how consistent they are for each individual from one administration to another, from one scorer to another, and from one set of items to another. A measure is said to have a high reliability if it produces similar results under consistent conditions. Reliability is a necessary but not sufficient condition for validity (Crocker & Algina, 2008). As such, an evaluation conclusion cannot be defended as valid if it is based on unreliable information. Information can be unreliable to the extent that it contains unexplained contradictions and inconsistencies or if different results would be obtained under subsequent yet similar information collection conditions. In classical test theory, reliability is defined as the consistency or reproducibility of scores. Inconsistencies in scores may be attributed to two types of measurement errors: random measurement error and systematic measurement error.

Random measurement error affects an individual's score because of purely chance happenings. Random measurement error in a large group of observations is not of major concern because it can affect different individuals' score in both positive and negative directions, and thus be cancelled out in the long run. **Systematic measurement error** consistently affects an individual's scores because of some particular characteristics of the persons or test that are unrelated to the construct being measured. Systematic error tends to accrue across examinees and should be of great concern.

The goal of any measurement procedure is to identify a person's true score using his or her observed score, which is expressed as:

$$X = T + E$$

where X is the observed score, T is the true score, and E is the measurement error (Guilford, 1936). The equation shows that a person's observed score is equal to his or her true score plus measurement error. Stated in another way, measurement error is the discrepancy between a person's observed score and true score.

The degree of reliability is represented by a reliability coefficient. The reliability coefficient is a numerical index of reliability, typically ranging from 0 to 1.

A number closer to 1 indicates high reliability. A low-reliability coefficient indicates more error in the assessment results, a reliability coefficient of .00 indicates that all measurement variation is attributed to error, whereas a reliability coefficient of 1.00 indicates no measurement error. The closer a reliability coefficient is to 1.00, the more confident an evaluator can be that a measurement is an accurate representation of a person's true score. For example, if a reliability coefficient is .90, then about 90% of the variance in the observed score is due to variability in true scores, whereas about 10% is due to error. A commonly stated rule of thumb is that reliability may be considered good or acceptable if the reliability coefficient is .80 or above. However, in some situations a somewhat lower level is about all one can obtain and is acceptable for the type of decision to be made based on the study's results. This could be the case when the employed instrument is one of several instruments being utilized; when variation of measures obtained with the instrument is very small; and when the decision to be made based on the set of measures entails low risk. In other situations, that may involve life and death—such as the test of a manned rocket's readiness for launching—a reliability estimate of .80 clearly would be unacceptable. Hence, an evaluator must exercise careful judgment in determining an instrument's acceptable level of reliability.

Three ways to obtain a reliability coefficient are the test–retest method, the equivalent-forms method, and the internal-consistency method. The **test–retest method** involves administering the same test twice to the same group, with a certain time interval between the two administrations. A reliability coefficient is then calculated to indicate the relationship between the two sets of scores obtained. When the **equivalent-forms method** is used, two different but equivalent (also called alternate or parallel) forms of an instrument are administered to the same group of individuals during the same time period, followed by calculating a reliability coefficient between the two obtained sets of scores. There are several **internal consistency methods** for estimating reliability, all of which require only a single administration of an instrument. The split-half procedure involves scoring two halves (usually odd items vs. even items) of a test separately for each person and then calculating a correlation coefficient for the two sets of scores. The reliability coefficient is calculated using the Spearman–Brown prophecy formula. A simplified version of the formula is

Reliability of scores on total test =

$$\frac{(2 \times \text{reliability for } \frac{1}{2} \text{ test})}{(1 + \text{reliability for } \frac{1}{2} \text{ test})}$$

If an evaluator obtained a correlation coefficient of .70 for half of the test by comparing one half of the test items to the other half, then the reliability of scores for the total test would be:

$$\text{Reliability of scores on total test} = \frac{(2 \times .70)}{(1 + .70)} = .82$$

Evidently, the reliability of an instrument can be increased by the addition of more items, provided they are similar to the original ones. The other commonly used **internal consistency methods** are the Küder–Richardson approaches, including KR20 and KR21 and the coefficient alpha. Both can be obtained with most statistical software packages such as SPSS and SAS. More recently, Padilla and Zhang originated a new internal consistency measure, the Bayesian coefficient alpha, which enjoys all the advantages of the traditional coefficient alpha as well as the benefits of Bayesian methods (Padilla & Zhang, 2011). Evaluators can choose to ensure the reliability of their instruments with one or more of these types of reliability measures. Other developments in psychometric and measurement theory, such as the generalizability theory (Cronbach, Gleser, Nanda, & Rajaratnam, 1972) and item response theory (IRT), provide alternative ways of estimating reliability; interested readers are referred to Brennan (2001), de Ayala (2009), and Embretson and Reise (2000).

Many evaluations involve the use of raters to collect information about a program, such as when raters use a rubric to grade a teaching excerpt. Multiple raters may grade the same excerpt differently even if they use the same rubric. Thus, interrater reliability is needed to characterize the consistency or lack thereof among the scores given by different raters. Various models of interclass correlation coefficients can be used to assess the extent to which raters provide consistent estimates about what they observe, rate, code, or judge. Interested readers are referred to Davey, Gugiu, and Coryn (2010) for a comparison of **interrater reliability** coefficients and formulas for calculating them. Evaluators are advised to determine which forms of reliability are most appropriate to their evaluation study and make proper assessments. To ensure reliable information, evaluators should strive to reduce and document the amount of error variance and its impact on an evaluation's information and conclusions.

Meeting the Information Management Standard

This standard states, "Evaluators should employ systematic information collection, review, verification, and storage methods" (Joint Committee, 2011, p. 193). Many mistakes can occur in any of the information collection and handling activities, such as collecting, scoring, coding, recording, organizing, filing, releasing, analyzing, and reporting information. Evaluators should ensure that information is collected systematically, reviewed and verified regularly to eliminate errors, and stored properly for ease of use and confidentiality. Collected information should be subjected to reviews and verifications for accuracy. An evaluation's information should be regularly and closely checked so that it is free of errors. The evaluator might need to develop a database to house collected information for efficient and controlled access and use. There should be specific plans and assignments regarding who will collect the information, from whom, and when, where, and how they will collect it. Interviewers should conduct interviews following protocols, coders should code the information according to clear specifications, and those charged to manage the information should store and secure data and draft reports against unauthorized access. The lead evaluator should analyze the information in accordance with sound principles of analysis, making sure that reports are clear, free of mistakes, and delivered only to authorized recipients.

Caveats Regarding the Meeting of Standards

Often, evaluation assignments have practical constraints that make it difficult for evaluators to fully meet all of the standards associated with sound information collection. For example, frequently there are no preexisting instruments that are demonstrably valid for collecting the needed information. Consequently, evaluators often have to create their own instruments and do so in a limited time period, with constricted resources. Developing sound information collection instruments is technically demanding and time-consuming and often requires the expert work of a well-trained psychometrician. Also, evaluators rarely have sufficient time and resources to carry out a full sequence of developing, pilot-testing, reformulating, norming, and validating new instruments, a process that could require years of painstaking and costly work.

In the real world of time- and resource-constrained evaluation assignments, evaluators often have to make do with less than optimal information collection procedures. They may construct new instruments as systematically as they can or adaptively use existing available instruments that may have only marginal validity for the particular study. Rather than gathering new information, they may rely on existing information that they deem to be basically acceptable. One valuable piece of advice is that evaluators should employ multiple information sources and multiple information-gathering procedures and instruments and compare and contrast the different sets of results. Such contrasts of multiple information findings can confirm or raise questions about the consistency and validity of the obtained information. Moreover, the evaluators should forthrightly report inadequacies in the obtained information, as well as the related findings and conclusions. Basically, evaluators should do whatever is feasible to increase the sensibleness and defensibility of their findings, conclusions, and judgments (Bamberger, Rugh, & Mabry, 2012). Many practical guidelines for acting on this advice are found throughout the Joint Committee (1994, 2011) *Program Evaluation Standards,* especially those discussed in this section.

Common Information Collection Procedures

Together, the seven standards we have discussed provide guidance for ensuring that an evaluation's information will reliably, validly, and usefully answer the client group's questions and fully assess the subject program's merit and worth. Evaluators should study the full texts of the information collection standards that appear in the Joint Committee (1994, 2011) *Program Evaluation Standards* and regularly apply them in designing and carrying out their evaluations.

Also, we stress again that evaluators can greatly enhance their evaluations by employing multiple information sources and multiple data collection procedures. Such practices provide a wide scope of information and enable checks and balances across the different sets of information that are keyed to the same questions. Employing multiple information sources and procedures is especially important when it is not feasible to fully validate a single information collection procedure or instrument.

Table 9.3 displays commonly used data collection procedures and the areas of information needs each of these procedures often serves. The row headings list 20 information collection procedures commonly used by evaluators, and the column headings are the seven areas of information needs drawn from the context, input, process, and product evaluation of the CIPP Model. The X's placed in the table reflect our judgments of which procedures are generally applicable to which information needs. The evaluator can use a blank version of this matrix to summarize an information collection plan by placing X's in cells that signify which procedures they have chosen to meet selected information (from those categories arrayed across the matrix's top). Different evaluators would insert their own X's in the matrix, depending on the information requirements of their particular evaluation assignments and the extent to which they need to employ multiple measures. Such a display provides a visual summary of (1) the information collection procedures that will be applied to address selected information needs and (2) the extent to which the evaluation will employ multiple measures to address the different evaluation needs.

Documents

Stufflebeam and Coryn (2014) recommend that evaluators start the information collection process by identifying and assessing potentially relevant existing information. Starting with a good understanding of existing information has many clear advantages. It can help identify which information needs are addressed and which will contribute to the scope of utilized information, avoid recollecting information that already exists, decrease the information, thereby creating a burden for respondents, and produce cost savings for the evaluation. As with information still to be collected, existing information should be assessed against and held to meet standards of accuracy, relevance, and propriety. In identifying the potentially relevant existing information, the evaluator should consult with the client to identify and access such information and take whatever steps are required to safeguard the rights of human subjects associated with the information.

Many types of existing information can be useful in an evaluation, and much but not all of this information is likely to be found at the program site. To help readers brainstorm the wide range of preexisting information that might be helpful in serving evaluative purposes, we offer Table 9.4. The table's two columns, respec-

TABLE 9.3. A Cross Display of Information Collection Procedures and Areas of Information Needs

Information Collection Procedures	Context Evaluation: Program context and needs	Input Evaluation: Program plan and competing approaches	Process Evaluation: Program activities and costs	Product Evaluation: Program reach to targeted recipients	Product Evaluation: Program outcomes	Product Evaluation: Program sustainability	Product Evaluation: Program transportability
Documents	X	X	X	X	X	X	
Literature review	X	X			X	X	X
Tests	X				X	X	
Interviews	X	X	X	X	X	X	X
Traveling observers			X	X	X	X	X
Site visits	X	X	X	X	X	X	X
Surveys	X	X	X	X	X	X	X
Focus groups	X	X	X	X	X	X	X
Hearings	X	X	X	X	X	X	X
Public forums	X			X	X	X	X
Observations			X	X	X		
Case studies			X	X	X	X	X
Goal-free study					X	X	X
Self-assessment	X		X		X	X	X
Delphi	X	X	X	X	X	X	X
Rating scales					X		
Debates	X	X					
Log diaries						X	X
Video records	X		X		X		
Photography	X		X		X		

Note. From Stufflebeam and Coryn (2014). Copyright © 2014 Daniel L. Stufflebeam and Chris L. S. Coryn. Adapted by permission.

TABLE 9.4. Preexisting Information Examples

Internal to a Program	External to a Program
— Statistics on participants	— Area demographic information
— Needs assessment reports	— Consumer reports
— Mission statement	— Census data
— Strategic plan	— Books
— Institutional records	— Journal articles
— Program proposal	— Encyclopedias
— Program budgets	— Magazines
— Program status updates	— Newspaper
— Program evaluation reports	— Court records
— Minutes of meetings	— Laws and statutes
— Staff résumé	— police reports
— Program financial records	— Real estate records
— Accounting reports	— Chamber of commerce records
— Audit reports	— Accreditation standards
— Log of visitors	— Accreditation records
— Test reports	— State standards
— Correspondence	— State achievement test reports
— Students attendance records	— National achievement test reports
— Students graduation records	— Polls
— Students discipline records	— National survey reports
— Hospital records	— State survey reports
— Registration information	— Local survey reports
— School admission records	— National data sets
— College graduation records	— State data sets
— Local data sets	— White House reports
— Traffic reports	— Congressional records
— Local news reports	— Department of Education reports
— Insurance records	— Professional association reports
— Police records	— Health Department reports
— News releases	— Internet sites
— Other: _____	— Other: _____

Note. From Stufflebeam and Coryn (2014). Copyright ©2014 Daniel L. Stufflebeam and Chris L. S. Coryn. Adapted by permission.

tively, list documents and information that are often internal and external to the program.

Literature Review

Literature review gathers existing information for evaluation purposes and can add scholarly credibility to an evaluation. In the context of program evaluation, a literature review is an investigation of a body of literature that pertains to evaluation questions or procedures. Such a review can, for example, identify questions, procedures, and findings of similar evaluations; illuminate characteristics of the subject program's history and environment; help answer the evaluation's questions, especially those that assess the program's context and plan; and possibly identify research findings pertaining to the treatment and outcome variables involved in the program to be evaluated.

Literature review usually starts with a specific question. For example, in the planning period, the evaluator might want to focus the literature review on identifying what procedures and instruments have been used to assess preservice teachers' need for the service-learning experience. When trying to answer a substantive question, one might want to find out what impacts similar service-learning projects have had on preservice teachers. The evaluator might begin by doing an informal exploratory search of the literature to get a general feeling for how much information there is. Subsequently, the evaluator may specify the search parameters, such as (1) literature published within a set time period; (2) information from certain types of sources, such as refereed journals, evaluation reports, doctoral dissertations, and official government reports; and (3) documents containing certain keywords. Then the evaluator can use an appropriate Web search engine to identify documents meeting these search criteria.

Using the World Wide Web (WWW), an evaluator can find information on almost any topic with just a few clicks of the mouse button. Google Scholar or the Librarians' Index to the Internet uses software programs (also known as *spiders* or *Web crawlers*) that search the entire Internet, looking at millions of websites and then indexing all of the words on them. The search results obtained are usually ranked in order of relevancy. The evaluator then needs to systematically review and wade through the obtained documents to identify pertinent responses to the question of interest. He or she would study the results from the review to identify areas of agreement and contradiction. Additionally, the evaluator would look at references in the documents carefully, then obtain and study additional relevant documents that were not already in the original set. Finally, the evaluator could analyze and synthesize all of the obtained information and combine it with other information to form a coherent answer to the question of interest. For an example of a comprehensive literature review, see this book's appendix, which contains a comprehensive review of literature related to the CIPP Model.

Observation

Some evaluation questions can be answered by observing how a program actually operates and what it produces. Program evaluators observe and report on such program activities as the program's staff meetings, meetings with program stakeholders, special events, participation by beneficiaries, and so on. Those conducting the observations may be the evaluator; traveling observers or resident observers assigned to systematically observe and record program activities; specially contracted observers, such as goal-free evaluators; program staff members who agree to make and record observations; or selected program beneficiaries who agree to make and record observations. In general, such observers may be partitioned into participant observers and nonparticipant observers.

In **participant observation**, members of the program's staff or beneficiaries take on the role of observing program activities and reporting on what they observe. Participant observation occurs when an assigned observer participates fully in the program being observed, makes written records of what is observed, and provides feedback to the lead evaluator. Generally, a participant observer may be given a list of program aspects to observe and describe; a list of key questions to address; an outline for writing reports; specifications regarding the number and timing of needed reports; criteria to be met in producing credible, useful reports; and strict guidelines related to protecting the rights of program staff and beneficiaries.

In **nonparticipant observation**, observers carry out similar tasks but are not members of either the program staff or the beneficiary group. These observers are members of the evaluation team or specially contracted observers. Nonparticipant observation involves the observer sitting on the sidelines and not participating in the activities being observed. Under such an observation assignment, the program participants know that observations are being made and who is making them.

In some evaluations, nonparticipant observer assignments may be relatively unstructured; for example, the observer might simply be instructed to observe the program's implementation, make notes about what is observed, and at a future time respond to the evaluator's questions about the program. The evaluator is wise to entrust this latter type of observation to an experienced, skilled, highly perceptive observer. Relatively unstructured observation is best employed when the evaluator wants to uncover possible features of the program, as it actually operates, that may be unexpected and considerably at variance with the program's objectives and plan of operation.

For both participant and nonparticipant observers, the evaluator should provide at least a minimum structure for carrying out the observations. The structure for observations should be keyed to the program's objectives and key activities and the evaluation's main questions. Additionally, the structure for observations should include guidelines for meeting professional standards of utility, feasibility, propriety, accuracy, and accountability, and especially should include safeguards for protecting the privacy rights of program staff members and beneficiaries. In general, observations for an evaluation should not report on the activities of named staff members and beneficiaries but on how the program actually operates, what barriers it faces, how the barriers are addressed, what variations are evident across different applications of the program's plan, what the program achieves, and what possible positive and negative side effects eventuate. The evaluator should specifically instruct observers to adhere to a given protocol for observations that, at a minimum, lay out the timing and frequency of required observations, the program aspects to observe, the questions to be addressed, and the required reports.

Covert versus **overt observations** are highly sensitive options for the evaluator to consider. In covert observation, the observer is akin to a spy on a program whose identity and observation efforts are kept secret. For ethical reasons, we are, in general, opposed to the practice of covert observation in program evaluations. Observing people and reporting their behaviors secretly without their knowledge or permission can violate ethical standards of evaluation, especially in evaluations of elementary and secondary school programs, where parental permission is essential. This practice can also undermine the evaluation's credibility, especially if and

when the surreptitious observer is exposed—an all too likely occurrence.

We advise the evaluator to inform the program's participants as to who the participant observer is, what will be observed, and what measures will be taken to protect their rights, especially to privacy. Overt participant observation removes ethical concerns by openly identifying the observers' identity. To address the possibility that overt observation may cause program staff and beneficiaries to behave differently when their behaviors are being recorded, we recommend that the observation period be relatively long so that program staff and beneficiaries come to see the observers as a nonthreatening part of the "woodwork." Accordingly, we advise the observers to be as unobtrusive and noninterfering as they can. By openly identifying observation plans so that interested program staff and beneficiaries can review them, the evaluator helps to build stakeholders' respect for the total evaluation process. Overall, we strongly advise against the practice of covert observation in program evaluations and posit that careful planning and execution of aboveboard observations can overcome attendant threats to validity.

We grant that in some assignments covert observation may be defensible. Such assignments include, for example, a store's secret shopper observers and an airline's selected passengers who serve as undercover evaluators of the services that airline service personnel deliver. Notably, these two examples are outside the normal practice of program evaluation.

Much of the previous discussion assumes that the observer will adhere to the principles and procedures of **naturalistic observation**, which involves observing people in their natural settings. The observer does not manipulate variables to control any aspects of the activities and simply observes and records what goes on as things naturally occur. The activities between a caregiver and babies under care are probably best evaluated through naturalistic observation.

When using observation as a means of collecting evaluation information, the evaluator should be aware of the **observer effect** and **observer bias**. The observer effect refers to the fact that the presence of an observer can have considerable effect on the behavior of those being observed and hence on the outcome of an evaluation. The observer can arouse curiosity and cause a lack of attention to the task at hand. A novel observer who records such behavior might let the inaccurate information distort the evaluation results. An effective way of getting around the reactivity problem is to stay around long enough to get people used to the observer's presence. The observer may want to spend some time in the setting before starting to record observations to enable people to become accustomed to their presence and go about their usual activities.

The observer's focus in observing program activities can also influence the behaviors of those being observed if the observer specifically cues program participants to the types of behaviors they are monitoring. For example, an observer recording people's courtesy may influence those being observed to act more politely than usual if the observer states what behavior is being observed. Thus, we advise observers not to apprise program staff or beneficiaries of the specific behaviors being studied. Instead, it is sufficient to inform program personnel that the observations are focused on the program's operations.

Another threat to the validity of observational information is observer bias, which refers to the possibility that certain characteristics or ideas of the observers may bias what they "see." It is argued that no matter how carefully the observers try to remain impartial, their observations will likely possess some degree of bias. All observers should try to do all they can to control their bias, which can be done in several ways. They could spend a large amount of time at the site to get to know their subjects and environment well. They could collect a large amount of information to check their perceptions against what the information reveals. They could collect information from a variety of perspectives using a variety of formats to help capture the complexity of the setting. They could prepare detailed field notes and try to reflect on their own subjectivity as a part of the field notes. They could work in teams to check their observations against those of others. All of these moves can help the observers reflect on how their own attitudes may influence what they perceive.

Interviews

Interviewing is another main technique that evaluators use to collect qualitative information. Interviewing involves carefully asking relevant questions and is an important means of checking the accuracy of impressions gained through observations. Interviews can provide valuable information about people's ideas, experiences, opinions, attitudes, values, and thoughts. Fetterman (1998) believes that interviewing is the most important information collection technique a qualitative researcher can employ.

Evaluators may consider three main types of **interviews**: structured, semistructured, and informal. The formal techniques of **structured** and **semistructured interviews** use a series of questions designed to elicit specific answers from respondents. The structure of these interviewing approaches enables the evaluator to obtain responses to standardized questions and subsequently compare the different responses. Such responses may come from different respondents and from different times of the interviews. These types of interviews can be helpful in gathering information to test certain assumptions about how the program is supposed to operate, as well as hypotheses about program outcomes.

Informal interviews have much less structure than structured and semistructured interviews. On the surface, they resemble casual conversations. They do not involve any standardized questions or specified sequence of when they are asked. The main purpose of informal interviews is to enable key persons with some role in the program to freely express what they know and think about the program. Although informal interviews may appear to be easy to conduct, they are, in fact, difficult to do well. The interviewer must be skilled in giving prompts that stimulate respondents to open up about what they know and think about a program. He or she must also be skilled in asking follow-up questions and in asking questions multiple times, but in different ways, so as to be able to compare the respondent's different answers to similar versions of a question. The interviewer must also be able, tactfully, to keep the respondent focused on the interview's main focus and, as needed, must be proficient in extinguishing long, drawn out responses that are not informative. He or she must also be a good recorder of what is learned. Above all, the interviewer must be an excellent listener.

Issues of privacy and even ethics can become something of concern in interviews. Interviewers are often faced with difficult decisions as the interview progresses regarding questions such as: Is the question too personal? Should I dig deeper into how the respondent feels about this issue? Is it more appropriate to refrain from probing further about the individual's response? How do I establish a climate of ease while trying to learn some sensitive detail about the respondent's association with the program? How can I dissuade the respondent from violating the other person's privacy or from slandering the person? How can I tactfully remain neutral when the respondent expresses a particular position regarding a controversial argument?

A skillful interviewer ought to first and foremost establish an atmosphere of trust and mutual respect. He or she should also begin with nonthreatening questions to put the respondent at ease and can then gradually pose more sensitive and probing questions.

Patton (2002) categorized six types of questions, all or any of which can be asked during an interview: background/demographic questions, knowledge questions, experience/behavior questions, opinion/values questions, feelings questions, and sensory questions. Background/demographic questions are those routine types of questions regarding background information about the respondents. Knowledge questions gather factual information that respondents hold. Experience/behavior questions pertain to what the respondents are doing or have done; these questions aim to elicit descriptions of experiences, behaviors, or activities that could have been observed. Opinion/values questions target respondents' judgments concerning some topic or issue. Questions pertaining to feelings gauge how respondents emotionally react to certain program aspects or other things (e.g., they may have considerable interest in the aspect or none at all).

Fraenkel, Wallen, and Hyun (2015, pp. 452–454) discussed a set of important guidelines for all interviews; among them are:

- Respect the culture of the group being interviewed.
- Respect the individual being interviewed.
- Be natural.
- Develop an appropriate rapport with the participant.
- Ask the same question in different ways during the interview.
- Ask the interviewee to repeat an answer or statement when there is some doubt about the completeness of a remark.
- Vary who controls the flow of the communication.
- Avoid leading questions that lead the participants to respond in a certain way.
- Don't ask dichotomous questions (questions that permit a yes–no answer) when you are trying to get a complete picture.
- Ask only one question at a time.
- Listen actively.
- Don't interrupt.

Focus Groups

A **focus group** isn't just a collection of readily available people who are convened to talk about whatever comes into their minds. The focus group is a special type of group in terms of its purpose, size, composition, and deliberations (Krueger & Casey, 2009). A focus group session should be focused and managed to obtain a carefully selected group's responses to a set of predetermined questions.

In program evaluations, a focus group's purpose is to select, convene, and engage a group of about 7–10 stakeholders to address key questions related to the evaluation. The selected group may be drawn from beneficiaries, program staff, community members, or other interested groups with relevant perspectives on the subject program. Example questions for the session may include: What are the most important questions to be addressed by the evaluation? What audiences are most important for receiving and acting on the evaluation's findings? What are important potential uses of the findings? What are the most important needs to be addressed by the subject program? How important and appropriate are the program's stated goals? What barriers should be anticipated and addressed in carrying out the program's plan? What are the credibility and significance of the evaluation's findings? How can the obtained evaluation findings best be applied? What arrangements and resources are needed to make optimal use of the evaluation's findings?

Evaluators should consider conducting focus group interviews when they are looking for the range of ideas or perceptions that people have about something related to the subject program; when they are trying to understand differences in perspectives between groups or categories of people; when they are trying to uncover factors that influence opinions, behavior, or motivation; when they want useful advice to emerge from the group; and, especially, when they are seeking ways to assure the evaluation's constructive impacts. Focus groups can also be used to judge program plans and materials, help gather information needed to design quantitative instruments, or shed light on quantitative data already collected. In applications of the CIPP Model, focus group sessions with selected groups of intended users of findings are especially useful for obtaining perspectives on the credibility and potential utility of the final report and how best to secure uses of the findings.

Focus groups provide an interactive environment where members can hear, ponder, reflect on, and comment on ideas and judgments expressed by other members of the group. Focus groups work well when participants feel comfortable, respected, and free to give their opinions without being judged. The coordinator should create an environment that permits and encourages participants to share perceptions and points of view and to feel free to disagree without being disagreeable. The coordinator should not pressure group members to reach consensus when clear disagreements are evident in exchanges between group members. The coordinator should manage the session so that all members have equitable opportunities to contribute, no one dominates the discussion, and the available time for the session is used efficiently.

When planning focus group sessions, the evaluator should decide what types of people could render the needed information. In some focus group efforts, the evaluator might engage several different types of people, such that the information acquired reflects a wide range of different, key perspectives. A given focus group might be organized to reflect the composition of the intended audience as a whole, or it might include persons who share the same type of perspective (e.g., school district administrators, program staff members, or beneficiaries). The evaluator might employ only one focus group or several. For example, if the evaluator is seeking to determine how different groups could constructively apply the findings from an evaluation of a self-help housing project, he or she might empanel several different groups with varying interests in the findings. These might be groups of co-builders, project staff members, construction contractors, local school teachers, area business personnel, local lenders, local employers, area law enforcement, local fire service personnel, local parks and recreation personnel, and/or local clergy.

A focus group's main purpose is to understand rather than make inferences. Although a group's members could be chosen randomly for a population, representativeness is not necessarily the primary factor in selecting the group's members. The primary aim should be to compose a group that is likely to deliver incisive responses to the focus group questions or whose members are in especially advantageous positions to make effective use of the evaluation's findings.

Within marketing research, the traditionally recommended size for a focus group is 10–12. However, we believe the ideal size of a focus group for program evaluations is 7–10. In our experience, focus groups with

more than 10 people are usually too large to control and to secure equitable participation by all members of the group.

Regarding the number of needed focus groups, Krueger and Casey (2009) recommend, as a rule of thumb, empanelling between three or four focus groups for each type or category of individuals. This recommendation must be taken with a grain of salt because the needs and resources of different evaluations can vary enormously. Once the evaluators have conducted the first three or four group sessions, they can determine if they have reached saturation in what can be learned from the particular type of group. If not, Krueger and Casey advise them to engage more such groups. By engaging three to four groups of the same type, the evaluator can examine the extent to which key findings are consistent across groups and are thus dependable for incorporation into evaluation reports. In this regard, the information analyst looks for stable patterns and themes across groups. For large-scale, well-resourced evaluations, we see value in the Krueger and Casey advice that researchers should replicate focus group sessions with each type of group until the quest to identify stable trends and patterns in perceptions has succeeded or has clearly failed.

In the evaluation of an academic support program for college students with special learning needs, it was important to hear the reactions of students with special learning needs who had completed the program, as well as the parents, mentors, and staff members who were involved in the program. Furthermore, it was helpful to compare and contrast the responses of these different groups. Since the evaluator believed feedback from the college students and their parents would be most useful for the evaluation, she placed emphasis on getting information from them. She engaged three focus groups of college students, two groups of parents, two groups of mentors, and one group of staff and university administrators. Figure 9.2 shows the multicategory design for this focus group study.

A focus group's success is heavily dependent on the quality of questions asked. Because the focus group is a social experience, the questions addressed to the group should be conversational and oriented to creating and maintaining a free-flowing, informal exchange. The questions should be clear, short, easy to state, free of jargon and technical terms (unless the group is conversant with such terms), and often open-ended. Different categories of questions are used at different stages dur-

Group 1: Students	○ ○ ○
Group 2: Parents	○ ○
Group 3: Mentors	○ ○
Group 4: Staff	○
Group 5: University administrators	○

FIGURE 9.2. Multicategory design for a focus group study (○ represents focus group).

ing the focus group session, usually following an order, such as that shown in Figure 9.3.

Obviously, a competent moderator is critical to a focus group's success. The moderator's role is to frame questions, foster participation by all members of the group, listen carefully to participants' responses, ask follow-up questions, respect disagreements among the members, and document lessons learned. The moderator should have a clear and unwavering understanding of the focus group session's purpose and must communicate clearly, listen carefully, be attentive to inputs from all group members, be nondefensive, and be respectful and totally civil. The coordinator must be highly skilled in managing group processes.

Effective focus group sessions are systematic information collection activities. Accordingly, such sessions should meet the requirements of competent information collection and documentation. Capturing the lessons learned can include: memory that is written up later, field notes, flipcharts, audio recording, video recording, and computer-based rapid transcripts. Effective steps should be taken to document the inputs received and verify that the written account is an accurate account of what the group members actually said. The documentation should be subjected to systematic content analysis and written up in a succinct report that is tailored to assist the evaluator's decision making and production of evaluation reports.

Focus group findings can be used to advise decision making before, during, or after a project or program.

Focus groups are often useful for evaluators to lay the groundwork for subsequent surveys. Evaluators can use focus groups to learn about language, concepts, and factors that are amenable to inclusion in a survey instrument. Subsequently, the evaluator can develop or select meaningful instruments that allow for larger samples and statistical analysis. Evaluators can also use focus groups following other data collection activities to help interpret findings and chart recommendations for later action. A potential problem that can seriously threaten the trustworthiness of focus group deliberations is the case in which one or more members totally dominate the discussion and successfully suppress input from other members. A skilled moderator can and should act to minimize such counterproductive, stifling influence and should invite and welcome inputs from all group members. All group members should be encouraged and welcomed to reflect on and express their views without pressure or intimidation by other group members.

Traveling Observers and Resident Researcher

The **traveling observer (TO) information collection technique** began in the mid-1970s at The Evaluation Center of Western Michigan University (Stufflebeam & Coryn, 2014) and has been applied in many of The Evaluation Center's evaluations. The TO is a field researcher who is trained and assigned to conduct preliminary investigations in advance of subsequent primary evaluations by a panel of experts or the evaluation's lead investigator. Before undertaking the fieldwork, the TO develops and secures approval of a detailed Traveling Observer Handbook for systematically carrying out the TO assignment. The employment of a traveling observer according to an explicit protocol is a method in that, as in naturalistic inquiry, the observer is the instrument.

The TO travels from project site to project site to contact and establish rapport with project personnel and other potential data providers; collect preliminary information, especially concerning project implemen-

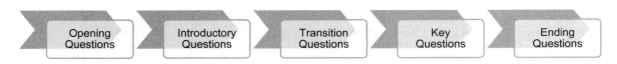

FIGURE 9.3. The sequence of focus group questions.

tation and outcomes; and work out a plan for a follow-up site visit by an expert team. The TO provides the expert team with orientation information prior to the team's site visits and gives the needed support during these visits. The TO usually spends considerably more time on the sites than the expert team does, and his or her work not only increases the efficiency of the expert team, but also saves money for a sizable portion of the needed field research. The resident researcher technique is a variation of the TO technique. It is simply the application of the TO approach at a single site instead of multiple sites.

A specially tailored Traveling Observer Handbook is an essential aspect of the TO technique. The TO develops this manual based on the design for the evaluation plus the TO assignment. Figure 9.4 is a sample table of contents for a Traveling Observer Handbook.

Advocate Teams Technique

The Advocate Teams Technique (ATT) was created at The Evaluation Center when the center was housed at The Ohio State University (Stufflebeam & Coryn, 2014, pp. 325–326, 551). It was developed in 1969 to help the Texas-based Southwest Regional Educational Laboratory identify and assess alternative strategies for serving the education needs of migrant children and ultimately allocate $10 million to support the operationalization and application of the top-ranked strategy. The ATT offers a systematic way to identify and assess competing strategies for addressing high-priority needs and problems and is keyed directly to a decision-making group's desire for creative solutions to high-priority needs and problems. It is particularly helpful in program planning and allocation of funds when different groups have sharply different predilections about what approach should be adopted and funded. Through application of the ATT, the evaluator can exploit the biases of opposing groups by developing alternative plans that incorporate the competing positions and then comparing, contrasting, and judging them via a systematic, fair input evaluation process.

Proper application of the ATT involves the 15 main steps displayed in Table 9.5.

Other Techniques

We want to reiterate that it is very important for evaluators to employ multiple techniques to collect information from multiple sources. We advise evaluators to consider and make effective use of the information collection techniques reviewed here and also to be resourceful in searching broadly for other techniques that are relevant to their evaluation's information requirements. Some of these techniques or approaches were discussed in detail in Stufflebeam and Coryn (2015), including the Success Case Method (Chapter 6), case study evaluation (Chapter 12), and goal-free evaluation (Chapter 14). Other useful techniques—including surveys, rating scales, **data mining**, needs assessment, visual methodologies, cost analysis, and ethnography—are covered extensively in many research and evaluation methods textbooks (e.g., Bickman & Rog, 2009; Davidson, 2005; Fitzpatrick, Sanders, & Worthen, 2011; Fraenkel, Wallen, & Hyun, 2015; Margolis & Pauwels, 2011; Rossi, Lipsey, & Freeman, 2004).

Creating an Information Collection Table

Sound information collection is central to the success of any evaluation. Compiling and managing an information plan is a complex enterprise. Its contents may include a diversity of information, information collection procedures, information sources, information collectors, and times for information collection. Consequently, it can be easy for the evaluator to lose track of all aspects of the information collection plan. Accordingly, evaluators need an efficient way to organize and keep track of the various facets of their information collection plans.

Creating an information collection table and sharing it among project staff and designated information collectors can be especially helpful for communicating and managing details of the information collection plan. Information collection tables can display some or all of the following: project objectives, information collection tools, information sources, information collection timing, information collectors, and special notes.

Table 9.6 is a product evaluation information collection table that has been used by the evaluator of a mathematics teacher professional development project. As part of the product evaluation, the evaluator planned to collect information to assess the attainment of four project objectives: increasing teacher content knowledge, increasing student's achievement, improving classroom instruction, and developing partnerships. The evaluator listed indicators, corresponding instruments, sources for obtaining the information, and times for information collection activities.

1. **The Traveling Observer Assignment**
   1.1. Summary of the TO job description
   1.2. Protocols for contacting project personnel and obtaining needed permissions and cooperation
   1.3. Key evaluation standards to be met, especially Human Rights and Respect and Clear Reporting
   1.4. Key questions to be addressed by the TO
   1.5. Services to be provided to the site visit team
   1.6. Time frame for the TO assignment
   1.7. Required reports
   1.8. Budget for TO expenditures
   1.9. Tools, such as cameras and tape recorders for the TO work
   1.10. Arrangements for providing insurance coverage for the TO's work
   1.11. Rules concerning professional behavior expected
   1.12. Criteria for judging TO reports
   1.13. Rules about communicating and disseminating findings

2. **The subject project**
   2.1. Brief description
   2.2. Map showing project location(s)
   2.3. Contact persons and their addresses, phone numbers, and e-mail addresses
   2.4. Schedule of key project events

3. **The site visitors to be served**
   3.1. Evaluation team members and their addresses, phone numbers, and e-mail addresses
   3.2. Members of the site visit team and their addresses, phone numbers, and e-mail addresses

4. **TO work plan**
   4.1. Schedule for TO site visits to project sites
   4.2. Documents to be collected and content analyses to be performed
   4.3. Interviews to be conducted
   4.4. Photographs to be taken
   4.5. Briefing materials to be developed and presented to the site visit team
   4.6. Schedule and location for meetings with the site visit team
   4.7. Agendas for briefing sessions with site visitors
   4.8. Plan of data-gathering activities for the site visit team
   4.9. Rules for processing information and keeping it safe
   4.10. Arrangements for housing and providing meals for the site visit teams
   4.11. Arrangements for rental cars or other modes of transportation
   4.12. Issues that may arise and what to do about them

5. **TO tools**
   5.1. Tentative outlines for TO reports
   5.2. Interview protocols
   5.3. Expense report forms
   5.4. Diary for logging TO activities
   5.5. Evaluation standards attestation form
   5.6. Letter of introduction, provided by the lead evaluator
   5.7. Letter of instruction, provided by the project director

FIGURE 9.4. A sample table of contents for a Traveling Observer Handbook.

TABLE 9.5. Advocate Teams Techniques Tasks

1. The evaluation client stipulates a target group of beneficiaries and identifies objectives to be achieved in meeting this group's needs.

2. The evaluator discusses with the client and other stakeholders their predilections about what different project strategies might be effective for addressing the needs of the targeted beneficiaries.

3. The evaluator compiles and/or collects relevant background information, including especially relevant needs assessment information, and creates an information bank with relevance to the tasks of developing project strategies and writing advocate team reports.

4. The evaluator reaches agreement with the client on the program strategies to be developed or at least the perspectives from which competing strategies should be developed.

5. The evaluator and client work out specific criteria for judging the acceptability and excellence of competing project strategies.

6. The evaluator establishes an advocate team, usually comprised of three to five relevant experts, for each program strategy to be developed.

7. The evaluator provides each team with the subject objectives, the supporting bank of relevant information concerned especially with the target group's needs, the criteria to be referenced in judging and ranking the competing advocate team reports, the general approach to be worked up—or, alternatively, the perspective from which the team is to create and write up a new program strategy, an outline for writing up their proposed program strategy, clerical assistance, office materials, a place to conduct their work, and a deadline for producing the report.

8. Each advocate team then meets in isolation from the other team(s), reviews the needs assessment data, obtains and studies other relevant information, brainstorms toward working out the main elements of the project strategy.

9. Ultimately, the team fleshes out the strategy they have developed into an operational plan, makes sure it is responsive to the stipulated assessment criteria, and writes their advocate team report.

10. In consultation with the client, the evaluator establishes an independent, metaevaluation panel whose members collectively include relevant substantive perspectives and evaluative expertise.

11. The evaluator then engages the metaevaluation panel to evaluate the advocate teams' proposals against the predetermined criteria and rank them on overall merit.

12. The evaluator presents the advocate team reports and the independent assessments and ranking of them to the client group.

13. The client group chooses a strategy for implementation or assigns a convergence team to merge the best features of the competing plans into a hybrid plan.

14. The evaluator may then develop a plan and budget for pilot-testing and possibly strengthening the selected strategy.

15. The client group either moves forward with the pilot testing of the selected strategy or may move directly to implement it without pilot testing.

TABLE 9.6. A Product Evaluation Information Collection Table

Objective of Project	Indicators	Data Source	Collection Timing
1. Increasing teacher content knowledge			
Increase content knowledge of the number and operations and algebraic thinking concepts detailed in the Common Core State Standards (CCSS).	Improvement of teachers' scores on content knowledge test: Diagnostic Mathematics Assessments for Elementary Teachers *http://louisville.edu/education/centers/crmstd/diag-math-assess-elem* North Carolina Teacher Evaluation Standard III: Teachers know the content they teach	Teachers	Pre- and posttest for each cohort in July and again in May of the following year *Pre–postcomparison of North Carolina Teacher Evaluation Standard III: Teachers know the content they teach*
Increase understanding of the Standards for Mathematical Practice in the CCSS.	Teachers' self-report of knowledge of mathematical practices and how they are evident in their classrooms	Teachers	Postinterviews (subset of teachers)
Increase self-efficacy in mathematics teaching.	Increased ratings on the Mathematics Teaching Efficacy Beliefs Instrument *http://web.mnstate.edu/trn/TRNweb/mtebi.pdf*	Teachers	Pre–postmeasure for each cohort in July and again in May of the following year
2. Increasing student achievement			
Increase student mathematics achievement.	Improved scores on grades K–2 Interview Assessments (AMC Anywhere)	K–2 students of participating teachers	Quarterly
	Improved scores on grades 3–8 end-of-grade tests	Grades 3–8 students of participating teachers	Prior-year and present-year scores
Demonstrate student use of mathematical practices—specifically mathematical modeling and explanation.	Evidence of student use of explanations and modeling in classroom lessons and on student work	Teachers Project Team	Classroom observations and student work from common tasks teachers do with students, quarterly
3. Improving classroom instruction			
Increase teachers' access to high-challenge tasks that align to the CCSS.	Teachers' analysis of currently used tasks for cognitive demand and alignment with the CCSS	Teachers Project Team	Collection of high-demand tasks at each grade level for the standards in the number and operations and algebraic thinking domains of the CCSS, ongoing
Increase teachers' use of strategies to promote student discourse.	Evidence of teacher use of strategies to support student explanations North Carolina Teacher Evaluation Standard IV: Teachers facilitate learning for the students	Teachers Project Team	Pre–postclassroom observations *Pre–postcomparison of North Carolina Teacher Evaluation Standard IV: Teachers facilitate learning for the students*

(continued)

TABLE 9.6. *(continued)*

Objective of Project	Indicators	Data Source	Collection Timing
Increase focus on the use of data for instructional decision making and planning.	Observations of teachers' use of data	Teachers Project Team	Pre–postclassroom observations; quarterly grade-level discussions during professional development as teachers discuss recommendations for next steps based on student data from individual student interviews and work
4. Developing sustainable partnerships			
Develop a mutual understanding of the needs of all partners and the resources to meet those needs.	Partners' report of connections, communication, and support	Teachers' Project Team	Management meetings
Establish a pipeline in middle grades mathematics to local STEM industries.	Inclusion of mathematical applications used by local industries in tasks/lessons developed by teachers	Teachers' industry partners	Lesson plans; classroom observations
Develop classroom teachers leaders who can lead and support district mathematics initiatives.	Records of leadership activities completed by teacher leaders	Teacher Leaders Project Team	Logs of coaching and other leadership activities

Organizing Collected Information

The amount and types of evaluation information collected for an evaluation can be vast in quantity and thus difficult to manage. It requires careful and methodical organization. The evaluator needs to develop a data management plan and arrange for equipment, facilities, materials, and personnel needed to process, update, and control the evaluation information. An important word of precaution before we proceed is "confidentiality." That is, evaluators must ensure that confidentiality requirements are strictly met at all times. This means that only authorized personnel can access and use the information. Evaluation information files should be kept in locked filing cabinets in a locked office and controlled by a designated evaluation team member who has been IRB trained and fully understands the confidentiality requirements for the project information. When data are transferred from one site to another, the evaluator must apply measures to ensure that evaluation information will not leak out. Moreover, the evaluator should be aware that certain cloud file storage and transfer methods are not secure.

When making information organization decisions, evaluators must keep data analysis needs in mind. For example, if a set of data will be analyzed using statistical software SPSS, then it is best to enter, organize, and update these data in SPSS. As another example, in a repeated measures design, the evaluator must assign an identifier to each participant so that the person's subsequent responses can be linked to her or his previous responses. In fact, it is almost always essential to use an identifier. For security reasons, the identifier should not be easily associated with the person. Identifiers to avoid especially include the person's name, social security number, birth date, address, phone number, and email address.

For each set of information, evaluators need to follow systematic steps in organizing and managing it to ensure its accuracy and security. Some information, such as video recordings, must be transcribed for later analysis. Some information needs to be coded, and some needs to be keyed into a computer. It is good practice to save the information in its original format, even after it has been transferred to another format, so that the evaluators and other pertinent parties can go back and recheck information for accuracy. Those who carry out the information-related work must be trained to ensure accuracy, and the evaluator regularly checks their work for accuracy.

The evaluator needs to establish a functional system to file, control, and retrieve information that directly reflects the evaluation's structure. When making information organization decisions, the evaluator should keep in mind structural aspects of the evaluation. In relation to the CIPP Model, these may include context, input, process, and product evaluations, as well as evaluation client groups, evaluation questions, evaluation staff members, information collection instruments, and evaluation reports. Additional identifiers may be the evaluation's different time periods. It is recognized that there is not one system that would suit the information management needs of all evaluations. The following general categories are useful for consideration:

- *Focusing of the evaluation*: task order or RFP, the proposal, the contract, the budget, IRB records, evaluation standards and criteria, key participants' correspondence records, relevant background reports, literature, evaluation schedule.

- *Information collection*: methods and data collection instruments, sampling plans, information sources, information-gathering protocols, information collection assignments, information collection personnel training, information collection schedule.

- *Information analysis*: analysis plans, synthesis plans, analysis assignments, rubrics, instrument users' manuals.

- *Reporting*: reporting plans, reporting schedule, draft reports, final reports, stakeholders' feedback on draft reports, technical appendices, multimedia materials for presentations.

- *Follow-up of reports*: feedback workshops, focus groups, conferences, publications.

- *Metaevaluation*: standards for information collection, standards attestation, independent reviews.

Creating a database may be necessary for some evaluations, especially if the evaluation involves a large amount of data or will need to track the evaluand over time. A considerable amount of planning is needed to make a database work the way it should. The evaluator or the data analyst should give clear directions to data management personnel regarding the appropriate computer software, data entering, coding, checking, verifying, recording, and updating, to ensure that the database is created, maintained, and useful.

Summary

Collecting sound information from reliable sources is essential to the success of all evaluations. To form complete, sound, and valid judgments of a program's merit and worth, evaluators should obtain a sufficient range and depth of pertinent, appropriate, and reliable information. The Joint Committee (1994, 2011) provides authoritative standards and systematic guidelines for collecting, validating, and using evaluative information. Evaluators are advised to familiarize themselves with these standards and regularly apply them. These standards and guidelines can help evaluators determine what information to collect and from what sources, uphold the rights of human participants, understand a program's context, describe program operations, apply appropriate sampling methods, ensure the reliability of evidence, validate data collection instruments, efficiently organize and maintain obtained information, and maintain the integrity of the information.

Due to practical constraints in almost all program evaluations, evaluators have to utilize less-than-perfect information collection instruments and procedures. To counter this weakness, evaluators are advised to employ multiple methods to collect multiple types of information from multiple sources to allow for cross-checks in their pursuit of consistent, dependable findings. Even so, they are still obligated to report the limitations of the information they obtain. This chapter has identified some of the wide-ranging qualitative and quantitative information collection techniques and approaches that are applicable in program evaluations.

REVIEW QUESTIONS • • • • • • • • • •

1. What are the main questions to be answered in each of the following types of evaluation: context, input, process, and product?

2. Make a matrix that includes illustrations of quantitative and qualitative information that would be relevant in conducting a context evaluation to help develop goals for a school's project to improve student attendance.

3. List and define generic criteria that could be used to judge and rank alternative strategies for improving a school's student attendance.

4. Develop a response to the following question:

What information and associated information collection methods would be especially relevant for determining and judging the outcomes of an elementary school's project to improve students' use of computers?

5. This chapter discussed the Joint Committee standards for guiding and assessing information collection in an evaluation. Explain the relevance of each of the following standards to the information collection task: Relevant Information, Human Rights and Respect, Explicit Program and Context Descriptions, Defensible Information Sources, Valid Information, Reliable Information, and Information Management.

6. Develop a two-by-four matrix of quantitative and qualitative information collection methods by context, input, process, and product evaluations and provide in each cell an example of a key information requirement and associated information collection method.

7. Considering that a dominant person can have undue influence on a focus group's results, what moves can a skilled moderator make to assure that all participants have equal opportunities to express their views.

8. List two common types of interviews and give your views of guidelines for effectively conducting each type.

9. List and explain at least three ways to control observer bias when conducting observations.

10. Why is it advisable for evaluators to employ multiple information collection methods?

11. What are the basic steps you would take to validate a data collection instrument to be used in a program evaluation?

12. In what ways are literature reviews useful in program evaluations? List what you see as guidelines for conducting a sound literature review.

13. What is the traveling observer technique? How is it used in program evaluations and for what purposes?

14. Summarize the Advocate Teams Technique. Explain its use in program evaluations that apply the CIPP Model.

15. Explain the focus group procedure and identify three ways it can be used in program evaluations.

CHAPTER 10

Analyzing and Synthesizing Information

"Answering an evaluation's questions and judging the subject program requires competent analysis and synthesis of relevant, valid information."

This chapter explains how to analyze quantitative and qualitative information and how to synthesize information to form bottom-line conclusions regarding a program's merit and worth. Key topics include foundational concepts that undergird sound analysis and synthesis; quantitative and qualitative analysis procedures that are especially useful in analyzing information obtained in context, input, process, and product evaluations; explanations and illustrations for selected procedures; the computer analysis utility known as SPSS; templates for displaying analysis results; and guidelines for synthesizing quantitative and qualitative analyses.

Overview
• •

The Joint Committee on Standards for Educational Evaluation (2011) states, "Accurate analyses are required for sound reasoning to conclusions. Accurate analyses allow information to be aggregated and reduced, described, summarized, and understood, and its limitations to be made explicit in the context of specific evaluation questions and uses. Without technically adequate analyses, sound reasoning is undermined" (p. 202). In addition to conducting sound analyses, evaluators should also be skilled in synthesizing analysis results to arrive at defensible, bottom-line conclusions. It is patently clear that sound processes of information analysis and synthesis are vital to an evaluation's success.

Many textbooks on evaluation treat the topics of analysis and synthesis of information lightly and only advise readers to consult textbooks on statistics and qualitative research. In this chapter we identify, explain, and give examples of quantitative and qualitative analysis techniques that are especially applicable in program evaluations. We also explain how to synthesize both types of analysis findings to answer a client group's evaluation questions and reach solid conclusions about a subject program's effectiveness and overall value.

This chapter's key parts include the conceptual underpinnings of analysis and synthesis' quantitative and qualitative analysis techniques that have particular applicability to the CIPP Model; detailed discussions of selected analysis techniques; computer-assisted analysis using SPSS; ways to convey data graphically; and guidelines for synthesizing analysis and synthesis results.

Among this chapter's specific topics are types of information, basic inferential statistics, nonparametric data analysis techniques, t-tests, chi-square tests, analysis of variance (ANOVA), multivariate analysis of variance (MANOVA), how to calculate effect sizes, how to choose between nonparametric tests and parametric tests, how to compute descriptive statistics using SPSS, procedure for assessing normality using the Explore function in SPSS, and computer software for qualitative data analysis. The chapter's 15 appendices contain material of use in dealing with the nuts and bolts of analysis. We hope that readers will find this chapter to be a convenient reference and practical guide to useful analysis and synthesis procedures and tools.

Before proceeding with this chapter's main topics, we want to state a caveat. Evaluators should use analysis procedures and tools selectively to answer an evaluation's questions and support bottom-line conclusions about the subject program's merit and worth. Evaluators should not apply sophisticated analysis procedures and tools to display one's technical repertoire, as sometimes has happened in evaluations. Such off-the-mark behavior is unlikely to impress the evaluation's users and may well discredit the evaluator as lacking the competence and maturity to directly and efficiently address the client group's evaluation questions.

Foundational Concepts of Analysis and Synthesis

To effectively carry out evaluations, the evaluator needs a clear understanding of the conceptual underpinnings of analysis and synthesis, including those summarized in this section.

Goals of Analysis and Synthesis

Basically, **information analysis** is a process of inspecting, **cleaning**, transforming, and modeling information, with the goal of describing characteristics and patterns, highlighting useful information, identifying themes and patterns, and assessing **statistical significance** and practical significance. The purpose of **information synthesis** is to draw together analysis results and deliver well-founded conclusions.

Types of Information

The two broad categories of information to be analyzed and synthesized are quantitative and qualitative. Quantitative information is expressed in numbers, whereas qualitative information is typically expressed in narrative text, photographs, or video clips.

Quantitative information is often used to measure an entity's amount of something; examples are a student group's average achievement test scores at the beginning and end of an instructional program, and the number of men and women who attended a town hall meeting. Quantitative information may pertain to a small sample of subjects, a very large sample, or a total population.

Qualitative information, on the other hand, may consist of an in-depth description and incisive examination of a particular entity, such as a theatrical play, or, as another example, distillation and interpretation of recorded exchanges in a town hall meeting. Qualitative information is often used to describe a situation or gain insight into a particular practice—for example, a transcript of a focus group session. Qualitative information typically has the form of written narrative, images, or video or sound recordings.

Descriptive Statistics and Inferential Statistics

Just as the two basic acts of evaluation are description and judgment, the main divisions of analysis are descriptive statistics and inferential statistics.

Data analysis usually starts with **descriptive statistics**. These may include frequency counts; percentages; percentiles; quartiles; **measures of central tendency**, including mean, median, and mode; **measures of dispersion**, such as range, variance, and standard deviation; a measure of a **distribution**'s skewness; and a measure of the distribution's peakness, that is, kurtosis. When the evaluator wants to convey the essential characteristics of a set of data, he or she can arrange the data into an interpretable form, such as a frequency distribution or a graphical display. Descriptive statistics such as mean, median, and mode let the evaluation audience know where the majority of the scores are; while quartiles, standard deviations, and variances let the audience know how spread out the scores are.

Inferential statistics are intended to make inferences (educated conclusions) about population parameters based on measures obtained from a random sample of the population and based on certain assumptions. To make an inference from a random sample to the parent population, the evaluator performs calculations to develop powerful arguments about what would be learned if the whole population was measured. The analysis tools used to make such inferences include measures of central tendency and dispersion, significance tests (also known as hypothesis tests), and **confidence intervals**.

Type I and II Errors

In the process of concluding whether an observed difference between experimental and control group means is real or only due to random error, the evaluator typically will set up and conduct a test of statistical significance. Such a test's purpose is to judge the acceptability of a hypothesis (H1) that the observed difference is only due to sampling error. To reach a defensible judgment in the matter, the evaluator sets an alpha level of, for example, .05. Such an alpha level denotes the upper bound on the probability of accepting the observed difference as real when in fact it is due to random error. In this case, across a large sample of studies using the same treatment conditions, dependent measures, and alpha level, the evaluator would expect to mistakenly judge an observed difference as real less than 5% of the time. This kind of mistake is known as a type I error. The probability of making such an error is dictated by where the evaluator sets the alpha level of significance. By setting a small alpha level, such as .01, the evaluator minimizes the type I error of wrongly judging an observed difference to be real and can be reasonably confident that the observed difference is real and not due to sampling error.

However, the smaller one sets the alpha level (to designate the region of type I error), the greater the probability of making a type II error. A type II error occurs when the decision rule does not reject H1 (the hypothesis of no statistically significant difference between the observed means), although a certain alternative H2 (a hypothesis of a certain level of true difference between the observed means) is true. The region of type II error for a given alternative hypothesis is designated as beta. The potential size of a type II error depends on both the preset alpha level of significance and one's particular alternative hypothesis (H2).

Sometimes the risk associated with making a type II error is so important that the evaluator is justified in setting a large alpha level and accepting a relatively high level of risk of making a type I error while minimizing the risk of making a type II error. We can see the logic of trade-offs between types I and II errors in people's ordinary decisions in their daily lives. For example, consider a case where a person—whose car broke down on a seldom-traveled country road that is adjacent to a frozen-over river—needs to cross the river to get help from a service station that he sees on the other side of the river. Because he knows the nearest bridge is 5 miles upstream, this person wants to save time by simply walking across the frozen river. However, the ice might not be sufficiently thick to support the person's weight. For this person, the type I error would be wrongly deciding that the river's ice is too thin to support a walk across the river, with the consequence of needlessly walking to the distant bridge, crossing it, and then walking the additional 5 miles to the service station. The type II error would be in erroneously deciding that the ice is sufficiently thick to support a walk across the river. Clearly, in this case the type II error is much more important than the type I error; to avoid this potentially disastrous mistake, the person would be prudent to walk the needed ten-plus miles to get safely to the service station on the river's other side. This decision to avoid the risk of falling through thin ice into the freezing river could be a life-saving choice.

Type I and type II errors are defined in Table 10.1.

The concepts of type I error and type II error are important in evaluation work because sometimes small differences between control group and treatment group outcome measures are of practical importance. If the evaluator sets a very small alpha level (e.g., .01), a small but practically important difference between treatment and control group means might be rejected. A stark example is that early investigations of the possible link between cigarette smoking and lung cancer applied small alpha levels and rejected small but critically important indications of a causal link between tobacco use and lung cancer. The investigators in these early studies failed to reject the H1 hypothesis that cigarette smoking did not cause lung cancer. Failure to accept the subsequently validated H2 hypothesis linking cigarettes to lung cancer proved to be a very serious type II error. One can only wonder how many lives might have been saved if this highly important type II error had been investigated and avoided much sooner than it was.

Qualitative Analysis

Qualitative analysis refers to the systematic examination of representations of experiences, performances, characteristics, or other descriptions presented in narra-

TABLE 10.1. Definitions of Type I and Type II Errors

Decision	True State of Affairs	
	H1 is true (i.e., the observed difference between means is only due to sampling error).	H1 is false and H2 is true (i.e., the observed difference between means is real [coinciding with H2] and is not due to sampling error).
Reject H1 Accept H2	Type I error	No error
Do not reject H1 Do not accept H2	No error	Type II error

tive or other symbolic but not numerical form. Qualitative analysis characterizes the essence or central focus of a set of qualitative information, draws out patterns and key themes, looks for consistency or contradictions, examines intensity, and, in general, assesses the information's relevance to answering an evaluation's questions.

Among the useful publications on qualitative analysis are the following: Birks, Chapman, and Francis (2008); Butler-Kisber (2010); Chenail (2010); Corbin and Strauss (2007); Creswell (2013); Denzin and Lincoln (2011); Fetterman (2010); Fielding and Lee (1998); Golafshani (2003); LaCompte and Goetz (1982); Leninger (1985); Miles and Huberman (1984); Morse (1991); Patton (2008); Straus (1987); and Tesch (1990).

Quantitative Analysis

Analyzing quantitative information involves summarizing and examining one or more sets of numerical data. Such an analysis usually is done to assess the correlation between the two sets of data or to identify and assess differences between indicators from the two sets (often termed main effects), such as means, medians, or modes. In more sophisticated examinations, the analysis may search out and assess means (known as **simple effects**) that may be different for subgroups in a study's sample. **Quantitative analysis** uses numerical methods to ascertain size, magnitude, amount, and the like, and can aggregate and summarize numerical information. The main aims of quantitative analyses are to determine and display experience, performances, characteristics, or other descriptions modeled by or summarized by ordered numerical systems. Culminating analyses to determine the significance of findings involves tests of significance and/or employment of confidence intervals.

In general, quantitative analysis of numerical data embodies the field known as statistics. The basic aims of statistical analyses are to describe the data obtained from a random sample of a population—especially its mean and standard deviation—and to infer what the true measures would be if the total population was measured. Thus, statistics can be divided into two broad branches: descriptive statistics and inferential statistics, as displayed in Figure 10.1 and explained below. Descriptive statistics describe and summarize a sample (and sometimes the population). Inferential statistics make inferences (educated conclusions) about population parameters based on measures obtained from a sample of the population and based on certain assumptions.

Quantitative information appears in four types of measurement scales:

1. *Nominal:* values merely name the category to which the object under study belongs (e.g., gender).

2. *Ordinal:* measures of objects are ranked from top to bottom to reflect each object's quality or status compared to the others (for example, rankings of the overall assessed quality of 4-year colleges in the United States), but the distances between adjacent objects are not necessarily equal.

3. *Interval:* the scale has no exact 0, but the distances between points on the scale are equal. (e.g., temperatures).

4. *Ratio:* values have an absolute 0 and equal intervals (e.g., weights).

Readers may consult a wealth of excellent publications on the wide range of available quantitative analysis techniques. Among others are Cook and Campbell (1979); Edmonds and Kennedy (2013); Glass, Wilson,

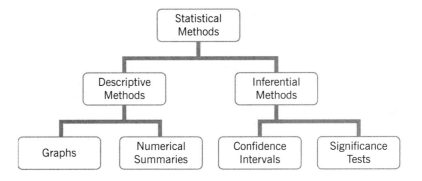

FIGURE 10.1. Types of statistical methods.

and Gottman (2008); Hopkins and Glass (1978); Jaeger (1990); Raudenbush and Bryk (2002); Shadish (2010); Wiersma and Jurs (2005); and Winer (1962).

Synthesis

The culminating synthesis step in an evaluation involves combining quantitative and qualitative analysis results to form clear, defensible conclusions. Basically, such conclusions should provide well-founded, actionable answers to the evaluation's questions as well as judgments of the subject program's merit and worth. Generally, the synthesis should address the evaluation's questions with succinct quantitative analyses and buttress these analyses with qualitative information that add meaning to the quantitative analyses. Often the evaluator can illuminate the meaning of quantitative analyses by buttressing them with such qualitative information as stakeholders' testimony. A useful approach to synthesizing quantitative and qualitative information may be found in Scriven's (1994) classic article, titled "The Final Synthesis."

Given the preceding set of basic principles of analysis and synthesis, we next provide an overview of specific procedures that are especially useful in program evaluations that apply the CIPP Model.

Analysis Procedures of Particular Use in Context, Input, Process, and Product Evaluations

Context, input, process, and product evaluations serve different purposes, typically involve different types of information, and, accordingly, require different analysis procedures. Table 10.2 is an advance organizer for this chapter's coverage of qualitative and quantitative analysis procedures. The table identifies a selected set of qualitative and quantitative analysis procedures and denotes (with X's) those that we see as especially applicable to analyzing information obtained from context, input, process, and product evaluations.

Analysis Procedures of Use in Context Evaluations

As discussed in Chapter 9, context evaluation collects information using such procedures as document review, interviews, surveys, site visits, hearings, study of individual cases, focus groups, time series studies, and diagnostic tests. To analyze the information gathered from such procedures, the evaluator will almost always find particularly useful the qualitative analysis technique of content analysis. Depending on the particular context evaluation, the evaluator may find it useful to analyze photographs of the program's environment and/or to systematically study filed information on a sample of individuals to be served by the program. In the latter case, the evaluator should look into individuals' records only after obtaining appropriate approvals. In context evaluations that seek to determine why an existing program is failing, the evaluator might adopt and apply the logic and methods of the pathologist's forensic analysis procedures or the modus operandi method employed by detectives.

In analyzing the information obtained from a context evaluation, the evaluator likely will also need to apply a range of quantitative methods. These methods could include calculations of: scores, rankings, ratings,

TABLE 10.2. Judgments of Selected Qualitative and Quantitative Methods' Main Applicability to Context, Input, Process, and Product Evaluations

Methods	Context Evaluations	Input Evaluations	Process Evaluations	Product Evaluations
Qualitative				
Content analysis	X	X	X	X
Photographic displays	X		X	X
Case descriptions	X		X	X
Logic model analysis		X		X
Forensic analysis	X			X
Goal-free analysis				X
Detective style, modus operandi analysis	X			X
System analysis	X	X		
Quantitative				
Scores, frequency counts, ranks, and ratings	X	X	X	X
Descriptive statistics (mean, median, mode, range, variance, standard deviation, skew, kurtosis)	X	X		X
Percentages and percentile ranks	X		X	X
Cross break tables	X	X		X
Questionnaire analysis	X		X	X
t-test	X			X
Chi-square test		X		X
Mann–Whitney *U* test	X			X
ANOVA				X
ANCOVA				X
Cost analysis		X	X	X
Trend analysis	X			X
MANOVA				X
Discriminant function analysis				X
Effect size analysis				X
Correlations and multiple correlation	X			X
Factor analysis				X
Epidemiological analysis	X			

and trend lines; means, medians, and modes; variances and standard deviations; percentages and percentiles; correlations; *t*-tests, Mann–Whitney tests; and, in health-related studies, epidemiological searches for the underlying causes of a disease. If a questionnaire has been administered to obtain stakeholder inputs, the evaluator could usefully apply a relevant computer program to analyze the questionnaire results.

In an evaluation of the effectiveness of the Motivate, Adapt and Play (MAP) project (Davis, Zhang, & Hodson, 2010), in order to determine whether there was a need for a physical activity program, the evaluators first conducted a context evaluation to examine the physical fitness levels of elementary-age students with intellectual disabilities in the area county. They analyzed the results of a literature search and concluded that (1) U.S. children were less fit than European children, (2) children with disabilities were especially at risk for poor health as a result of sedentary lifestyles, and (3) sedentary behavior in children with intellectual disabilities likely was influenced by insufficient motor or physical fitness because competence in movement is crucial to activity participation.

The evaluators also collected quantitative information to assess whether weight is associated with the fitness level of elementary-aged students with learning disabilities. The fitness measures were selected from the Brockport Physical Fitness Test (BPFT) because this test battery had been validated for study of students with learning disabilities (Winnick & Short, 1999). Five measures were chosen to assess health-related fitness: (1) body mass index (BMI), (2) the 16-meter modified Progressive Aerobic Cardiovascular Endurance Run (PACER) to measure cardiovascular endurance, (3) the modified curl-up test of abdominal strength and endurance, (4) the modified pull-up test to measure arm strength, and (5) the back-saver sit-and-reach (BSSR) test to measure flexibility.

The evaluators used SPSS procedures to obtain descriptive statistics on all five fitness measures (see Appendix 10.1) and compared the results to the FITNESSGRAM and BPFT's age-specific and gender-specific standards. The results are reported in Table 10.3. The percentages of participants who met the healthy standards are listed in the "satisfactory" column, and the percentages of participants who did not meet the standards are listed in the "unsatisfactory" column.

The average BMI of the 26 students was 19.95, a value that is close to the heavier end of the healthy

fitness zone based on the FITNESSGRAM standard. When compared to the FITNESSGRAM healthy fitness zones, roughly 19% of the students were overweight, 7% of the students were "at risk," 67% had healthy weight, and 4% were underweight. Therefore, a total of 33% had unhealthy weight and 67% had healthy weight (see Table 10.3). The 15 students ages 10–11 (because BPFT has standards for only these ages) were assessed using the BPFT standard in addition to the FITNESSGRAM standard; a total of 33% of them had unhealthy weight, while 67% had healthy weight.

To investigate whether the observed differences between students with healthy weights and those with unhealthy weights were statistically significant, a Mann–Whitney test (Mann & Whitney, 1947) was conducted to compare students with unhealthy weights and those with healthy weights regarding their performance on each of the five fitness measures (Table 10.4). The Mann–Whitney test was used instead of the commonly known *t*-test because the Mann–Whitney test is a nonparametric test that is appropriate when the sample size is small and the shape of the underlying data distribution is unclear.

The results of this study of the physical fitness levels of children with intellectual disabilities strongly indicated low fitness levels in comparison to the healthy standards set for typical students (Meredith & Welk, 2010), as well as the healthy standards for students with

TABLE 10.3. Participants' Fitness Performance Compared to FITNESSGRAM and BPFT Standards

Measures	Standards	Satisfactory (%)	Unsatisfactory (%)
BMI	FITNESSGRAM	67	33
	BPFT	67	33
PACER	FITNESSGRAM	7	93
	BPFT	60	40
Modified curl-up	FITNESSGRAM	42	58
	BPFT	33	67
Modified pull-up	FITNESSGRAM	23	77
	BPFT	13	87
BSSR	FITNESSGRAM	65	35
	BPFT	60	40

TABLE 10.4. Healthy versus Unhealthy Weight Fitness Comparisons Using the Mann–Whitney U Test

Measures	Group	N	Mean	Mann–Whitney U	p
PACER	Healthy	18	12.67	53.5	.30
	Unhealthy	8	8		
Modified curl-up	Healthy	18	12.5	50	.07
	Unhealthy	8	5.13		
Modified pull-up	Healthy	18	3.44	34	.02*
	Unhealthy	8	0.25		
BSSR right	Healthy	18	10.31	52.5	.28
	Unhealthy	8	8.43		
BSSR left	Healthy	18	9.91	53.5	.30
	Unhealthy	8	8.80		
Pedometer steps	Healthy	18	3862.30	56	.37
	Unhealthy	8	3419.87		

Note. The asterisk (*) indicates statistical significance at the alpha = .05 level.

disabilities (Winnick & Short, 1999). In all of the fitness measures obtained, high percentages of students were below the recommended minimum standards.

As already noted, 33% of the students in the study had unhealthy weight according to the FITNESS-GRAM and the BPFT standards. By the FITNESS-GRAM standard for typical students, 93% of the participants did not meet the standard for the PACER, 58% performed below the modified curl-up standard, 77% were not able to complete the minimum number of modified pull-ups, and approximately 35% did not meet the criteria for the BSSR. Similarly, by the BPFT standard for children with ID, 40% of the participants did not meet the standard for the PACER, 67% performed below the modified curl-up standard, 87% were not able to complete the minimum number of modified pull-ups, and approximately 40% did not meet the criteria for the BSSR.

The context evaluation concluded that there was a serious and urgent need to institute effective measures to promote physical activity among elementary students with intellectual disabilities.

Analysis Procedures of Use in Input Evaluations

When conducting an input evaluation, the evaluator needs to identify and assess competing program strategies and subsequently do a close analysis of the operational plan for the selected program strategy.

The information initially obtained in input evaluations includes program assessment criteria, alternative program strategies, the narrative description of each identified strategy, their projected costs, and ratings of each strategy. Following evaluation of the strategies and selection of one of them, the additional input evaluation information may include the selected program strategy, a logic model of the selected strategy, the operational plan for carrying out the strategy, provisions for internal and external evaluation, the budget, and the contract.

Accordingly, those conducting input evaluations need to employ both qualitative and quantitative analysis techniques. The qualitative techniques may include content analysis and examination of the staff's logic model (if one was developed), while the fundamental quantitative analysis will be in the form of summaries and breakouts of costs, as well as ratings of each strategy against preestablished criteria.

The main purposes of input evaluations are (1) to identify and assess system capabilities, alternative program strategies, and the chosen strategy's procedural design, budget, schedule, staffing, and stakeholder involvement plans and (2) to help assure that the selected inputs are responsive to beneficiaries' assessed needs and targeted program goals. Qualitative information analysis procedures, including content analysis and system analysis, can be especially useful in input evaluations. Quantitative analysis procedures often utilized in input evaluation include scores, means, medians, ranks, ratings, standard deviations, and cost analysis. Input evaluations that include field tests of competing alternative program approaches may usefully include chi-square tests, *t*-tests, and analyses of variance. One of the most useful analysis techniques is the **cross-break table**. One version has criteria listed down the side, options listed across the top, and some form of rating or judgment in the matrix's cells. Another version has options listed down the side, columns of strengths and weaknesses listed across the top, and brief explanations in the cells. Systematic content analysis is useful in closely examining the program's operational plan and associated budget, especially prior to submitting the plan in the form of a proposal for funding.

Analysis Procedures of Use in Process Evaluations

Process evaluation aims to identify or predict defects in the procedural design or its implementation; provide information for preprogrammed implementation decisions; affirm activities that are working well; and record and judge procedural events and activities. The information obtained for process evaluation often includes staff meetings, progress reports, expenditure reports, implementation evaluation reports, activity records, minutes of meetings, photographic records, beneficiary feedback, staff interviews, oversight personnel interviews, media releases, program website, program **listserv**, program newsletter, videotapes of program events, audiotapes, and/or field notes.

Quantitative and qualitative analysis procedures of use in analyzing process-related information may include frequency counts, content analysis, photographic analysis, various descriptive statistics, ratings, analysis of case material for selected subjects, questionnaire analysis, and cost analysis.

Analysis Procedures of Use in Product Evaluations

Product evaluation identifies intended and unintended outcomes; relates them to goals and assessed needs and to context, input, and process information; and judges the program's quality, worth, probity, equity, cost, safety, and significance.

The information gathered to answer the product evaluation questions may include milestone reports, main effects, side effects, goal-free evaluation reports, beneficiary judgments, staff self-assessments, expert judgments, external evaluation reports, observer reports, photographic records, contrast to similar projects, sustainability potential, transportability potential, accomplishment reports, program website, program listserv, program newsletter, focus groups, program hearing, diagnostic test results, survey results, rating scale results, achievement test results, organizational databases, and videotapes of observable benefits for intended beneficiaries.

An arsenal of quantitative and qualitative analysis procedures can be utilized to analyze this large variety of information for product evaluation. To analyze narrative and other qualitative evidence of program outcomes, the evaluator may use such qualitative analysis procedures as content analysis, photographic analysis, analysis of individual cases, and conceptual analysis to model how the program operated. Relevant quantitative methods for analyzing product evaluation information may include scores, frequency counts, ratings, t-tests, chi-square, trend analysis, and cost analysis, among others.

Overview of Commonly Used Statistical Procedures

An annotated list of statistical procedures commonly used in evaluation is displayed in Table 10.5. In the sections that follow, we present details of quantitative analysis procedures that are especially useful in applications of the CIPP Model.

Figure 10.2 provides a visual breakdown of the main measures of central tendency and dispersion/variation. Subsequently, we provide detailed explanations of these and related statistics.

Measures of Central Tendency

Mean

A **mean** is the arithmetic average computed by summing all the values in the dataset and dividing the sum by the number of data values. For a finite set of data with measurement values $X_1, X_2, \ldots, X_n$ (a set of n numbers), the mean is defined by the formula $(X_1 + X_2 + \ldots + X_n)/n$, or

$$\bar{X} = \frac{\sum X_i}{n}$$

Median

A **median** is the middle number in the dataset ($n/2$), when arranged in ascending order (small to large). If there are odd numbers of observation, then the median is the $(n + 1)/2$th ordered value. If there are even numbers of observation, then median is the average of the two middle values.

Mode

A **mode** is the data point that has the highest frequency (maximum occurrence). Mode is not a measure of central tendency. If the data are roughly symmetric and there are no outliers, the mean and median are roughly

TABLE 10.5. A List of Statistical Procedures Commonly Used in Evaluation

- **Descriptive statistics**: count (frequencies), minimum, maximum, percentage, mean, mode, median, range, interquartile range (IQR), standard deviation, variance, ranking
- **Visualizing categorical data**: frequency table, bar chart, pie chart
- **Visualizing numerical data**: stem-and-leaf plot, histograms, bar graphs, line graphs, scatterplots, boxplots
- **Basic inferential statistics**:
  - ▪ Comparison on categorical variable: **chi-square test**
  - ▪ Comparison on numerical variables:
    - ○ **t-test** (for comparisons between two datasets)
      - □ Independent-samples t-test
      - □ Dependent-samples t-test (correlated t-test)
    - ○ **ANOVA** (for comparisons among three or more groups or datasets)
      - □ Within-subjects ANOVA (comparisons of the same subjects under different conditions)
      - □ Between-subjects ANOVA (comparisons among different groups of subjects)
      - □ Split-plot ANOVA (aka mixed-design ANOVA; test for differences between two or more independent groups while subjecting participants to repeated measures)
    - ○ **ANCOVA** (for comparisons among three or more groups or datasets using a covariate)
    - ○ **MANOVA** (for comparisons on two or more outcome variables among three or more groups or datasets)
  - ▪ Correlational (test for association)
    - ○ **Pearson's r** (parametric, for numerical data)
    - ○ **Spearman's correlation** (nonparametric, for ordinal-type data)
    - ○ **Regression** (criterion is numerical)
    - ○ **Multiple regression** (criterion is numerical, multiple predictors)
    - ○ **Logistic regression** (criterion is categorical)
    - ○ **Multiple logistic regression** (criterion is categorical, multiple predictors)
    - ○ **Discriminant function analysis** (multiple regression equivalence for categorical criterion)
    - ○ **Factor analysis** (determine whether many variables can be described by a few factors)
    - ○ **Path analysis** (test the likelihood of a causal connection among three or more variables)
    - ○ **Structural equation modeling** (explore and possibly confirm causation among several variables)
- **Nonparametric techniques**
  - ▪ **Mann–Whitney U test** (nonparametric alternative to the t-test for analyzing ranked data)
  - ▪ **Kruskal–Wallis one-way analysis of variance** (when there are two or more independent variables to compare)
  - ▪ **Sign test** (to analyze two related samples)
  - ▪ **Friedman two-way analysis of variance** (when two or more related groups are involved)

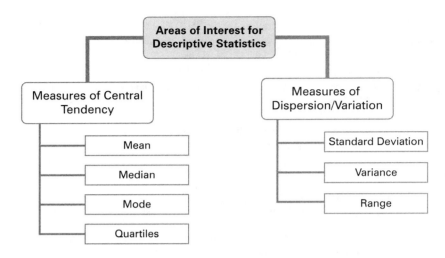

FIGURE 10.2. Breakout of main statistics of central tendency and dispersion/variation.

the same and the mean is usually used. For skewed data, the median is often used because it is resistant to outliers, whereas the mean is affected by such outliers.

Quartile Rank

A **quartile rank** is any of the three values that divide a dataset, ordered from highest to lowest values into four equal parts, so that each part/quartile represents one-fourth of the dataset.

- The first quartile (designated Q1) represents the lowest 25% of data, with the top value in this subset being labeled as the 25th percentile.
- The second quartile (designated Q2) represents the 25% of data that falls between the 25th and 51st percentiles, with the 50th percentile marking the top of the bottom half of the data.
- The third quartile (designated Q3) represents the 25% of data that falls between the 50th and 76th percentiles, with the 75th percentile marking the top of the bottom three-quarters of the data.
- The fourth quartile (designated Q4) represents the top 25% of the data.

The difference between the upper and lower quartiles is called the *interquartile range*.

Characterizations of Samples

Descriptive statistics N, Minimum, Maximum, Mean, Standard Deviation, Skewness, and Kurtosis describe the characteristics of a sample. **Skewness** provides an indication of **symmetry** of the distribution, and **kurtosis** provides information about the distribution's **"peakness."** If the distribution is perfectly normal, then Skewness and Kurtosis should be 0. The data distribution information can be used in parametric statistical techniques.

Measures of Dispersion

Standard Deviation

A **standard deviation** can be interpreted as the average distance of the individual observations from the mean. The standard deviation of the population is represented as σ. The standard deviation of the sample is represented as s:

$$s = \sqrt{\frac{\sum_{i=1}^{n}(x_i - \bar{x})^2}{n-1}}$$

where s is the standard deviation of the sample, x_i is the value of each variable in the dataset, x bar represents the mean, n is the total sample size, and $\sum$ stands for summation—that is, it says that we need to take the sum of "x_i – x bar" for all values of x.

Variance

A **variance** is defined as the square of a standard deviation. Variance of the population is represented as "σ times σ" or σ squared. Variance for the sample is represented as "s times s" or s squared:

$$s^2 = \frac{\sum_{i=0}^{n}\left(x_i - \overline{x}_i\right)^2}{n-1}$$

where s stands for standard deviation of the sample, x_i is the value of each variable in the dataset, x bar represents the mean, n is the total sample size, and $\sum$ stands for summation—that is, it says that we need to take the sum of "x_i – x bar" for all values of x.

Range

A **range** is defined as the difference between the largest and smallest values in a dataset. The *interquartile range* (IQR) is the range between the first quartile and the third quartile. Thus, the IQR contains 50% of the data. ValueMax stands for the highest (maximum) value in the dataset, and ValueMin stands for the lowest (minimum) value in the dataset.

Obtaining Descriptive Statistics Using SPSS

SPSS is a point-and-click statistical software that is easy to use even for people who are not advanced in statistical software utilization. It can be used for most statistical procedures, and descriptive statistics are the most basic ones. To obtain the descriptive statistics for the overweight and healthy weight elementary students with learning disabilities, the SPSS procedure for descriptive statistics was used (see Appendix 10.1).

Visualizing Quantitative Information

Graphically presenting evaluative information in frequency tables, bar charts, and pie charts is usually the first step in data analysis and can be a powerful and straightforward way to show an evaluation's audience the participants' performance levels on various variables. As a result, graphical presentation has been employed in many evaluation studies that applied the CIPP Model.

Visualizing Categorical Data

An evaluator needing to gain an understanding of the breakout of a categorical variable, such as the gender of the participants, and seeking to help the audience visualize and appreciate its meaning could follow the SPSS procedure for graphs presented in Appendix 10.2. A bar graph uses vertical bars to represent the data. The X-axis represents the grouping variable (e.g., gender), and the Y-axis represents frequency of occurrence.

Visualizing Numeric Data

Evaluators often use **graphs** to help the audience visualize numeric data. The ways to visually present numeric data frequently include stem-and-leaf plot, histograms, bar graphs, line graphs, scatterplots, and boxplots.

Stem-and-Leaf

Stem-and-leaf is a device for presenting quantitative data in a graphical format, similar to a histogram, to assist in visualizing the shape of a distribution. A stem-and-leaf plot can be regarded as a special table where each data value is split into a "stem" (the first digit or digits) and a "leaf" (usually the last digit). The evaluator (Zhang) for a Math Science Partnership (MSP) project followed the procedures in Appendix 10.3 to create a stem-and-leaf plot for a numerical variable, teachers' math content knowledge (variable name: Knowledge) during a context evaluation.

Histograms

Histograms are used to display the distribution of a single continuous variable, such as "math content knowledge." It can generate separate histograms for different groups (e.g., male/female). See the example histogram in Appendix 10.4, which was created through use of SPSS.

Bar Graphs

Bar graphs can visually display the numerical variable of interest, such as math content knowledge, by groups of participants, such as male and female teachers (variable, "gender"), and age group (variable, "age group"). See Appendix 10.5 for applicable SPSS procedures.

Line Graphs

Line graphs allow evaluators to inspect the mean scores of a continuous variable across a number of different values of a categorical variable (e.g., time 1, time 2, time 3). Line graphs are also useful for graphically exploring the results of ANOVA. Line graphs are provided as an optional extra in the output of ANOVA. In the MSP project example, the evaluator could look at the trend in content knowledge of female and male teachers prior to the MSP project, during the project, and after the project (see Appendix 10.6).

Scatterplots

Scatterplots are used to explore the relationship between two continuous variables (e.g., age and income). It is a good idea to generate scatterplots before calculating correlations. The scatterplots indicate whether the subject variables are related in a linear or curvilinear fashion. Only linear relationships are suitable for correlational analyses. The scatterplot will also indicate whether the variables are positively correlated (high scores on one variable are associated with high scores on the other) or negatively correlated (high scores on one variable are associated with low scores on the other). The scatterplot indicates the strength of the relationship between two variables (a cigar shape with definite clumping of scores around an imaginary straight line indicates a strong relationship). During the input evaluation, the evaluator for the MAP project looked at the relationship between students' numbers of steps and their BMI (Davis, Hodson, et al., 2010). See the SPSS procedure for scatterplots that was followed in Appendix 10.7. The generated scatterplot indicates the strength of the correlation between steps and BMI scores. Be advised that a scatterplot does not give definitive answers about a correlation's strength. Accordingly, one typically needs to calculate the appropriate statistic. If there is no indication of a curvilinear relationship, then it is okay to calculate a Pearson product–moment correlation.

Boxplots

Boxplots are useful for evaluators to display the distribution of scores on a variable. As shown in Figure 10.3, the distribution of scores is represented by a box and

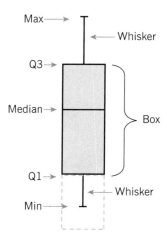

FIGURE 10.3. A boxplot.

whiskers. Each box contains 50% of the cases, and the line inside the box represents the median. The whiskers go out to the variable's largest and smallest values. The outliers appear as little circles with the ID number of the case attached. Boxplots can also be used to compare the distributions of two groups of scores, such as male and female students' pacer scores. Boxplots indicate variability in scores within each group and allow visual inspection of the differences between groups. See Appendix 10.8 for SPSS procedures for creating boxplots.

Basic Inferential Statistics

t-Tests

The **t-test** is a parametric statistical test used to see whether a difference between the means of two samples is significant. There are two forms of t-tests: independent-samples t-tests and dependent-samples t-tests.

Independent-Samples t-Tests

Independent-samples t-tests are used to assess whether there is a statistically significant difference between the means of two randomized, independent samples. Such a test is used to compare the mean scores, on some continuous variable, for two different groups of participants: for example, male and female (variable: gender). Refer to Appendix 10.9 to carry out the SPSS procedures for independent-samples t-tests.

Dependent-Samples t-Tests

A dependent-samples t-test—also referred to as t-test for correlated observations, within-subjects t-test, or paired-samples t-test—is used to assess whether the t-statistic obtained from a single sample's set of paired difference or gain scores is statistically significant. In such a test, each subject serves as her or his own control. An example of this type of test is seen in a hypothetical case in which an evaluator would carry out a t-test for correlated observations to determine whether a group of soldiers attained better post-course rifle range scores than those they earned prior to reading and being instructed in the contents of a marksmanship manual. In this example, the evaluator would compare the obtained t-statistic to a preset level of statistical significance (e.g., .05).

This type of t-test is frequently used when one has only one group of subjects and collects data from them on two different occasions or under two different conditions. Pretest/posttest experimental designs are an example of this type of situation. This approach is also used when one has matched pairs of participants (i.e., each person is matched with another on specific criteria, such as age). One of the pairs is exposed to intervention and the other is not. Scores on a continuous measure are then compared for each pair. Paired-samples t-tests can also be used when one measures the same person in terms of his or her response to two different questions and both questions are rated on the same scale. Refer to Appendix 10.9 for the SPSS procedure for the paired-samples t-test.

In the MAP project evaluation example, the evaluator compared the participants' posttest scores and pretest scores on each fitness measure with a paired-samples t-test (see Table 10.6).

Effect Size Analysis

Effect size analyses examine the magnitude of an identified effect. Below we explain this concept in relation to t-tests for independent samples and correlated samples.

Effect Size Analysis for Independent-Samples t-Test

The results from an independent samples t-test may tell us that the difference in the two sets of scores was unlikely to occur by chance; that is, they are significantly different from each other. However, such an analysis

TABLE 10.6. Paired-Samples t-Test of Student Performance before and after the MAP Program (N = 25)

Measures	Assessment	Mean	SD	t	df	p	ES (d)
BMI	Before	19.96	5.92	.056	24	.956	.01
	After	19.94	5.71				
PACER	Before	10.28	11.72	2.69	24	.013*	.55
	After	13.24	10.89				
Modified curl-up	Before	7.12	11.80	2.089	24	.048*	.42
	After	12.64	10.55				
Medicine ball throw	Before	101.52	73.92	2.081	24	.048*	.42
	After	129.08	80.02				
Sit-and-reach right	Before	23.08	7.49	4.278	24	.000*	.882
	After	27.10	8.67				
Sit-and-reach left	Before	21.86	7.84	5.329	24	.000*	1.07
	After	26.68	8.07				

Note. N = 25. The asterisk (*) indicates statistical significance. ES, effect size; d, Cohen's d.

does not tell us the magnitude of the difference. One way to determine the magnitude of the difference is to calculate an effect size. There are multiple different effect size statistics, the most commonly used being the eta squared. Eta squared can range from 0 to 1 and represents the proportion of variance in the dependent variable that is explained by the independent variable. SPSS does not provide eta-squared values for t-tests. However, it can be calculated using the information provided in the output:

$$\text{Eta squared} = t^2/[t^2 + (N1 + N2 - 2)]$$

Then compare the obtained eta-squared value to Cohen's criterion for eta squared (Cohen, 1988, pp. 284–287): 0.01 = small effect, 0.06 = moderate effect, and 0.14 = large effect.

Effect Size Analysis for Paired-Samples t-Test

Although the results from the paired-samples t-test tell us that the difference in the two sets of scores was unlikely to occur by chance—that is, they are significantly different from each other—they do not tell us how much the difference is—that is, the magnitude of the intervention effect. One way to gain an understanding of the magnitude of the effect is to calculate an effect size, eta squared:

$$\text{Eta squared} = t^2/[t^2 + (N - 1)]$$

Compare the obtained eta-squared value with Cohen's criterion for eta squared (Cohen, 1988, pp. 284–287): 0.01 = small effect, 0.06 = moderate effect, and 0.14 = large effect.

Chi-Square Test

A **chi-square test** for independence is used when evaluators wish to explore the relationship between two categorical variables, each with two or more categories. Evaluators may use such a test to examine whether a statistically significant difference exists between observed and expected frequencies within one or more categories. For example, an evaluator might use a chi-squared test to test the hypothesis that the percentages of a community's residents with no high school diploma, a high school diploma, or a college degree are the same as was the case in the community a decade ago.

Here is another example an evaluator might ask: Is there an association between gender and drinking alcohol? In other words, are males more likely to be alcohol drinkers than females?

This evaluator would need two categorical variables, with two or more categories in each:

- Gender (male/female)
- Drinker (yes/no)

And the lowest expected frequency in any cell should be 5 or more. Refer to Appendix 10.11 to carry out the SPSS procedures for the chi-square test for independence.

Once the output is obtained, in the "Chi-Square Tests" table,

- Look at the Pearson chi-square value and the sig. value for significance.
- For a two by two table, use the Continuity correction (Yates' correction) values instead of the Pearson chi-square values.

In the "Symmetric Measures" table, look at the effect size phi coefficient, and compare its value to Cohen's (1988) criteria of 0.10 for small effect, 0.30 for medium effect, and 0.50 for large effect.

Analysis of Variance

Analysis of variance (ANOVA) is used to determine if statistically significant differences exist among means of three or more sets of scores. We use t-tests to compare the scores of two different groups or conditions. In many evaluation situations, however, we are interested in comparing the mean scores of more than two groups. In these cases, we would use ANOVA, which compares the variance between the different groups (believed to be due to the independent variable) to the variability within each of the groups (believed to be due to chance). The ANOVA F-statistic is a ratio of the between-group variance to the within-group variance:

$$F = MS_{\text{between}}/MS_{\text{within}}$$

A large F is evidence *against* H_0, since it indicates that there is more difference between groups than within groups.

Between-subjects ANOVA, also called between-groups ANOVA, should be used when there are different participants in each of the groups. Within-subjects ANOVA, often known as repeated-measures ANOVA, is used when you are measuring the same participants under different conditions or at different time points.

Why Not Multiple t-Tests?

- The major problem is that the *t*-tests are not independent of one another. (If *A* is significantly better than *B,* and *B* is better than *C,* then we already know that *A* is better than *C.*)
- The lack of independence with multiple *t*-tests results in unknown type I error rate (no longer 0.05). The probability of committing at least one type I error in an analysis is called the experiment-wise error rate (EER) or family-wise error rate (FWR). ANOVA is an attempt to maintain the FWR at a known (acceptable) level.
- The number of *t*-tests needed increases geometrically as a function of the number of groups, which makes analysis cognitively difficult. ANOVA organizes and directs the analysis, allowing easier interpretation of results.

Assumptions of ANOVA

- *Independence:* The score for any particular subject is independent of the scores of all other subjects; that is, it provides a unique piece of information about the treatment effect.
- *Normality:* The scores within each treatment population are normally distributed. ANOVA is robust to departures from normality, although the data should be symmetric.
- *Homogeneity of variances:* The variances of scores in each treatment population are equal.

One-Way ANOVA

One-way ANOVA involves one independent variable (referred to as a factor), which has a number of different levels. These levels correspond to the different groups or conditions. For example, in comparing the effectiveness of three different methods of instruction on students' reading scores, there is one factor (teach-ing method) with three levels (e.g., whole class, small group, and self-paced). The dependent variable is a continuous variable (reading scores). In a between-subjects design, different individuals are assigned to different groups (one level of independent variable). In a within-subjects design: all the participants are exposed to all levels of the conditions.

One-Way Between-Groups ANOVA

One-way between-groups ANOVA involves one categorical independent (grouping) variable with three or more levels (groups) and one continuous dependent variable. In the example, is there a difference in depression scores for white, black, and Hispanic participants? The independent variable is "ethnicity" (white, black, Hispanic), and the dependent variable is "depression" (depression scores). The SPSS procedures provided in Appendix 10.12 can be used to perform a one-way between-subjects ANOVA with **post-hoc tests**.

In the SPSS Output, the "descriptives" table gives information about each group. Always check this table first. The test of homogeneity of variances explores whether the variance in scores is the same for each of the three groups. In the "Test of Homogeneity of Variance" table, check the **significance** value (sig.) for Levene Statistic. If sig. >.05, then the data did not violate the assumption of homogeneity of variance, and you can use the results in the ANOVA table. However, if Levene Statistic sig. < .05, then use the results in the table headed "Robust Tests of Equality of Means" (Welch and Brown-Forsythe) because the data violated the homogeneity of variance assumption.

The ANOVA table provides the values for sum of squares, df, Mean Square, F, and sig. If sig. <= .05, there is a significant difference somewhere among the mean scores on your dependent variable for the three groups. You can then look at the "Multiple Comparisons" table in the output to see the results of the post-hoc tests. Under the "Mean Difference" column, anything with an * means that the two groups being compared are significantly different from one another at the $p < .05$ level.

Calculating Effect Size

SPSS does not generate effect size for this analysis, but it can be calculated using the information provided in the ANOVA table. The formula is

$$\text{Eta squared} = \frac{\text{Sum of squares between groups}}{\text{Total sum of squares}}$$

We can then compare the obtained eta squared to Cohen's criteria: 0.01 as a small effect, 0.06 as a medium effect, and 0.14 as a large effect (Cohen, 1988, pp. 284–287).

One-Way Within-Group ANOVA with Post-Hoc Tests

For product evaluation, evaluators often need to compare the performance of participants before, during, and after an intervention, and find out which mean scores differ significantly. This can be done with a one-way within-group ANOVA with post-hoc tests. In a one-way within-group (repeated measures) ANOVA, each subject is exposed to two or more conditions or measured on the same continuous scale on three or more occasions.

Example evaluation question: Is there a change in participants' reading efficacy over the 3 years of the reading intervention? In this example, there is one independent variable (Categorical) (e.g., year 1, year 2, year 3) and one dependent variable (continuous) reading efficacy scores at year 1, 2, and 3: efficacy1, efficacy2, efficacy3. See Appendix 10.13 for the procedure for one-way within-group (repeated measures) ANOVA used in this example.

In the SPSS output, the descriptive statistics provide information on the means, standard deviations, and the N. We need to look at the output table with the heading "Mauchly's Test of Sphericity" to check the sphericity test results. The univariate statistic requires sphericity. The sphericity assumption requires that the variance of the population difference scores for any two conditions are the same as the variance of the population difference scores for any other two conditions. When the sphericity asssumption is violated (sig. <= .05), we need to look at the multivariate ANOVA results instead of the univariate ANOVA results.

In the "Multivariate Tests" table, Wilks' lambda is commonly reported. Sig. <= .05 indicates significance, and we can conclude that there is a statistically significant effect for time: there was a change in reading efficacy scores across the 3-year periods of reading intervention.

A significant result from the ANOVA analysis suggests that there is a difference somewhere among your sets of scores (year 1, year 2, year 3). The "Pairwise Comparisons" output table tells you which pair of time

points differs significantly. "Mean Differences" with an * next to it represents that the pairs being compared are significantly different.

Two-Way Between-Groups ANOVA

Two-way means that there are *two independent variables* (e.g., age, gender), and one dependent variable (e.g., confidence), *Between-groups* indicates that different subjects are in each of the groups. There are two **main effects**: comparing the means of the various levels of an independent variable. Each independent variable has its own main effect (e.g., main effect of age, main effect of gender). There is one possible **interaction effect**, which reflects the effect associated with the various combinations of two independent variables (e.g., the influence of age on confidence levels depends on whether you are male or female). Two-way between-groups ANOVA can test the main effect for each independent variable and explore possible interaction effects.

Example evaluation question: Do self-confidence levels differ across age group and gender? In this example, there are two independent variables: Age (age group) and Gender (gender). There is one dependent variable: self-confidence (confidence). See Appendix 10.14, the SPSS procedure for two-way between-groups ANOVA.

In the SPSS output table labeled "Descriptive Statistics," we can look at the mean, standard deviations, and N for patterns. Then we look at "Levene's Test of Equality of Error Variances" table; if sig. > .05, it indicates the equality of variance assumption was not violated.

In the "Tests of Between-Subjects Effects" table, first, check if there is a significant interaction effect (sig. <= .05) (e.g., the influence of age on self-confidence levels depends on whether you are male or female). If you find a significant interaction effect, you should interpret the interaction effect and should not interpret the main effect. If interaction effect is not significant, then you can interpret the main effects.

Effect Size for Two-Way Between-Groups ANOVA

The effect sizes for two-way between-groups ANOVA are directly provided in the SPSS output, under the "partial eta squared" column. The output table labeled "Multiple Comparisons" tells you where the differences occur. Only look at this table if you have obtained a significant main effect or interaction effect. In the "Multiple Comparisons" table, a mean difference value marked with an * indicates a significant difference on the dependent variable (e.g., self-confidence) between two comparison groups at the .05 level.

Analysis of Covariance

Analysis of covariance (ANCOVA) is an extension of ANOVA. It allows evaluators to explore differences between groups while statistically controlling for an additional continuous variable(s) (covariates). The **covariate** is a variable that we suspect may be influencing scores on the dependent variable. SPSS uses the regression procedure to remove the variation in the dependent variable that is due to the covariate(s) and then performs analysis of variance. By removing the influence of the additional variable(s), ANCOVA can increase the power or sensitivity of the F-test. When covariate scores are available, we have information about differences between treatment groups that existed before the experiment was performed. ANCOVA uses linear regression to estimate the size of treatment effects given the covariate information. The adjustment for group differences can either increase or decrease, depending on the dependent variable's relationship with the covariate.

ANCOVA can be particularly useful for two-group pretest–posttest design (comparing the impact of two different interventions, taking before and after measures for each group). Also, it works for situations when it is impossible to randomly assign participants into different groups, but instead have to use existing groups (existing classes of students).

To choose appropriate covariates, one should have a good understanding of the theory and existing research. The covariates should be continuous variables, measured reliably, and correlate significantly with the dependent variable. Ideally, choose a small set of covariates that are only moderately correlated with one another, so that each contributes uniquely to the variance explained. Covariates must be measured before the treatment is performed to prevent covariate scores from being influenced by the treatment.

Assumptions of ANCOVA

The assumptions of ANCOVA include all three assumptions common to ANOVA and four assumptions specific to ANCOVA:

- Independence: An individual's scores on the covariate and dependent variable are independent of all other subjects.
- Normality: For an individual with the same score on the covariate in the same group, the dependent variable has a normal distribution.
- Homogeneity of variances
- Linear regression (between the dependent variable and covariate)
- Homogeneity of regression coefficients
- Independence of covariate and treatment
- Reliability of covariate (Cronbach's alpha > .70)

Performing One-way ANCOVA

Example research question: Is there a difference in the Math Anxiety test scores for the math skills-building group (group 1) and the anxiety counseling group (group 2) while controlling for their pretest scores on this test? In this example, there are three variables:

- One independent categorical variable with two or more levels or conditions (group 1 = math skills building, group 2 = anxiety counseling)
- One dependent continuous variable (Math Anxiety Test posttest score)
- One continuous covariate (Math Anxiety Test pretest score)

See Appendix 10.15 for the detailed processes and procedures for checking assumptions and performing a one-way ANCOVA in SPSS.

Analysis of Associations

In contrast to analysis procedures for examining differences between measures for two or more groups are a set of procedures for examining association, especially correlation between sets of data. We summarize the main tests for examining associations below.

Pearson's r

Pearson's r, also known as the Pearson product-moment correlation coefficient, is a measure of the linear correlation (dependence) between two numerical variables X and Y, giving a value between +1 and –1 inclusive, where 1 is total positive correlation, 0 is no correlation, and –1 is total negative correlation. It is widely used in the sciences as a measure of the degree of linear dependence between two variables. It was developed by Karl Pearson (1857–1936) in the 1880s.

Spearman's Correlation

Spearman's correlation, or Spearman's rho, is a nonparametric measure of statistical dependence between two ranked variables. Named after Charles Spearman (1863–1945) and often denoted by the Greek letter ρ, it assesses how well the relationship between two variables can be described using a monotonic function. If there are no repeated data values, a perfect Spearman correlation of +1 or –1 occurs when each of the variables is a perfect monotone function of the other. Spearman's coefficient is appropriate for both continuous and discrete variables, including ordinal variables.

Regression

Regression analysis is a statistical process for estimating the relationships among variables. More specifically, regression analysis helps you understand how the typical value of the dependent variable (or "criterion variable") changes when any one of the independent variables is varied, while the other independent variables are held fixed. Most commonly, regression analysis estimates the conditional expectation of the dependent variable given the independent variables—that is, the average value of the dependent variable when the independent variables are fixed. In all cases, the estimation target is a function of the independent variables called the regression function. In regression analysis, it is also of interest to characterize the variation of the dependent variable around the regression function, which can be described by a probability distribution.

Multiple Regression

Multiple regression is an extension of simple linear regression. It is used when we want to predict the value of a numerical outcome variable based on the value of two or more other variables (predictors). For example, you could use multiple regression to understand whether exam performance can be predicted based on IQ, study time, test anxiety, school attendance, and gender. Multiple regression also allows you to determine the overall

fit (variance explained) of the model and the relative contribution of each of the predictors to the total variance explained.

Logistic Regression

Logistic regression analysis is a widely used analysis procedure that is similar to linear regression analysis except that the outcome is dichotomous (e.g., success/failure or yes/no or died/lived). That is, logistic regression is a regression model where the dependent variable (DV) is categorical. Cases with more than two categories are referred to as multinomial logistic regression, or, if the multiple categories are ordered, as ordinal logistic regression. For example, we could use simple logistic regression to understand whether pass/fail on an exam can be predicted based on study time. Logistic regression was developed by statistician David Cox in 1958.

Other Quantitative Information Analyses

In the previous sections, we explored the use of basic and commonly used quantitative information analyses. Beyond those, there are some basic, intermediate, and advanced quantitative analysis procedures that we would like to briefly introduce here. Detailed coverage of these procedures can be found in many statistical books (e.g., Agresti & Finlay, 1997; Borenstein, Hedges, Higgins, & Rothstein, 2009; Cohen, 1988; Fraenkel & Wallen, 2011; Freund & Simon, 1997; Hancock & Mueller, 2010; Hosmer & Lemeshow, 2000; Grissom & Kim, 2005; Myers & Well, 2003; Pallant, 2010; Sheskin, 2007; Zhang & Algina, 2008, 2011).

Mann–Whitney U Test

The **Mann–Whitney U test** is a nonparametric alternative to the t-test used when a researcher wishes to analyze ranked data. It is a test of the null hypothesis that two samples come from the same population against an alternative hypothesis, especially that a particular population tends to have larger values than the other. It can be applied on unknown distributions contrary to a t-test, which has to be applied only on normal distributions, and it is nearly as efficient as the t-test on normal distributions. The Wilcoxon rank-sum test is not the same as the Wilcoxon signed-rank test, although both are nonparametric and involve summation of ranks.

Multivariate Analysis of Variance

Multivariate analysis of variance (MANOVA) is an extension of the analysis of variance when you have more than one dependent variable. These dependent variables should be related in some way, or there should be some conceptual reason for considering them together. MANOVA compares the groups and lets you know whether the mean differences between the groups on the combination of dependent variables are likely due to chance. To do this, MANOVA creates a new summary dependent variable, which is a linear combination of each of the original dependent variables. Readers are referred to Pallant (2010) for more information about MANOVA and how to conduct MANOVA analysis.

Multiple Logistic Regression

While simple logistic regression analysis refers to the regression application with one dichotomous outcome and one independent variable, **multiple logistic regression** analysis applies when there is a single dichotomous outcome and more than one independent variable (more than one predictor). For example, we could use logistic regression to understand whether pass/fail on an exam can be predicted based on IQ, study time, test anxiety, school attendance, and gender.

Discriminant Function Analysis

Discriminant function analysis is a statistical analysis to predict a categorical dependent variable (called a grouping variable) by one or more continuous or binary independent variables (called predictor variables). The original dichotomous discriminant analysis was developed by Sir Ronald Fisher (1890–1962) in 1936. It is different from an ANOVA or MANOVA, which is used to predict one (ANOVA) or multiple (MANOVA) continuous dependent variables by one or more independent categorical variables. Discriminant function analysis is useful in determining whether a set of variables is effective in predicting category membership. Discriminant analysis is used when groups are known a priori (unlike in cluster analysis). In simple terms, discriminant function analysis is classification—the act of distributing things into groups, classes, or categories of the same type. Moreover, it is a useful follow-up procedure to a MANOVA, instead of doing a series of one-way ANOVAs, for ascertaining how the groups differ on the composite of dependent variables.

Factor Analysis

Factor analysis is a statistical method used to describe variability among observed, correlated variables in terms of a potentially lower number of unobserved variables called factors. For example, it is possible that variations in four observed variables mainly reflect the variations in two unobserved variables (called latent variables). Factor analysis searches for such joint variations in response to unobserved latent variables. The observed variables are modeled as linear combinations of the potential factors, plus "error" terms. The information gained about the interdependencies between observed variables can be used later to reduce the set of variables in a dataset. Factor analysis is related to principal component analysis, but the two are not identical. Latent variable models, including factor analysis, use regression modeling techniques to test hypotheses producing error terms, while principal component analysis is a descriptive statistical technique.

Principal Component Analysis

Principal component analysis (PCA) is a technique used to emphasize variation and bring out strong patterns in a dataset. It is often used to make data easy to explore and visualize. PCA involves a mathematical procedure that transforms a number of (possibly) correlated variables into a (smaller) number of uncorrelated variables called principal components. The first principal component accounts for as much of the variability in the data as possible, and each succeeding component accounts for as much of the remaining variability as possible.

Path Analysis

Path analysis is a straightforward extension of multiple regression. Its aim is to provide estimates of the magnitude and significance of hypothesized causal connections between sets of variables. Path analysis is used to describe the directed dependencies among a set of variables. This includes models equivalent to any form of multiple regression analysis, factor analysis, canonical correlation analysis, discriminant analysis, as well as more general families of models in the multivariate analysis of variance and covariance analyses (MANOVA, ANOVA, ANCOVA). In addition to being thought of as a form of multiple regression focusing on causality, path analysis can be viewed as a special case of structural equation modeling—one in which only single indicators are employed for each of the variables in the causal model. That is, path analysis is structural equation modeling with a structural model, but no measurement model. Other terms used to refer to path analysis include causal modeling, analysis of covariance structures, and latent variable models.

Structural Equation Modeling

Structural equation modeling (SEM) is a family of statistical methods designed to test a conceptual or theoretical model to explore and possibly confirm causation among several variables. Some common SEM methods include confirmatory factor analysis, path analysis, and latent growth modeling. The term *structural equation model* most commonly refers to a combination of two things: a measurement model that defines latent variables using one or more observed variables, and a structural regression model that links latent variables together. The parts of a structural equation model are linked to one another using a system of simultaneous regression equations. SEM is widely used in the social sciences because of its ability to isolate observational error from measurement of latent variables.

Kruskal–Wallis One-Way Analysis of Variance

The **Kruskal–Wallis one-way analysis of variance** (named after William Kruskal [1919–2005] and W. Allen Wallis [1912–1998]) is a nonparametric method for testing whether samples originate from the same distribution, and its parametric equivalent is one-way ANOVA. It is used for comparing two or more samples that are independent and that may have different sample sizes, and it extends the Mann–Whitney U test to more than two groups. When rejecting the null hypothesis of the Kruskal–Wallis test, then at least one sample stochastically dominates at least one other sample. The test does not identify where this stochastic dominance occurs or for how many pairs of groups stochastic dominance obtains. Dunn's test would help analyze the specific sample pairs for stochastic dominance. Since it is a nonparametric method, the Kruskal–Wallis test

does not assume a normal distribution of the residuals, unlike the analogous one-way analysis of variance.

Sign Test

The **sign test** is a statistical method to test for consistent differences between pairs of observations, such as the weight of subjects before and after treatment. Given pairs of observations (e.g., weight pre- and posttreatment) for each subject, the sign test determines if one member of the pair (such as pretreatment) tends to be greater than (or less than) the other member of the pair (posttreatment). The paired observations may be designated x and y. For comparisons of paired observations (x,y), the sign test is most useful if comparisons can only be expressed as $x > y$, $x = y$, or $x < y$. If, instead, the observations can be expressed as numeric quantities ($x = 7$, $y = 18$), or as ranks (rank of $x = $ 1st, rank of $y = $ 8th), then the paired t-test or the Wilcoxon signed-rank test will usually have greater power than the sign test to detect consistent differences.

Friedman Two-Way Analysis of Variance

The **Friedman two-way analysis of variance** is a nonparametric statistical test developed by the U.S. economist Milton Friedman (1912–2006). Similar to the parametric repeated measures ANOVA, it is used to detect differences in treatments across multiple test attempts. The procedure involves ranking each row (or block) together, then considering the values of ranks by columns. Applicable to complete block designs, it is thus a special case of the Durbin test. The Friedman test is used for one-way repeated measures analysis of variance by ranks. In its use of ranks, it is similar to the Kruskal–Wallis one-way analysis of variance by ranks. The Friedman test is widely supported by many statistical software packages.

We turn now to the important topic of how to choose between a parametric test and a nonparametric test.

Choosing between a Nonparametric Test and a Parametric Test

Most evaluators are more familiar with parametric analyses than nonparametric analyses. **Nonparametric tests** are also called distribution-free tests because they don't assume that your data follow a specific distribution. Generally, one should use nonparametric tests when the data don't meet the assumptions of the parametric test, especially the assumption about normally distributed data. But there are additional considerations. It also should be kept in mind that the parametric analysis tests group means, while nonparametric analysis tests group medians.

Reasons to Use Parametric Tests

Parametric tests can perform well with skewed and non-normal distributions if one satisfies the sample size guidelines shown in Table 10.7. Parametric tests can also perform well when the spread of each group is different. While nonparametric tests don't assume that one's data follow a normal distribution, they do have other assumptions that can be hard to meet. For nonparametric tests that compare groups, a common assumption is that data for all groups must have the same spread (dispersion). If your groups have different spreads, the nonparametric tests might not provide valid results. On the other hand, if you use the two-sample *t*-test or one-way ANOVA, you can simply go to the Options subdialog in SPSS and uncheck *Assume equal variances*. Voilà, you are good to go even when the groups have different spreads! Importantly, parametric tests usually have more statistical power than nonparametric tests. Thus, you are more likely to detect a significant effect when one truly exists.

Reasons to Use Nonparametric Tests

First, if your area of study is better represented by the median, then you should use nonparametric tests. For example, the center of a skewed distribution, like income, can be better measured by the median where 50% are above the median and 50% are below. If you

add a few billionaires to a sample, the mathematical mean increases greatly even though the income for the typical person doesn't change.

Second, in this case the sample size is very small. If you do not meet the sample size guidelines for the parametric tests and are not confident that the data are normally distributed, it is best to use a nonparametric test. When your sample is very small, it might not even be possible to ascertain the distribution of the data because the distribution tests would lack sufficient power to provide meaningful results. In this **scenario,** the investigator is in a tough spot, with no valid alternative. Nonparametric tests have less power to begin with, and it is a double whammy when, on top of that, the sample size is very small!

Third, if you have ordinal data, ranked data, or outliers that can't be removed, then it is best to use a nonparametric test. Typical parametric tests can only assess continuous data, and the results can be significantly affected by outliers. Conversely, some nonparametric tests can handle ordinal data, ranked data, and not be seriously affected by outliers. You should be sure to check the assumptions for the nonparametric test because each one has its own data requirements.

Procedures for Analyzing Qualitative Information

Qualitative information is commonly collected and highly useful in CIPP evaluations. Qualitative analysis is often needed in all of the context, input, process, and product evaluations. Formal qualitative data analysis became a practice in the early 20th century (Johnson & Christensen, 2000). The process of qualitative data analysis involves making sense out of text and image data. Data analysis begins early in a qualitative study. The evaluator alternates between data collection and data analysis (meaning from raw data). Creswell (2014) explains that qualitative data analysis "involves preparing the data for analysis, moving deeper and deeper into understanding of the data (some qualitative researchers like to think of this as peeling back the layers of an onion), representing the data, and making an interpretation of the larger meaning of the data" (p. 183). It is an ongoing process that involves continual reflection about the data, asking analytic questions, and writing memos throughout the study (Creswell, 2013).

Creswell (2014) sees qualitative data analysis as an ongoing process involving continual reflection about the data, asking analytic questions, and writing memos throughout the study. He goes further by saying that

TABLE 10.7. Sample Size Guidelines for Parametric Tests

Parametric Analyses	Sample Size Guidelines for Non-normal Data
One-sample *t*-test	Greater than 20
Two-sample *t*-test	Each group should be greater than 15.
One-way ANOVA	• If you have two to nine groups, each group should be greater than 15. • If you have 10 to 12 groups, each group should be greater than 20.

"qualitative data analysis is conducted concurrently with gathering data, making interpretations, and writing reports" (p. 184).

While many qualitative data reported in journal articles and books are of a generic form of analysis, recently many researchers have gone beyond this generic analysis to add a procedure within the specific strategies of qualitative inquiry:

- Grounded theory has systematic steps (Corbin & Strauss, 2007) that involve generating categories of information (open coding), selecting one of the categories and positioning it within a theoretical model (axial coding), and then explicating a story from the interconnection of these categories (selective coding).

- Case study and ethnographic research involve a detailed description of the setting or individuals, followed by analysis of the data for themes or issues (Stake, 1995; Wolcott, 1994).

- Phenomenological research utilizes the analysis of significant statements, the generation of meaning units, and the development of an essence description (Moustakas, 1994).

- Narrative research uses re-storying the participants' stories using structural devices such as plot, setting, activities, climax, and denouement (Clandinin & Connelly, 2000).

Despite the existing analytic differences based on the type of strategies, qualitative inquiries largely use a general procedure, and an ideal situation is to blend the general steps with the specific research strategy steps. Creswell (2014, pp. 185–186) urges researchers to look at qualitative data analysis as following steps from the specific to the general and as involving multiple levels of analysis (pp. 185–186).

• *Step 1. Organize and prepare data for analysis.* This involves transcribing interviews, optically scanning materials, typing up field notes, or sorting and arranging the data into different types depending on the sources of information.

• *Step 2. Read through all the data.* A first step is to obtain a general sense of the information and to reflect on its overall meaning. What general ideas are participants expressing? What is the impression of the overall depth, credibility, and use of the information?

Sometimes qualitative researchers write notes in margins or start recording general thoughts about the data at this stage.

• *Step 3. Begin detailed analysis with a coding process.* Coding is the process of organizing the material into chunks or segments of text before bringing meaning to information (Rossman & Rallis, 1998, p. 171). It involves taking text data or pictures gathered during data collection, segmenting sentences (or paragraphs) or images into categories, and labeling those categories with a term. Often, a term is based on the actual language of the participant (called an *in vivo* term). The detailed guidance for the coding process provided by Tesch (1990) engages researchers in a systematic process of analyzing textual data (see Table 10.8).

Bogdan and Biklen (1992, pp. 166–172) suggested the types of codes to look for in a qualitative database:

- Setting and context codes
- Perpectives held by subjects
- Subjects' ways of thinking about people and objects
- Process codes
- Activity codes
- Strategy codes
- Relationship and social structure codes
- Preassigned coding schemes

• *Step 4. Use the coding process to generate a description of the setting or people as well as categories or themes for analysis. Description* involves a detailed rendering of information about people, places, or events in a setting. Researchers can generate codes for this description. This analysis is useful in designing detailed descriptions for case studies, ethnographies, and narrative research projects. Then use the coding to generate a small number of themes or categories, perhaps five to seven categories for a research study. These themes are the ones that appear as major findings in qualitative studies and are often used to create headings in the findings sections of studies. They should display multiple perspectives from individuals and be supported by diverse quotations and specific evidence.

Beyond identifying the themes during the coding process, qualitative researchers can do much with themes to build additional layers of complex analysis.

TABLE 10.8. The Eight-Step Coding Process Recommended by Tesch

1. **Get a sense of the whole.** Read all the transcript carefully. Perhaps jot down some ideas as they come to mind.

2. **Pick one document** (i.e., one interview)—the most interesting one, the shortest, the one on the top of the pile. Go through it, asking yourself, "What is this about?" Do not think about the substance of the information but its underlying meaning. Write thoughts in the margin.

3. **When you have completed this task for several participants, make a list of all topics.** Cluster together similar topics. Form these topics into columns, perhaps arrayed as major topics, unique topics, and leftovers.

4. **Now take this list and go back to your data.** Abbreviate the topics as codes and write the codes next to the appropriate segments of the text. Try this preliminary organizing scheme to see if new categories and codes emerge.

5. **Find the most descriptive wording for your topics and turn them into categories.** Look for ways of reducing your total list of categories by grouping topics that relate to each other. Perhaps draw lines between your categories to show interrelationships.

6. **Make a final decision on the abbreviation for each category and alphabetize these codes.**

7. **Assemble the data material belonging to each category in one place and perform a preliminary analysis.**

8. **If necessary, recode your existing data.**

Note. Excerpted from Tesch (1990, pp. 142–145).

For example, researchers interconnect themes into a storyline (as in narratives) or develop them into a theoretical model (as in grounded theory). Themes are analyzed for each individual case and across different cases (as in case studies) or shaped into a general description (as in phenomenology). Sophisticated qualitative studies go beyond descriptions and theme identification and into complex theme connections.

• *Step 5. Advance how the description and themes will be presented in the qualitative narrative.* The most popular approach is to use a narrative passage to convey the findings of the analysis. This might be a discussion that mentions a chronology of events, the

detailed discussion of several themes (complete with subthemes, specific illustrations, multiple perspectives from individuals, and quotations) or a discussion with interconnecting themes. Many qualitative researchers also use visuals, figures, or tables as adjuncts to the discussions. They present a process model (as in grounded theory), advance a drawing of the specific research site (as in ethnography), or convey descriptive information about each participant in a table (as in case studies and ethnographies).

• *Step 6. A final step in data analysis involves making an interpretation or meaning of the data.* Asking "What were the lessons learned?" captures the essence of this idea (Lincoln & Guba, 1985). These lessons could be the researcher's personal interpretation, couched in the understanding that the inquirer brings to the study from her or his own culture, history, and experiences. It could also be a meaning derived from a comparison of the findings with information gleaned from the *literature* or *theories*. In this way, authors suggest that the findings confirm past information or diverge from it. It can also suggest new questions that need to be asked—questions raised by the data and analysis that the inquirer had not foreseen earlier in the study.

These steps can be easily applied and widely useful to CIPP evaluations: for example, analysis of diverse information from a context evaluation to assist in setting goals and priorities; in-depth contrast of competing strategies in an input evaluation; a retroactive, in-depth characterization of the process followed in a completed project in a process evaluation; and pulling together, analysis and synthesis of all of the obtained context, input, process, and product evaluation to produce in culminating summative evaluation.

Computer Software for Qualitative Data Analysis

For large amounts of qualitative data, the evaluator may want to use an appropriate qualitative data analysis computer program. Basic to these programs is use of the computer as an efficient means of storing and locating qualitative data. Although the researcher still needs to go through each line of text (as in transcriptions) and assign codes, applying a relevant computer program can make this process faster and more efficient than hand coding.

Some of the proprietary qualitative data analysis software programs that are currently popular among users are: NVivo (Windows; Mac OS), MAXQDA (Windows; Mac OS), QDA Miner (Windows), ATLAS.ti (Windows; Mac OS and iPad announced), Coding Analysis Toolkit (CAT), and CAQDAS (Computer Assisted Qualitative Data Analysis Software). The free/open source software include Aquad (GPL licence, since version 7) (Windows), Cassandre (Java-based), Computer Aided Textual Markup & Analysis (CATMA), Compendium (Windows; Mac OS; Linux), ELAN (Java-based for Windows; Mac OS; Linux), FreeQDA (GPL2; Java-based), LibreQDA (AGPL3 license; Web-based), QDA Miner Lite, proprietary license, free version with reduced functionality (Windows), RQDA (Windows; Mac OS; Linux), TAMS Analyzer (Open source; Mac OS), and Transana for audio and video data (GPL2; release packages for purchase) (Windows; Mac OS; Linux).

Among these computer programs, the following merit special mention:

- MAXQDA (*www.maxqda.com*). This excellent program from Germany helps researchers systematically evaluate and interpret qualitative texts.
- Atlas.ti (*www.atlasti.com*). This is another great program from Germany that enables researchers to organize text, graphic, audio, and visual data files, along with coding, memos, and findings, into a project.
- NVivo (*www.qsrinternational.com*). This PC-based program from Australia combines the great features of the popular software program N6 (or Nud.ist) and NVivo concept mapping.
- HyperRESEARCH (*www.researchware.com*). Available for PC or MAC, this is an easy-to-use qualitative software package enabling users to code, retrieve, build theories, and conduct analyses of the qualitative data.

Synthesizing Information

Information synthesis is central to the Joint Committee's Justified Conclusions and Decisions standard (2011), and it requires evaluators to weave the evaluation's value base, information, and analyses into a unified set of conclusions. Each of the quantitative and qualitative analyses presented above can provide information needed for the evaluator to form judgments regarding some individual aspect(s) of the subject program or the total program. Once evaluators have all of the pieces of evaluation information analyzed, they need to proceed to the next important step: synthesizing information to reach bottom-line conclusions. These bottom-line conclusions have serious effects and social consequences because the evaluation audiences often use them not only to judge a program's quality and worth, but also to make important decisions regarding the program's future. Therefore, evaluators must derive their conclusions carefully and support the conclusions with sound evidence(s), and those conclusions should adequately address the audience's information needs and the full set of evaluation questions.

Based on our experience, we offer the following nine recommendations regarding information synthesis:

- Base evaluation conclusions on all pertinent information collected, sound information analyses, and defensible information synthesis.
- Consider both the main effects and the side effects of the program in order to reach the evaluation's conclusions.
- When contradictory results are presented by quantitative and qualitative analyses, consider how central each of these analyses is to the evaluation's bottom-line questions and how each piece of information should be weighted.
- When the results of the information analyses warrant, present bottom-line conclusions as well as plausible alternative conclusions, and offer reasons for presenting these alternative conclusions.
- To offer a justified statement of a program's merit, worth, significance, and probity, forthrightly present your best judgment but do not speculate and be careful but not overly cautious.
- Provide the audience with complete information regarding the bases for the evaluation's conclusions, including audience information needs, evaluation questions, evaluation design, program process, information collection, and information analyses.
- Engage representative stakeholders to review the conclusions and provide their feedback regarding the conclusions' clarity and credibility.

- Inform the audience of any ambiguous findings and conclusions and advise them to be mindful when applying those.
- Support the evaluation synthesis with a technical appendix or technical report that details the evaluation, information, and analyses.

Summary

Information analysis is central to an evaluation's main task of answering evaluation questions and judging a program's merit, worth, significance, and probity. In this chapter, we talk in detail about how to analyze and synthesize quantitative and qualitative information.

In analyzing qualitative data, evaluators may want to follow the general steps for qualitative data analysis given by Creswell (2014). These steps facilitate the search for trends, patterns, and themes in the qualitative information and help elaborate and explain quantitative findings. The chapter identifies a range of computer programs to facilitate both quantitative and qualitative analyses.

Within the quantitative data analysis category, we presented step-by-step guides on descriptive statistics, data visualization, and commonly used inferential statistics. These quantitative data analysis procedures allow us to inspect the behavior of participants, detect increases/decreases in the measures of behavior over time, examine the differences within people or groups, and identify connections between or among two or more variables. All of these can help us make judgments regarding the target evaluation program.

To synthesize information and render bottom-line conclusions, evaluators need to identify the bases for interpreting findings, such as beneficiaries' needs, objectives, standards, norms, the program's previous costs and performance, costs and performance of similar programs, and judgments by experts and program stakeholders. The chapter stresses the importance of taking into consideration all pertinent information, both quantitative and qualitative, and contrasting different subsets of qualitative and quantitative information to identify both corroborative and contradictory findings. The chapter's practical suggestions in this vein include embedding quantitative information within a qualitative narrative or embedding interview responses and other qualitative findings in the discussion of quantitative findings.

REVIEW QUESTIONS • • • • • • • • • • •

1. What are basic definitions and cogent examples of quantitative information and qualitative information?

2. What are the four types of scales of quantitative data and an example of each one?

3. What is the essential difference between descriptive statistics and inferential statistics?

4. What are the steps you would follow in analyzing a set of quantitative information?

5. In either qualitative analysis or quantitative analysis, why is it important to begin the analysis process by exploring the information?

6. Define type I error and type II error and give an example that shows the conflict between the two.

7. Give an example in which an independent-samples *t*-test should be used and an example in which the paired-samples *t*-test should be used.

8. What is the difference between ANCOVA and ANOVA? In what type of situation would you use ANCOVA?

9. What factors should you consider when choosing between parametric and nonparametric statistical analyses?

10. Summarize the steps you would follow to analyze a set of interview data.

11. What process would you follow in coding qualitative information?

12. What is a general definition of the synthesis task in an evaluation?

13. What do you see as a useful set of steps in carrying out a sound synthesis of sets of quantitative analyses and qualitative analyses in an evaluation?

APPENDIX 10.1. SPSS Procedure for Descriptive Statistics for Continuous Variables (Pallant, 2010)

I. In SPSS, from the top menu click on "**Analyze**," then select "**Descriptive Statistics**," then select "**Descriptives**."

II. Click on the continuous variables for which you need to obtain descriptive statistics. Click on the arrow button to move them into the "**Variables**" box (e.g., pacer).

III. Click on the "**Options**" button. Make sure "**mean**," "**standard deviation**," "**minimum**," "**maximum**" are ticked and then click on "**skewness**," "**kurtosis**."

IV. Click on "**Continue**," and then click on "**OK**" (or click on "**Paste**" to save the syntax to the "**Syntax Editor**" for future use).

Syntax for This Procedure

```
DESCRIPTIVES
VARIABLES=pacer
/STATISTICS=MEAN STDDEV MIN MAX KURTOSIS SKEWNESS.
```

APPENDIX 10.2. Visualizing Categorical Data: SPSS Procedure for Frequency Tables, Bar Charts, and Pie Charts (Pallant, 2010)

I. In SPSS, from the top menu, click on "**Analyze**," then "**Descriptive Statistics**," then "**Frequencies**."

II. Move the categorical variable of interest (e.g., gender) into the "**Variables**" box.

III. Click on "**Charts**," select "**Bar charts**" (or "**Pie charts**," or "**Histograms**"), and "**Frequencies**."

IV. Click on "**Continue**."

V. Click on "**OK**" (or click on "**Paste**" to save the syntax to the "**Syntax Editor**" for future use).

Syntax for Creating Frequency Table and Bar Chart:

```
FREQUENCIES VARIABLES=gender
/BARCHART FREQ
/ORDER=ANALYSIS.
```

Syntax for Creating Frequency Table and Pie Chart:

```
FREQUENCIES VARIABLES=gender
/PIECHART FREQ
/ORDER=ANALYSIS.
```

APPENDIX 10.3. SPSS Procedure for Creating a Stem-and-Leaf Plot (Pallant, 2010)

I. From the top menu, click on "**Analyze**," then "**Descriptive Statistics**," then "**Explore**."

II. Then put the variable you would like to plot (e.g., Knowledge) into the "**Dependent List**" box.

III. Click on "**Plots**," and make sure that "**Stem-and leaf**" under "**Descriptive**" is checked.

IV. Click on "**Continue**," then "**OK**" (or click on "**Paste**" to save the syntax to the "**Syntax Editor**" for future use).

Syntax for This Procedure

```
EXAMINE VARIABLES=Knowledge
/PLOT BOXPLOT STEMLEAF
/COMPARE GROUPS
/STATISTICS DESCRIPTIVES
/CINTERVAL 95
/MISSING LISTWISE
/NOTOTAL.
```

APPENDIX 10.4. SPSS Procedure for Creating a Histogram (Pallant, 2010)

I. From the top menu click on "**Graphs**," then select "**Legacy Dialogs**," then choose "**Histogram**."

II. Click on the continuous variable of interest (e.g., Knowledge) and move it into the "**Variable**" box.

III. If you want to generate separate histograms for different groups (male teachers/female teachers), put the grouping variable (e.g., gender) in the "**Panel by:**" section. Choose "**Rows**" if you want the two graphs on top of one another, or choose "**Column**" if you want them side by side.

IV. Click on "**OK**" (or on "**Paste**" to save the syntax to the "**Syntax Editor**" for future use).

Syntax for This Procedure

```
GRAPH
/HISTOGRAM=Knowledge
/PANEL COLVAR=gender COLOP=CROSS.
```

APPENDIX 10.5. SPSS Procedure for Creating a Bar Graph (Pallant, 2010)

I. From the top menu, click on "**Graphs,**" then select "**Legacy Dialogs,**" then choose "**Bar.**" Click on "**Clustered.**"

II. In the "**Data in chart are**" section, click on "**Summaries for groups of cases,**" click on "**Define.**" Then in the "**Bars represent**" box, click on "**Other statistic**" (e.g., mean).

III. Click on the continuous variable of interest (e.g., Knowledge). This should appear in the box listed as "**Mean.**" This requests SPSS to provide the means on the variable for the different groups.

IV. Click on your first grouping variable (e.g., agegroup). Click on the arrow to move it into the "**Category axis**" box (X axis).

V. Click on another grouping variable (e.g., gender) and move it into the "**Define Clusters by:**" box. This variable will be displayed in the legend.

VI. If you wish to display error bars on the graphs, click on the "**Options**" button and click on "**Display error bars.**" Then select what you would like the bars to represent (e.g., confidence intervals).

VII. Click on "**Continue**" and then "**OK**" (or on "**Paste**" to save the syntax to the "**Syntax Editor**").

Syntax for This Procedure

```
GRAPH
/BAR(GROUPED)=MEAN(Knowledge) BY agegroup BY gender
/INTERVAL CI(95.0).
```

APPENDIX 10.6. SPSS Procedure for Creating a Line Graph (Pallant, 2010)

I. From the top menu, select "**Graphs,**" then "**Legacy Dialogs,**" then choose "**Line.**"

II. Click on "**Multiple.**" In the "**Data in Chart Are**" section, click on "**Summaries for groups of cases.**" Click on "**Define.**"

III. In the "**Lines represent**" box, click on "**Other statistic.**" Click on the continuous variable of interest (e.g., knowledge). Click on the arrow button. The variable should appear in the box listed as "**Mean**" (this requests SPSS to display the mean knowledge score for the different groups).

IV. Click on your first grouping variable (e.g., age group). Click on the arrow to move it into the "**Category Axis**" box. This variable will appear across the bottom of the line graph (X-axis).

V. Click on another grouping variable (e.g., gender) and move it into the "**Define Lines by:**" box. This variable will be displayed in the legend.

VI. If you wish to add error bars to your graph, click on "**Options**" button. Click on the "**Display error bars**" box and choose what you would like the error bars to represent (e.g., confidence intervals).

VII. Click on "**OK**" (or click on "**Paste**" to save the syntax to "**Syntax Editor**" for future use).

Syntax for This Procedure

```
GRAPH
/LINE(MULTIPLE)=MEAN(knowledge) BY agegroup BY gender
/INTERVAL CI(95.0).
```

APPENDIX 10.7. SPSS Procedure for Creating a Scatterplot (Pallant, 2010)

I. From the top menu, click on "**Graphs**," then on "**Legacy Dialogs**," and then choose "**Scatter/Dot**."

II. Click on "**Simple Scatter**" and then on "**Define**."

III. Click on your first variable (usually the dependent variable) (e.g., BMI), click on the arrow to move it into the "**Y axis**" box. This requests that variable BMI appear on the vertical axis.

IV. Move the other continuous variable (usually the independent variable) (e.g., steps) into the "**X axis**" box. This requests that variable steps appear on the horizontal axis.

V. Move the grouping variable (e.g., gender) into the "**Set Markers by:**" box. This asks SPSS to display males and females using different markers.

VI. Move the ID variable into the "**Label Cases by:**" box.

VII. Click on "**OK**" (or on "**Paste**" to save the syntax to "**Syntax Editor**" for future use).

Syntax for This Procedure

```
GRAPH
/SCATTERPLOT(BIVAR)=steps WITH bmi BY gender BY id (IDENTIFY)
/MISSING=LISTWISE.
```

APPENDIX 10.8. SPSS Procedure for Creating a Boxplot (Pallant, 2010)

I. From the top menu, click on "**Graphs**," then select "**Legacy Dialogs**," and then "**Boxplot**."

II. Click on "**Simple**," then in the **"Data in Chart Are"** section, click on "**Summaries for groups of cases**," and then click on "**Define**."

III. Move the continuous variables of interest (e.g., pacer) into the "**Variable**" box.

IV. Move your grouping/categorical variable (e.g., gender) into "**Category axis**" box.

V. Click on ID and move it into "**Label cases**" box. This requests SPSS to identify the ID number of any outliers (cases with extreme values).

VI. Click on "**OK**" (or on **Paste** to save the syntax to "**Syntax Editor**").

Syntax for This Procedure

```
EXAMINE VARIABLES=pacer BY gender
/PLOT=BOXPLOT
/STATISTICS=NONE
/NOTOTAL
/ID=id.
```

APPENDIX 10.9. SPSS Procedure for Creating Independent-Samples *t*-Test (Pallant, 2010)

I. From the top menu, click on "**Analyze**," then select "**Compare Means**," then "**Independent Samples T Test**."

II. Move the dependent (continuous) variable (e.g., pacer) into the "**Test variable**" box.

III. Move the independent variable (categorical) variable (e.g., gender) into the section labeled "**Grouping variable**."

IV. Click on "**Define groups**" and type in the numbers used in the dataset to code each group. In the current data, 1=males, 2=females; so, in the "**Group 1**" box, type 1, and in the "**Group 2**" box, type 2. If you cannot remember the codes used, right click on the variable name and then choose "**Variable Information**" from the pop-up box that appears to find out.

V. Click on "**Continue**" and then "**OK**" (or click on "**Paste**" to save the syntax to "**Syntax Editor**").

Syntax for This Procedure

```
T-TEST
GROUPS=gender(1 2)
/MISSING=ANALYSIS
/VARIABLES=pacer
/CRITERIA=CI(.95).
```

APPENDIX 10.10. SPSS Procedure for Creating Paired-Samples *t*-Test

I. From the top menu, click on "**Analyze**," then select "**Compare Means**," and then "**Paired Samples T test**."

II. Click on the two variables that you are interested in comparing for each subject (e.g., pacer1: pacer laps time 1, pacer2: pacer laps time 2) and move them into the box labeled "**Paired Variables**" by clicking on the arrow button.

III. Click on "**OK**" (or click on "**Paste**" to save the syntax to "**Syntax Editor**").

Syntax for This Procedure

```
T-TEST PAIRS=pacer1 WITH pacer2 (PAIRED)
/CRITERIA=CI(.9500)
/MISSING=ANALYSIS.
```

APPENDIX 10.11. SPSS Procedure for Creating Chi-Square Test for Independence (Pallant, 2010)

I. From the top menu, click on "**Analyze**," then **"Descriptive Statistics**," and then "**Crosstabs**."

II. Click on one of your variables (e.g., gender) to be your row variable and click on the arrow to move it into the box marked "**Row(s)**."

III. Click on the other variable to be your column variable (e.g., drinker) and click on the arrow to move it into the box marked "**Column(s)**."

IV. Click on the "**Statistics**" button, select "**Chi-Square**" and "**Phi and Cramer's V**." Click on "**Continue**."

V. Click on the "**Cells**" button. In the "**Counts**" box, make sure there is a tick for "**Observed**." In the "**Percentage**" section, click on the "**Row**," "**Column**," and "**Total**" boxes.

VI. Click on "**Continue**" and then "**OK**" (or click on "**Paste**" to save the syntax to "**Syntax Editor**").

Syntax for This Procedure

```
CROSSTABS
/TABLES=gender BY drinker
/FORMAT=AVALUE TABLES
/STATISTICS=CHISQ PHI
/CELLS=COUNT ROW COLUMN TOTAL
/COUNT ROUND CELL.
```

APPENDIX 10.12. SPSS Procedure for One-Way Between-Subjects ANOVA with Post-Hoc Tests (Pallant, 2010)

I. From the top menu, click on "**Analyze**," then select "**Compare Means**," then "**One-way ANOVA**."

II. Click on your dependent variable (e.g., depression), then click on the arrow button to move it into the box marked "**Dependent List**."

III. Click on your independent variable (e.g., ethnicity), then click on the arrow button to move it into the box labeled "**Factor**."

IV. Click the "**Options**" button and click on "**Descriptive**," "**Homogeneity of variance test**," "**Brown-Forsythe**," "**Welch**," and "**Means Plot**."

V. For "**Missing values**," select "**Exclude cases analysis by analysis**."

VI. Click on "**Continue**."

VII. Click on "**Post Hoc**," then click on "**Tukey**."

VIII. Click on "**Continue**" and then "**OK**" (or click on "**Paste**" to save the syntax to "**Syntax Editor**").

Syntax for This Procedure

```
ONEWAY depression BY ethnicity
/STATISTICS DESCRIPTIVES HOMOGENEITY BROWNFORSYTHE WELCH
/PLOT MEANS
```

APPENDIX 10.13. Procedure for One-Way Within-Group (Repeated-Measures) ANOVA (Pallant, 2010)

I. From the top menu, click on "**Analyze**," then "**General Linear Model**," then "**Repeated Measures**."

II. In the "**Within Subject Factor Name**" box, type in a name that represents your independent variable (e.g., Time). This is not an actual variable name, just a label you give your independent variable.

III. In the "**Number of Levels**" box, type the number of levels or groups (time periods) involved (in this example, it is 3).

IV. Click "**Add**." Then click on "**Define**."

V. Select the three variables that represent your repeated measures variable (e.g., efficacy year 1: efficacy1, efficacy year 2: efficacy2, efficacy year 3: efficacy3), click on the arrow button to move them into the "**Within Subjects Variables**" box.

VI. Click on the "**Options**" box. In the area labeled "Display," select the "**Descriptive Statistics**" and "**Estimates of effect size**." If you wish to request post-hoc test, select your independent variable name (e.g., Time) in the "**Factor**" and "**Factor Interactions**" section and move it into the "**Display Means for**" box. Select "**Compare main effects**." In the "**Confidence interval adjustment**" section, click on the down arrow and choose "**Bonferroni**."

VII. Click on "**Continue**" and then "**OK**" (or click on "**Paste**" to save the syntax to "**Syntax Editor**").

Syntax for This Procedure

```
GLM efficacy1 efficacy2 efficacy3
/WSFACTOR=Time 3 Polynomial
/METHOD=SSTYPE(3)
/EMMEANS=TABLES(Time) COMPARE ADJ(BONFERRONI)
/PRINT=DESCRIPTIVE ETASQ
/CRITERIA=ALPHA(.05)
/WSDESIGN=Time.
Output:
```

APPENDIX 10.14. SPSS Procedure for Two-Way Between-Groups ANOVA (Pallant, 2010)

I. From the top menu click on "**Analyze**," then "**General Linear Model**," then "**Univariate**."

II. Click on your dependent, continuous variable of interest (e.g., confidence) and click on the arrow to move it into the box labeled "**Dependent variable**."

III. Click on your two independent, categorical variables (gender, agegroup) and move these into the box labeled "**Fixed Factors**."

IV. Click on "**Options**." Click on "**Descriptive statistics**," "**Estimates of effect size**," and "**Homogeneity test**." Click on "**Continue**."

V. Click on "**Post Hoc**." From the Factors listed on the left-hand side, choose the independent variables(s) with 3 or more levels that you are interested in (e.g., agegroup), and click on the arrow to move it into the "**Post Hoc Tests for**" section. Choose the test you wish to use (in this case, **Tukey**). Click on "**Continue**."

VI. Click on the "**Plots**" button. In the "**Horizontal**" box, put the independent variable that has the most groups (e.g., agegroup). In the box labeled "**Separate lines**," put the other independent variable (e.g., gender).

VII. Click on "**Add**." In the section labeled "**Plots**," you should now see your two variables listed (e.g., agegroup*gender).

VIII. Click on "**Continue**" and then "**OK**" (or click on "**Paste**" to save the syntax to "**Syntax Editor**").

Syntax for This Procedure

```
UNIANOVA confidence BY gender agegroup
/METHOD=SSTYPE(3)
/INTERCEPT=INCLUDE
/POSTHOC=agegroup(TUKEY)
/PLOT=PROFILE(agegroup *gender)
/PRINT=ETASQ HOMOGENEITY DESCRIPTIVE
/CRITERIA=ALPHA(.05)
/DESIGN=gender agegroup gender*agegroup.
```

APPENDIX 10.15. SPSS Procedures for Checking Assumptions and Conducting One-Way ANCOVA (Pallant, 2010)

Procedure for Checking Linearity for Each Group

Step 1

I. From the top menu, click on "**Graph**," "**Legacy Dialogs**," and then select "**Scatter/Dot**."

II. Click on "**Simple Scatter**." Click on the "**Define**" button.

III. In the "**Y axis**" box, put your dependent variable (in this case, math anxiety time2: anxiety2).

IV. In the "**X axis**" box, put your covariate (e.g., math anxiety time1: anxiety1).

V. Click on your independent variable (e.g., group) and put in the "**Set Markers**" box.

VI. Click on "**OK**" (or click on "**Paste**" to save to "**Syntax Editor**").

(continued)

Syntax for This Procedure

Syntax for This Procedure

```
GRAPH
/SCATTERPLOT(BIVAR)=anxiety1 WITH anxiety2 BY group
/MISSING=LISTWISE.
```

Step 2

I. Once you have the scatterplot displayed, double-click on it to open the "**Chart Editor**" window.

II. From the menu, click on "**Elements**" and select "**Fit line at Subgroups.**" Two lines will appear on the graph representing line of best fit for each group.

III. Click on "**File**" and then "**Close.**"

In the output from this procedure, check the general distribution of scores for each of the groups. Does there appear to be a linear (straight-line) relationship for each group? What we don't want to see is an indication of a curvilinear relationship. If a curvilinear relationship is found, then we need to reconsider the use of this covariate, or try transforming the variable and repeating the scatterplot to see whether there is an improvement.

Procedure for Checking Homogeneity of Regression Slopes

From the top menu, click on "**Analyze,**" then "**General Linear Model,**" then "**Univariate.**"

I. In the "**Dependent Variables**" box, put your dependent variable (math anxiety time2: anxiety2).

II. In the "**Fixed Factor**" box, put your independent or grouping variable (type of class: group).

III. In the "**Covariate**" box, put your covariate (math anxiety time1: anxiety1).

IV. Click on the "**Model**" button. Click on "**Custom.**"

V. Check that the "**Interaction**" option is showing in the "**Build Terms**" box.

VI. Click on your independent variable (group) and then the arrow button to move it into the "**Model**" box.

VII. Click on your covariate (anxiety1) and then the arrow button to move it into the "**Model**" box.

VIII. Go back and click on your independent variable (group) again on the left-hand side (in the "**Factors and Covariates**" section). While this is highlighted, hold down the Ctrl key, and then click on your covariate variable (anxiety1). Click on the arrow button to move this into the right-hand side box labeled "**Model.**"

IX. In the "**Model**" box, you should now have listed your independent variable (group); your covariate (anxiety1); and an extra line of the form: covariate * independent variable (group*anxiety1). The final term is the interaction that we are checking for.

X. Click on "**Continue**" and then "**OK**" (or click on "**Paste**" to save the syntax to "**Syntax Editor**").

SPSS Syntax for This Procedure

```
UNIANOVA anxiety2 BY group WITH anxiety1
/METHOD=SSTYPE(3)
/INTERCEPT=INCLUDE
/CRITERIA=ALPHA(0.05)
/DESIGN=group anxiety1 anxiety1*group.
```

In the output from this procedure, titled "Tests of Between-Subjects Effects" table, the only value of interest is the significance level of the interaction term (shown as Group*anxiety1). If the Sig. level for this interaction is greater than .05, your interaction is not statistically significant, indicating that you have not violated the assumption of homogeneity of regression slopes.

(continued)

Procedure for One-Way ANCOVA

I. From the top menu click on "**Analyze**," then "**General Linear Model**," then "**Univariate**."

II. In the "**Dependent Variables**" box, put your dependent variable (math anxiety time2: anxiety2).

III. In the "**Fixed Factor**" box, put your independent or grouping variable (e.g., type of class: group).

IV. In the "**Covariate**" box, put your covariate (e.g., math anxiety time1: anxiety1)

V. Click on the "**Model**" button. Click on "**Full Factorial**" in the "**Specify Model**" section. Click on "**Continue**."

VI. Click on the **Options** button.

VII. In the top section labeled "**Estimated Marginal Means**," click on your independent variable (group).

VIII. Click on the arrow to move it into the box labeled "**Display Means for**." (This will provide you with the mean score on your dependent variable for each group, adjusted for the influence of the covariate.)

IX. In the bottom section of the "**Options**" dialogue box, choose "**Descriptive statistics**," "**Estimates of effect size**," and "**Homogeneity test**."

X. Click on "**Continue**" and then "**OK**" (or click on "**Paste**" to save the syntax to "**Syntax Editor**").

Syntax for This Procedure

```
UNIANOVA anxiety2 BY group WITH anxiety1
/METHOD=SSTYPE(3)
/INTERCEPT=INCLUDE
/EMMEANS=TABLES(group) WITH(anxiety1=MEAN)
/PRINT=ETASQ HOMOGENEITY DESCRIPTIVE
/CRITERIA=ALPHA(.05)
/DESIGN=anxiety1 group.
```

CHAPTER 11

Reporting Evaluation Findings

"Competent reporting is indispensable to effective evaluation."

This chapter provides practical advice and tools to help evaluators and their clients collaborate in competently informing a project's stakeholders about an evaluation's aims and procedures, its progress through the course of the evaluation, interim findings as they become available, conclusions, and ways to apply findings. Competent reporting is essential to ensure that credible, useful evaluation reports do not merely gather dust on shelves but instead assist the evaluation's audience to appraise a project's quality and worth, make sound project-related decisions, meet project accountability requirements, and retain lessons learned for future use. The chapter provides concrete advice and tools for competently reporting an evaluation's progress and findings and fostering informed use of conclusions.

Overview
. . . .

Timely, competent reporting of an evaluation's progress and findings is essential to securing an evaluation's impact. Competent reporting is a complex and challenging undertaking that requires sustained involvement of the evaluation's client and other stakeholders, as well as the evaluator. This chapter provides evaluators and their clients with practical advice and tools for addressing the requirements of competent reporting. The advice and tools are intended for selective application whether one is conducting formative evaluation of a project's context, inputs, process, and/or products or a holistic, summative evaluation of the project. The chapter's contents include the aims of evaluation

reporting; actions evaluators can take to achieve the aims; many practical checklists; advice for identifying and engaging an evaluation's intended users and determining their intended uses of findings; procedures for providing interim feedback; formats for writing a final report; a form for attesting to an evaluation's adherence to standards; ways to assist intended users to apply findings; warnings against issuing unsubstantiated recommendations; and alternative media for disseminating findings. The chapter explains the use of evaluation review panels, feedback workshops, and focus groups as effective ways to inform an evaluation's stakeholders about an evaluation's findings and engage them in applying the findings; the chapter also discusses the use of input evaluation as a technically sound way to follow up a completed project evaluation to identify and thoroughly assess alternative actions for responding to the project evaluation's conclusions.

What Are the Aims of Competent Reporting?

The aims of evaluation reporting are twofold: to promote and assist a project's success through delivering timely, valid, actionable feedback to the project's overseers and staff, and ultimately to inform the full range of members of the right-to-know audience about the completed project's quality and worth. Failure to achieve these basic aims of formative and summative reporting will erase or seriously limit an evaluation's prospects for beneficial impacts. In the face of failed reporting, the project's client and other stakeholders could justifiably judge the evaluation to be useless—or even worse than useless, given the time and resources that were wasted in conducting the evaluation. No matter how well an evaluation was carried out technically, if its intended users do not consider and apply the findings as appropriate, then the evaluation has failed. On the other hand, an evaluation would be judged successful to the extent that (1) the subject project staff received and effectively applied sufficient, sound evaluative feedback to continually guide and strengthen their project and (2) the project's funder and full range of other interested stakeholders ultimately used the final report to understand the project, judge its merit and worth, and take warranted actions. Clearly, competent formative and summative reporting are essential components of sound, impactful project evaluations.

What Actions Should Evaluators Take to Achieve the Aims of Competent Reporting?

In this section, we draw on our experiences in conducting and reporting many evaluations and metaevaluations to distill the actions that we believe evaluators will find useful in reporting and securing the impacts of their evaluation projects. The section presents a checklist of actions for informing a project's client and other stakeholders about all relevant aspects of an evaluation, including especially its findings. The end game of these actions is to foster and assist appropriate uses of the evaluation's findings. Such uses include defining project goals, planning project procedures, continually monitoring and strengthening project operations,

judging outcomes, and meeting accountability requirements. The recommended evaluator actions in reporting and securing the impacts of evaluation findings are presented in Checklist 11.1 (at the end of this chapter). The following section explains each item on the checklist.

1. Reach Agreement on the Client's Role in Reporting Evaluation Findings

As explained in Chapter 4, evaluation clients can and should play the role of evaluation-oriented leader in all aspects of an evaluation. This is especially true of the process of reporting evaluation progress and findings. At the outset of planning an evaluation, the evaluator should define with the client the role he or she will play in supporting the reporting process. Ideally, this role includes reaching agreement on standards for effective evaluation reporting; clarifying and prioritizing evaluation questions; defining the evaluation's audience; helping to develop a functional plan and schedule for reporting findings; helping to determine the most effective ways to convey evaluation findings to all parts of the evaluation's audience; engaging project stakeholders to help focus evaluations and critique draft reports; arranging for an external metaevaluation of the evaluation; planning and budgeting for the evaluator's assistance in facilitating stakeholders' uses of the final evaluation report; and throughout the evaluation process, engaging the project's decision makers and other stakeholders to make effective use of reports.

In many evaluations, the client engages in a learning process related to the particular evaluation being conducted and program evaluation in general. The evaluator can enhance the prospects for effective conduct of a particular evaluation and organizational-based evaluation in general by mentoring the client to learn and embrace key aspects of evaluation. Such aspects include:

- Standards for sound evaluations
- A concept of evaluation that stresses use of findings
- A climate to foster use of evaluation findings
- Trust and feasibility by negotiating formal evaluation agreements
- Meaningful identification and engagement of stakeholders as users of evaluation findings
- Stakeholder roles and associated procedures for reviewing draft evaluation reports

- The substantial advantages of employing a stakeholder evaluation review panel
- The range of typically important evaluation questions
- A practical, standards-based framework for evaluation
- Multiple ways of reporting evaluation findings
- The importance of institutionalizing and mainstreaming systematic evaluation
- Steps for developing a climate conducive to stakeholders' effective use of evaluation findings
- Roles of internal and external metaevaluation
- The organization's members understanding and valuing evaluation's most important purpose: not to prove but to improve
- The case for investing required resources in cost-effective evaluation processes

It is essential for the evaluator to have a full and frank discussion with the client at the outset of an evaluation to define and agree on the client's role in assuring that reports will be germane, ethical, timely, useful, and used appropriately. Through a well-defined role of evaluation-oriented leadership, the client can help the evaluator produce and deliver reports that the evaluation's intended users can and will employ to improve the project and meet its accountability requirements. In the following discussions of evaluation reporting checkpoints, we add specificity to the tasks that the evaluation client can carry out in the interest of securing maximal beneficial uses of evaluation reports.

2. Confirm Agreements on Standards for Effective Reporting

As explained in Chapter 6 on designing evaluations and as is supported in previous chapters, in planning an evaluation, the evaluator should reach an agreement with the client on the standards that will guide the evaluation, including the reporting of findings. In general, we have advocated that evaluators seek advance agreements with their clients that the Joint Committee on Standards for Educational Evaluation (2011) *Program Evaluation Standards* be adopted. These standards should be used to guide and govern all aspects of an evaluation and provide the criteria for assessing and judging the evaluation. As regards the reporting function, the following Joint Committee standards

are particularly applicable to the reporting functions of preparing, validating, and disseminating evaluation findings:

- *U2 Attention to Stakeholders.* Evaluators should devote attention to the full range of individuals and groups invested in the program and affected by its evaluation.
- *U5 Relevant Information.* Evaluation information should serve the identified and emergent needs of stakeholders.
- *U7 Timely and Appropriate Communicating and Reporting.* Evaluations should attend to the continuing information needs of their multiple audiences.
- *U8 Concern for Consequences and Influence.* Evaluations should promote responsible and adaptive use while guarding against unintended negative consequences and misuse.
- *P1 Responsive and Inclusive Orientation.* Evaluations should be responsive to stakeholders and their communities.
- *P3 Human Rights and Respect.* Evaluations should be designed and conducted to protect human and legal rights and maintain the dignity of participants and other stakeholders.
- *P4 Clarity and Fairness.* Evaluations should be understandable and fair in addressing stakeholder needs and purposes.
- *P5 Transparency and Disclosure.* Evaluations should provide complete descriptions of findings, limitations, and conclusions to all stakeholders, unless doing so would violate legal and propriety obligations.
- *P6 Conflicts of Interests.* Evaluations should openly and honestly identify and address real or perceived conflicts of interests that may compromise the evaluation.
- *A1 Justified Conclusions and Decisions.* Evaluation conclusions and decisions should be explicitly justified in the cultures and contexts where they have consequences.
- *A4 Explicit Program and Context Descriptions.* Evaluations should document programs and their contexts with appropriate detail and scope for the evaluation purposes.
- *A7 Explicit Evaluation Reasoning.* Evaluation reasoning leading from information and analyses to findings, interpretations, conclusions, and judgments should be clearly and completely documented.
- *A8 Communication and Reporting.* Evaluation communications should have adequate scope and guard

against misconceptions, biases, distortions, and errors.

- *E1 Evaluation Documentation*. Evaluations should fully document their negotiated purposes and implemented designs, procedures, data, and outcomes.
- *E2 Internal Metaevaluation*. Evaluators should use these and other applicable standards to examine the accountability of the evaluation design, procedures employed, information collected, and outcomes.
- *E3 External Metaevaluation*. Program evaluation sponsors, clients, evaluators, and other stakeholders should encourage the conduct of external metaevaluations using these and other applicable standards.

The preceding standards are both demanding and highly functional for helping evaluators and their client groups assure that evaluation reports and reporting will be pertinent, technically defensible, ethical, understandable, and usable to the benefit of subject projects. It behooves the evaluator to take effective steps to ensure that the client and other stakeholders understand and embrace the standards and acquire capacity to apply them in judging evaluation reports. The evaluator should remind the client and other users of the standards that their full texts, including practical guidelines, can be found in the Joint Committee (2011) *Program Evaluation Standards*.

3. Invoke Protections for the Rights of Human Subjects

In planning and carrying out the evaluation reporting function, the evaluator must observe reasonable safeguards to protect the rights of all parties to the evaluation. These include the persons whose work is being evaluated and others who might, in some way, be harmed because of the collection of evaluation information and release of findings. The rights of human subjects in evaluations are likely to include obtaining the informed consent of those who contribute information; obtaining confidentiality or anonymity assurances; protecting against intrusions into personal records; honoring the client organization's protocols for obtaining, storing, and retrieving sensitive personnel information; and safeguarding each participant's personal information and dignity. The evaluator should communicate with the client to define the rights of human subjects to be protected and to emphasize how the rights will be protected. In particular, before signing on to do an evaluation, we advise evaluators to search

out and solicit views about the projected evaluation of persons who might, in some way, be harmed because of the evaluation. Then the evaluator can make a rational decision to proceed or not with the evaluation or can negotiate with the client ways to prevent harm to the concerned parties. In many evaluation assignments, the client organization will possess formal criteria for safeguarding the rights of human subjects and establishing an institutional review board to apply the criteria in approving or rejecting research and evaluation proposals. At the outset of planning an evaluation, including especially its reporting component, the evaluator should determine if the projected client organization has an institutional review board. If such a board exists, the client should secure and complete the board's compliance materials and then fully honor them in carrying out the evaluation and reporting its findings.

4. Delineate Reporting Agreements

As explained in Chapters 6, 7, and 8, the evaluator will project in general terms—in the evaluation design, budget, and contract—what reports will be delivered, at what times, to what audiences, and at what locations. The evaluator and client necessarily will reach accord on general reporting plans at the evaluation's outset. Such initial provisions are necessary to launch a fully defensible, goal-directed evaluation that will have initial buy-in by the client and other project stakeholders and that will be adequately funded. However, many evaluations are formative and involve a dynamic, interactive process. Consequently, the planning of the reporting process needs to be ongoing and responsive to project stakeholders' evolving needs for pertinent, timely feedback. Accordingly, the evaluator and client should agree that they and, as appropriate, other project stakeholders should periodically review and update the evaluation reporting plan. Functionally, it is best to conduct such review and updating exchanges soon after the delivery of each interim report. The added advantage of ongoing review and planning of the reporting function is that through participation in this process the client and other involved stakeholders increasingly will develop interest and be predisposed to study and apply evaluation findings.

5. Define the Evaluation's Audience

Prerequisites for producing evaluation impacts are to define the evaluation's intended users and project the ways they would likely use the findings. With these determinations, the evaluator can focus data collection and evaluation reporting directly on the needs of the overall audience and the special needs of subparts of the audience.

As a first step in clarifying the evaluation's audience, the evaluator should communicate with the client to identify the persons and groups considered to be important potential users of evaluation findings. Subsequently, the evaluator should communicate with a representative sample of potential users of findings to hear how they would use the findings, what kinds of reports would be most useful to them, when the reports would be most useful, and any concerns they might have about the release of evaluation findings. With regard to the latter point, before agreeing to conduct an evaluation, we reiterate that we have found it important to seek out and hear from those who worry they would be harmed by the evaluation and then, as appropriate, to enact safeguards for assuring that the evaluation would be fair to all stakeholders. Advance efforts to identify the evaluation's stakeholders, learn how they would use findings, and address any of their concerns about the reporting of findings provide the evaluator with a foundation for appropriately planning data collection, developing responsive reports, and helping the intended users to make beneficial uses of findings.

Table 11.1 is a matrix designed to assist evaluators and their clients to identify intended users and uses of findings. We suggest that the evaluator use this matrix's row headings to identify persons to interview in the course of planning the evaluation's reporting function. Based on the interviews, the evaluator can keep track of users' intended uses of findings by considering the matrix's column headings and placing checkmarks in the appropriate cells of the matrix. We believe such a filled out matrix provides the evaluator with a useful heuristic device for planning what reports to provide to which groups of intended users, what contents should be in each report, and when they should be provided.

6. Develop and Periodically Update a Sound Reporting Plan

The evaluator must make many key decisions in planning how best to meet the evaluative needs of the overall audience and its segments. Such decisions include:

- Determining the client group's needs for different types of reports: context, input, process, product,

sustainability, transportability, and overall summative reports.

- Determining the full range of intended report recipients, their common evaluative information needs, and the specialized needs of different segments of the audience.

- Outlining the contents of projected reports, including evaluation questions, needed information, and analysis and synthesis of findings.

- Scheduling production and review of draft reports and planning to obtain prerelease reviews of the drafts.

- Scheduling the completion and delivery of each report.

- Projecting ways to follow up delivery of reports by helping recipients to closely consider findings and determine how best to apply the findings.

- Meeting regularly with the client throughout the evaluation to review and update the reporting plan as appropriate.

Clearly, the planning of the evaluation reporting function must be ongoing. Such planning should be informed by ongoing interactions with the evaluation's client and the other members of the evaluation audience. The reporting plan should be updated periodically to take account of intended client uses (or lack of use) of interim reports and their judgments of those reports' quality and utility and of how future reporting could be improved.

7. Budgeting and Contracting

The advice presented in Chapters 7 (budgeting) and 8 (contracting) has special relevance for reporting evaluation findings. Although evaluation budgets and contracts typically provide for interim reporting and the final report, they often lack specificity concerning a host of other reporting items. We strongly recommend that evaluators specifically negotiate at the evaluation's outset with their client an extensive range of reporting-related items. The following is a list of such items for the evaluator and client to discuss and negotiate as they finalize the evaluation's budget and contract:

- Client's role in the evaluation reporting process
- Bottom-line evaluation questions
- Schedule of interim and final reports

TABLE 11.1. Matrix for Identifying Potential Users of Evaluation Findings and Determining How They Intend to Use the Findings

Potential Users of Findings	Potential Uses of Findings					
	Project Oversight	Project Management	Project Execution	Project Funding	Project Accountability	Dissemination of Project Results
Project funder						
Evaluation client						
Project director						
Project staff						
Project advisory group						
Project beneficiaries						
Project parent organization administration						
Stakeholder evaluation review panel						
Project parent organization board						
Persons who might be harmed by the evaluation						
Interested outsiders						
Media						
Legislators						
Potential adopters of the project approach						
Foundations						
Libraries/information repositories						
Government agencies						
Professional societies						
Scientific community						
General public						
Other						

- Standards for judging reports
- Stakeholder engagement in reviewing draft reports
- Employing an evaluation stakeholder review panel
- Authority for editing reports
- Intended users and uses of each projected report
- Venues for reporting evaluation findings
- Media for conveying evaluation findings
- Agreements on who will disseminate reports and when and how they will do so
- Evaluator's follow-up assistance for helping report recipients apply findings
- Provision for an external metaevaluation
- Possibility of conducting a follow-up input evaluation to identify and thoroughly assess alternative ways to respond to the evaluation's findings
- Provision for periodic review and updating of the reporting budget and agreement

It is good business practice for the evaluator and client to clarify and document advance reporting-related budgetary and contractual agreements. Such agreements help assure the feasibility, propriety, accuracy, credibility, and effectiveness of evaluation reporting. From the client's perspective, such careful planning helps assure that the evaluation will secure maximum impact from the funds expended on the evaluation. Such advance planning assures the client and stake-

holders that evaluation reports will be trustworthy, timely, and actionable. Also, advance agreements on reporting matters provide a stable, vetted basis for settling any disputes that may arise in reporting evaluation findings. Throughout the remainder of this chapter, we will regularly refer to needs for advance budgetary and contractual agreements to provide a sound foundation for following through with effective evaluation practices.

8. Engage Stakeholders in the Reporting Process

It is a well-known axiom of change processes that meaningful engagement of stakeholders in a change process helps them understand the process, and, if the process is sound and in stakeholders' legitimate interests, endorse it and act on its products. The relevance of this truism for evaluation reporting is that evaluators should meaningfully engage members of the evaluation's audience in the evaluation process, including the process of developing and disseminating reports.

Table 11.2 is a matrix that displays the aims and approaches for meaningfully engaging an evaluation's stakeholders in the evaluation reporting process. The row headings are five aims of engaging stakeholders in the evaluation process, while the five column headings are strategies that we have found to be effective for engaging stakeholders and "co-opting" them (in the best sense of the word) to endorse and use evaluation findings. The X's in the matrix's cells reflect our judg-

TABLE 11.2. Matrix for Relating Stakeholder Engagement Aims to Stakeholder Engagement Strategies

Stakeholder Engagement Aims	Stakeholder Engagement Strategies				
	Sit In on Project Staff Meetings	Circulate Reporting Plans for Comment	Town Hall Meetings	Focus Groups	Evaluation Review Panel
Focus reports on the right questions.	X	X	X		X
Scrutinize and correct draft reports.					X
Deliver reports when they are needed.	X	X			X
Provide reports to the full range of rightful recipients.		X	X	X	X
Secure appropriate impacts of evaluation findings.	X		X	X	X

ments of each engagement strategy's relevance to the five stakeholder engagement aims. Following are brief discussions of what we mean by each of the five engagement strategies and how we judge their power for achieving the five stakeholder engagement aims.

8.1. Sitting In on Project Staff Meetings

Providing that the client agrees, the evaluator can find it valuable to sit in on project staff and/or organizational board meetings. Listening to the proceedings is a valuable source of information for projecting and meeting project stakeholders' future decisions and associated needs for evaluation information. Also, by being present in the meetings, the evaluator can respond, if and when asked, for updates on evaluation plans and schedules or even for collected and validated data that may be pertinent to current project-related issues and decision situations. In general, however, the evaluator and client should agree that, in attending meetings, the evaluator will play a low-key role (e.g., speaking only when spoken to).

In the 1960s, Dr. Howard Merriman demonstrated the power of sitting in on project-related meetings when he regularly attended meetings of the Columbus, Ohio, School District Board of Education. He reported to Stufflebeam that regular attendance at board meetings proved invaluable. Repeatedly, it gave Merriman and his evaluation team a heads up on what information the board would need to carry out its oversight role and to help them make future policy decisions pertaining to the district's nearly $7 million in federally funded projects. In this example, it was essential that the district's superintendent had suggested and authorized Merriman to sit in on the board meetings. In a sense, this was one way the superintendent made sure that the evaluation of district Elementary and Secondary Act (of 1965) projects would prove its worth in providing decision makers at all levels of the district with timely, relevant evaluative feedback. A rule of thumb we follow in our evaluations is that the evaluator should never go around a client and interact with a higher authority figure or group, unless the client approves of such contact.

8.2. Circulating Evaluation Reporting Plans for Comment

Because project evaluations are typically interactive and responsive to stakeholder needs, planning for reporting findings necessarily is an ongoing process. Drafting and circulating reporting plans for comment can serve the needs of both the evaluator and the evaluation's audience. It serves the evaluator by gaining feedback on the extent to which the draft reporting plan is, at the particular time, sufficiently anticipatory and likely to be responsive to the client group's needs for evaluative feedback. Circulating the reporting plans also serves the client group by giving them advance projections of the type of evaluative feedback they will receive and when they will receive it. Additionally, such circulation of plans and invitations for comment gives the client group a voice in improving reporting plans so that future reports will be germane to their needs and delivered when they need them.

8.3. Holding Town Hall Meetings

Midway in an evaluation, it can be advantageous to announce and hold an open forum or town hall meeting to inform interested persons about an evaluation's purpose, plan, and progress and to obtain stakeholder feedback targeted to strengthening the evaluation, including its plan for reporting findings. Such meetings can be useful to the evaluator for stimulating widespread interest in the evaluation; gaining a sense of who is interested in the evaluation, what questions they see as most important, and the nature and timing of reports that would best serve their needs; and fostering attendee interest in receiving, reading, and using future evaluation reports.

About 2 weeks before the meeting, the evaluator, in consultation with the client, should send out an announcement of the projected town hall meeting, including its intended audience, purpose, date, time, and location. In general, the announcement should indicate that all interested persons are welcome to attend. The announcement can be sent via direct mail to persons the client deems potentially interested in the evaluation and it can also be posted in relevant newsletters, newspapers, and websites.

The town hall meeting should be held in an auditorium of sufficient size to accommodate the intended audience. At the meeting's outset, a sign-up sheet should be circulated to enable persons interested in following the evaluation to provide their name and e-mail address. The evaluator should indicate that the meeting's deliberations will be documented and that a summary will be made available to all attendees, for example, through an e-mail message or in the evaluation's website. The website's address, if one is to be used, should be printed on the one-page agenda for the town hall meeting. The evaluator should circulate the agenda and briefly go over it. Basically, the agenda should include the evaluator's questions for response by the group (see below) and a closing section to include free response by attendees, the client's response to the meeting, and the evaluator's final summary. The evaluator should then introduce the evaluation's client and ask the client to make a brief statement about the evaluation's purpose and the importance of stakeholders' involvement to assure its utility.

To begin the substance of the town hall meeting, the evaluator should provide orientation on what is being evaluated, why, how, with what projected reports and intended impacts, and when the reports will be completed. The evaluator should indicate that those interested in addressing questions should raise their hand to be recognized and that as they are recognized they will be provided with a microphone to make sure their statements are heard by the chair and the other attendees. Then the evaluator should go over the questions for stakeholder inputs that appear on the agenda sheet. Examples of such questions follow:

- What are the most important questions for the evaluation?
- What are the most important uses of the evaluation's final report?
- When is the best time to deliver the final report?
- Beyond the projected final printed report, what other ways of conveying findings would be most useful?
- What are the most important audiences for the evaluation's findings?
- What are the evaluator's expectations regarding how the study's findings will be used?
- What could be done to strengthen the evaluation's prospects for producing beneficial impacts?

To stay within a reasonable time limit for the session, we advise the evaluator to allow approximately 8 minutes for responses to each question. The evaluator should manage the ongoing exchange to make sure that no one respondent dominates and that each person who wants to speak is given an opportunity to comment or raise questions. The evaluator should keep to a minimum her or his responses to audience questions and should emphasize that the meeting's main purpose is to hear from the attendees.

At the meeting's end, the evaluation's client should briefly react to what he or she heard and thank the attendees for their contributions. Finally, the evaluator should conclude the meeting by summarizing the main points heard in the meeting, indicating how the attendees' inputs will be used, thanking the participants for their participation, and reiterating that a summary of the meeting will be made available to those present. Also, the evaluator should express openness to receive further inputs—by e-mail, phone, or correspondence.

8.4. Engaging Stakeholders in Focus Group Sessions

The methodology of focus groups provides another valuable means of engaging stakeholders in an evaluation. In our use of this method, we engage a small group of stakeholders to study an evaluation report and deliberate about practical ways to respond to evaluation findings. We have employed focus groups primarily following the completion of a final evaluation report, with the purpose of engaging one or more groups of stakeholders to systematically examine the evaluation's findings and determine what they see as the best ways to apply the findings. Such applications of findings may include decisions regarding recycling and strengthening the project; recommendations for particular use of findings; perspectives on sustaining, disseminating, or terminating the project; or recommendation of a follow-up input evaluation.

In our experience, a focus group should include seven to ten members who represent the evaluation's intended users. The evaluator should consult with the client to select and recruit members of the focus group but should not necessarily confine selections to the client's recommended participants. It is important to engage a representative set of intended users in the focus group deliberations. The evaluator should reach agreement with the client that individual focus group members will not be linked to specific points in the eventual focus group report. Focus group members should be apprised of this guarantee of anonymity.

About a week in advance of the focus group session, the evaluator should provide the focus group members with the subject evaluation report, ask them to study it in advance of the session, and stress that the main objective of the focus group session is to identify and thoroughly discuss how the evaluation's intended users can best apply the evaluation's findings. The evaluator or another member of the evaluation team should chair the focus group session, arrange to have its deliberations documented, and keep the discussion moving and focused on the issue of evaluation use. Typically, our focus group sessions have required one and a half to two hours.

Following the focus group session, the evaluator should summarize the group's deliberations, conclusions, and recommendations in a report. In writing the focus group report, the evaluator should be careful to preserve the anonymity of individual focus group members regarding particular points in the report. The evaluator should deliver the report to the evaluation's client, other stakeholders she or he may designate, and the focus group members. The evaluator should then engage the client, as well as other persons he or she may want involved, in an in-depth discussion of the focus group results and how best to make use of them.

We have found the focus group procedure to be a practical, powerful means of engaging stakeholders to identify practical ways to apply evaluation findings. The advantages of the procedure are that it is easy to conduct, is a means to engage stakeholders meaningfully in deliberating how evaluation findings could best be used, focuses directly on the issues of evaluation use and impact, and provides the client group with concrete ideas about how best to apply findings, including the option of funding an input evaluation to identify and assess alternative follow-up actions.

8.5. Engaging an Evaluation Stakeholder Review Panel

We strongly advise evaluators and their clients to consider appointing an evaluation stakeholder review panel and interacting with the panel throughout the course of an evaluation. Such a panel should include representatives of the different segments of the evaluation's audience. Ideally, the evaluation's client should chair the panel. Its main purpose is to provide the evaluator with timely reviews of draft reporting plans and reports. The panel may also review draft evaluation tools and facilitate data collection (e.g., by encouraging other stakeholders to cooperate with the evaluator's data collection process). The panel's reviews should focus on and provide feedback regarding the accuracy, clarity, and utility of draft reports and other evaluation materials, as well as the feasibility of reporting plans. The evaluator should use the panel's inputs to finalize interim reports and the final report and, as applicable, to strengthen reporting plans. A key advantage of the evaluation review panel technique is that by virtue of panelists' engagement in reviewing and helping to as-

sure the soundness and utility of reports, the involved stakeholders are likely to understand and endorse the reporting process, trust the reports that they helped finalize, make effective use of the reports, and encourage other stakeholders to take the reports seriously.

However, the evaluator must make clear to the panelists that their main role is to assess reports for accuracy and clarity, assess reporting plans for feasibility, and address other questions from the evaluators. The client and evaluator should stress that the panel's role does not include redesigning the evaluation or rewriting findings. The evaluator and client should head off any possible negative aspects of empowering the review panel, such as possible moves by panel members to shift into the role of technical advisor or leak evaluation findings before reports have been finalized. The key to avoiding such pitfalls lies in the client and evaluator's joint effort to set clear rules for the panel's involvement before the evaluation begins and thereafter to enforce those rules.

A detailed example of the employment of an evaluation stakeholder review panel by the Hawaii State Department of Education in its evaluation of the state's teacher evaluation system may be found in Stufflebeam and Coryn (2014, pp. 597–599). In that application, the state superintendent of public instruction chaired the panel. Its other members included commanding officers of the state's two large military posts, an elementary school teacher, a middle school teacher, a secondary school teacher, the director of the state's teacher evaluation system, a member of the state board of education, the director of the area's federally supported educational research and development center, a dean of an area college of education, an educational measurement specialist, a data processing specialist, a representative of the state chamber of commerce, a representative of the National Association for the Advancement of Colored People, the majority leaders of the state's senate and house of representatives, a representative of one of the state's largest industries, two high school students, a parent with children in an elementary school and a middle school, a parent of a high school student, and the president of the state school district's teachers union. This panel's composition illustrates that such a panel should include the full range of perspectives of people who could be expected to be interested in seeing a subject project or system improved and who want to make sure that the evaluation of the project or system will be germane, fair, transparent, and accurate.

Checklist 11.2 (at the end of this chapter) delineates steps for setting up, interacting with, and utilizing feedback from a stakeholder review panel. The checklist succinctly defines the responsibilities of the panel chair, the evaluator, stakeholder panelists, and a recorder for effective application of the stakeholder evaluation review panel technique. We know, based on our experiences in applying the technique, that evaluators and their clients can find this checklist valuable for setting up stakeholder evaluation review panels and engaging them to help make evaluation reports as accurate, clear, and useful as possible. Moreover, we have found that such meaningful, impactful involvement of a representative group of an evaluation's stakeholders strongly prepares and inclines them to provide leadership to their peers for fostering effective use of evaluation findings.

9. Issue Formative Evaluation Reports

Consistent with the CIPP Model's orientation to project improvement, the evaluator should address the client group's needs for ongoing formative evaluation by providing timely, decision-oriented reports. To do so, the evaluator should maintain ongoing exchange with the client and other key decision makers and strive to anticipate and address their needs for evaluative feedback. Such needs typically will include context evaluation reports to assist goal formulation, input evaluation reports to assist the development of project plans, interim process and product evaluation reports to help guide and strengthen the implementation and effectiveness of project plans, and a final summative evaluation report to fully describe and assess a completed project's quality, cost-effectiveness, overall value, and importance.

9.1. Context Evaluation Reports

Reporting of context evaluation findings is especially important for helping a client group formulate sound project goals before the project is launched. Checklist 11.3 (at the end of this chapter) is a checklist of the types of information that evaluators should consider as they compile a useful context evaluation report. We believe client groups are well served when they receive timely context evaluation reports that convey the types of information reflected in Checkpoint 11.3. However, not every checkpoint is necessarily applicable to the preparation of every context evaluation report. Evaluators should exercise discretion and common sense in choosing those checkpoints that are germane to preparing a given context evaluation report.

We advise evaluators and their clients to use the preceding checklist to talk through what information would be most helpful to include in a context evaluation report. Then the evaluator should design, produce, and deliver a context evaluation report that directly addresses the agreed-upon context evaluation questions and that substantiates context evaluation conclusions with evidence based on relevant indicators. Such indicators may be selected and delineated based on Checklist 11.3. The context evaluation report should provide the data backdrop that the client group needs to develop and validate project goals.

A generic outline for a context evaluation report appears in Table 11.3. We reiterate that reporting evaluation is and should be a responsive, creative activity. Thus, the outline in Table 11.3 is intended as a heuristic device, not an iron-clad prescription.

9.2. Input Evaluation Reports

Given a client group's determination of project goals, the evaluator can provide immensely valuable service by conducting and reporting a well-conceived and conduct-

---

TABLE 11.3. Generic Outline for Context Evaluation Reports

Introduction

Purpose of the report, intended users, intended uses, criteria invoked, data gathered, evaluators involved, and methods employed

Characterization of the project's mission

Geographic area of service, intended beneficiaries, initial goals, and long-range aims

Explication and validation of the project mission

Identification and assessment of needs, assets, opportunities, barriers, and the initial project goals

Recommendations

Highlighting of areas for strengthening and clarifying the project's mission and goals

Employment of context evaluation criteria in the ensuing product evaluation

Confirmation that the projected product evaluation will examine project success against the assessed needs of the intended beneficiaries, how well the project overcame initial barriers to its success, and how well it took advantage of relevant assets and opportunities

ed input evaluation. Input evaluation reports are useful both for initially planning a project and—after the project is completed—for planning a follow-up project. In either case, the evaluator should prepare and deliver a succession of two types of input evaluation reports. The first (Tier 1 input evaluation report) is a report that identifies, delineates, and assesses alternative strategies for meeting assessed needs and achieving the project's stated goals that address those needs. The second (Tier 2 input evaluation report) is a follow-up, detailed input evaluation report that closely examines the project's delineated chosen strategy and associated management plan.

The initial, Tier 1 input evaluation report should begin by identifying alternative, competing strategies for achieving the project's goals. Evaluators and their client group can identify or formulate such strategies by reviewing relevant literature; visiting relevant, similar projects; or engaging two or more planning teams to independently generate competing strategies for the subject organization's achievement of the project's goals. The evaluator should subsequently produce and deliver an input evaluation report that assesses each competing strategy. The report that evaluates the competing strategies should provide information and judgments keyed to criteria such as:

- Responsiveness to assessed and targeted needs of the intended beneficiary group
- Promise for achieving the project's stated goals
- Potential to overcome any identified barriers to the project's success
- Potential to take advantage of relevant area assets
- Cost
- Potential to attract needed funding
- Rationale and sound logic
- Evidence of successful use elsewhere
- Fit with relevant existing programs
- Acceptability to stakeholders
- Political viability
- Staffing and training requirements
- Requirements for facilities and equipment
- Adaptability
- Feasibility for implementation
- Prospects for sustainability
- Prospects for transportability, if that is of interest to the client group

Table 11.4 contains a general outline for a Tier 1 input evaluation report.

Once the client group has used the Tier 1 input evaluation report to choose and delineate a project strategy, the evaluator should produce and deliver a second input evaluation report that closely examines the group's plan for operationalizing and carrying out the strategy. That Tier 2 input evaluation report should contain assessments of the plan in terms of such variables as:

- Operational objectives
- Realistic time line
- Support of the organization's policy board
- Arrangements for project oversight
- Appropriate and sufficient budget

TABLE 11.4. General Outline for a Tier 1 Input Evaluation Report

Introduction

Purpose of the report, intended audience, intended uses, approaches assessed, criteria for judging the approaches, methods employed, evaluators involved

Overview of competing approaches

Characterization of each competing approach in terms of distinguishing features, rationale, goals, main procedures, staffing requirements, facilities and equipment needs, cost, past applications, provisions for evaluation

Criteria for judging the approaches

Responsiveness to the project's targeted needs and goals, fit with the organization's other programs, adaptability, feasibility for implementation, acceptability to stakeholders, political viability, prospects for sustainability, fundability, projected cost-effectiveness, evidence of successful use elsewhere, adequate provision for formative and summative evaluation, potential for use in other settings, etc.

Judgment of the approaches

Qualitative assessment of each approach as well as quantitative ranking of the approaches

Discussion

Pros and cons of selecting one of the approaches versus merging the strong features of competing approaches

Next steps

Projection of steps required to operationalize whatever approach is chosen

- Protocols for expending project funds
- Arrangements for keeping fiscal records
- Arrangements for maintaining fiscal accountability
- Arrangements to house the project
- Supply of needed equipment
- Provisions for protecting the rights of human subjects
- Provisions for documenting project activities
- Arrangements for secure filing and retrieval of project records
- Assignment of a qualified project manager
- Adequate staffing
- Staff orientation and training provisions
- Technically sound and utilization-focused provisions for ongoing process and product evaluation
- Clear, realistic provisions for keeping stakeholders informed and involved
- Commitment and provisions to sustain the project if it succeeds
- Projection of and plans to ameliorate any identified threats to the project's success
- Provisions for maintaining a record of lessons learned

Client groups will find an incisive Tier 2 input evaluation report that closely assesses their plan for implementing a chosen project strategy, in terms of variables such as those listed above, to be immensely valuable for shaking down and refining their plan before putting it into operation. Moreover, the evaluator will find such a detailed input evaluation report valuable for conducting and reporting follow-up, interim process evaluation. In general, a Tier 2 input evaluation report should be structured as seen in Table 11.5.

9.3. Interim Process and Product Evaluation Reports

Once a project has been launched, the evaluation task turns to providing staff and other stakeholders, as appropriate, with an ongoing flow of process and product evaluative feedback for use in monitoring, strengthening, and documenting project operations and interim accomplishments. Typically, the evaluator conducts the process and product evaluations in concert. Process evaluation dominates in the early stages, especially

TABLE 11.5. General Outline for a Tier 2 Input Evaluation Report

Introduction

Purpose of the report, intended audience, intended uses, criteria invoked, evaluators involved, and methods employed

Characterization of the project plan

General description of the plan and reference to its full documentation

Assessment of the plan

Point-by-point judgment of the plan against detailed criteria, such as those listed above

Recommendations

Highlighting of key needs for strengthening the plan

Follow-up evaluation

Summary of the evaluator's plan to monitor the project's adherence to the input evaluation criteria

---

while the staff is shaking down the plan into actual operations, refining the plan, orienting and training staff, interacting with interested stakeholder parties, and sooner or later stabilizing activities. Throughout this process, the evaluator provides process evaluation reports both to assist project improvement and to document the actual process. Early on during project implementation, the evaluator devotes much less attention to the product evaluation's aims of identifying, assessing, and documenting achievement of goals. However, as the project matures. the evaluator increasingly searches out, assesses, and reports outcomes, both intended and unintended.

Basically, the interim process evaluation reports address questions such as the following:

- To what extent do actual project operations match the planned operations?
- Is the project on schedule?
- What if any implementation problems require staff attention?
- Do project staff members possess the attitudes and skills required to carry out their assignments?
- Are project staff members working well as a team?
- Is staff morale positive and functional?
- Is the project being efficiently and effectively managed?

- Does the project have what it needs in terms of materials, equipment, facilities, and funds?
- Are the project's staff members keeping stakeholders sufficiently informed about the project's progress?
- Is the project effectively engaging the intended beneficiaries and keeping them informed of what is being done to achieve the project's goals?
- Are stakeholders being effectively engaged to give meaningful feedback that staff can use to keep the project relevant to stakeholders' needs?
- Are staff members making effective use of stakeholder inputs?
- Is the project maintaining fiscal accountability?
- Is the project plan in need of revision and, if so, in what respects?

Once a project's staff has stabilized project activities and the project is working as intended, the evaluator increases her or his attention to reporting interim product evaluation findings. Interim product evaluation reports should address questions such as the following:

- Are the targeted needs of project beneficiaries being addressed and met?
- Are the project's goals being achieved?
- Are the project's results different or the same for different subsets of beneficiaries?
- What, if any, are the project's positive side effects?
- What, if any, are the project's negative side effects?
- To what extent are the project's interim accomplishments satisfactory?

Checklist 11.4 (at the end of this chapter) is a checklist for helping to guide the interim reporting of process and product evaluation findings. Clearly, obtaining and reporting interim process findings is at the heart of evaluation's role in project improvement. Documentation of such findings is also essential for helping interested parties learn what was actually done in the project that would account for the project's eventual success or lack of success. As the project matures, it becomes increasingly important for the evaluator to apprise the client group and stakeholders of how well the project is meeting the targeted needs of beneficiaries and achieving the stated goals. The main intent of Checklist 11.4 is to guide evaluators to do an effective job of issuing evidence-based interim process and product evaluation reports that help project client groups carry out effective projects.

10. Issue Summative Evaluation Reports

As appropriate, develop and deliver a comprehensive summative evaluation report and supporting documents. The summative report package should include:

- The main report, including an embedded executive summary, the evaluator's attestation of the extent to which the evaluation met the standards of the evaluation profession, and, as appropriate, the client's response to the evaluation
- A separate executive summary
- A backup technical report, unless sufficient technical appendices were included in the main report
- Any derivative, specially tailored reports
- Visual aids, such as PowerPoint slides, to support the client group's presentation of findings to stakeholder groups

The core of the main report should include, as applicable, sections on context, input, process, and product evaluation findings. It is noteworthy that in the summative evaluation report, the product evaluation component may be broken out by impact or **reach to the intended beneficiary** population, effectiveness in addressing beneficiaries' needs and achieving project goals, sustainability of positive results, and transportability of the assessed approach.

In preparing the final report, key its contents to the questions the users want answered, but also ensure that, in addition to addressing the stakeholders' questions, the final report thoroughly assesses the project's merit, worth, and significance. Write the main report, together with any shorter, derivative reports that may be required, directly and practically, and organize each one to help the audience's different segments attend directly to the findings that are of most use to them.

10.1. A Model Outline for Summative Evaluation Reports

Table 11.6 is a model outline for evaluators to consider in producing a final, summative evaluation report and its supporting components. A principle underlying the model outline is that a summative evaluation report should be organized to take account of the fact that dif-

TABLE 11.6. General Outline for a Final, Summative Evaluation Report

Cover

- Title of the evaluation, with subtitle, as appropriate
- Title of the project being evaluated
- Sponsor of the subject project
- Authors of the report

Executive summary

- A one-page overview denoting the project assessed, its goals, the evaluation's intended audience, the evaluator, the evaluation approach employed, main findings, and conclusions

Evaluation organization

- Name and address of the evaluation organization
- Principal evaluator(s)
- Evaluation period
- Date of the report

Contributor page

- Listing of the evaluation report's contributors and their respective roles

Project leaders

- Lead project administrator
- Relevant policy board members
- Key project staff members

Values page

- A captioned pithy representation of the subject project's stated values

Subject project

- Characterization of the project's intended beneficiaries, mission, goals, location, period under review, main methods, and staff

Audience for the report

- Intended users
- Intended uses

Tables

- Table of contents
- Tables of tables, figures, checklists, templates, and photographs

Prologue (origin of the evaluation)

- Who requested the evaluation, why, and for whom?
- Who are the evaluators, what are their perspectives and credentials, how did they approach the assignment?
- What is the subject project's title?
- What are the project's mission, goals, and approach?
- What are the evaluation's bottom-line questions?

Introduction (significance of the project and overview of the report)

- What needs and problems provide the focus for the project?
- How has this evaluation documented the project's approach and impacts?
- What are the evaluation's key audiences?
- How is the report organized to address differential information needs of different parts of the audience?

Part 1: Background of the project (descriptive and intended for the entire audience)

- What group initiated the project, when, and why?
- What are the project's goals?
- Who are the project's intended beneficiaries?
- What is the project's administrative structure?
- What is the social and political context in which the project operates?
- Photographic reprise to depict key aspects of the project's background.

Part 2: Project implementation (a strictly descriptive account, intended especially for those who might be interested in replicating the project's approach)

- Overview of the project
- Management and coordination
- Development of project protocols and procedures
- Collaborative arrangements
- Staff assignments
- Identification and involvement of specific project beneficiaries
- Delivery of project services to beneficiaries
- Metrics and data collection
- Funding
- Internal and external communication
- Review and revision of project goals and procedures
- Photographic reprise to depict key aspects of the project's operations

Part 3: Results (Evaluative and intended especially for oversight bodies and a wide range of interested audiences)

- Evaluation standards, purpose, audience, staff, budget, reports, process to apply findings, and provisions for metaevaluation
- Approach and methods for describing and judging the project's quality, worth, cost-effectiveness, and importance
- Context evaluation: Were the project's goals addressed to important assessed needs of the project's intended beneficiaries? Did the project effectively overcome barriers to meeting those needs? What, if any, were the relevant assets and funding opportunities that the project might have used?

(continued)

TABLE 11.6. *(continued)*

Part 3: Results *(continued)*

- Input evaluation: Was the project's approach maximally responsive to the project's goals and the assessed and targeted needs of the project's beneficiaries? Did the approach take advantage of relevant assets and opportunities?
- Process evaluation: Did the project's administrators and staff effectively implement the project's plan of action? Did the staff make needed improvements in the project plan?
- Impact evaluation: To what extent did the project reach and serve all of the intended beneficiaries? Were there instances of the project diverting resources and services to serve groups other than the targeted beneficiaries?
- Effectiveness evaluation: What were the extent and significance of the project's positive outcomes? What, if any, were the project's negative outcomes?
- Sustainability evaluation: To what extent are the project's successful practices and positive outcomes being sustained, or likely to be sustained?
- Transportability evaluation: To what extent has the project's approach been successfully adapted and applied elsewhere?
- Photographic reprise to highlight and make vivid the project's accomplishments

Conclusions (intended for all audiences)

- The project's notable strengths
- The project's notable weaknesses
- Key lessons learned
- Bottom-line assessment of the project's quality, cost-effectiveness, worth, and significance
- Photographic reprise depicting the evaluation's main message

Appendix (or separate technical report)

- References
- Evaluation agreement
- Project logic model
- Sampling procedures
- Key data sources and tools
- Data collection schedule
- Validity and reliability evidence
- Meeting agendas
- Information management procedures
- Data analysis procedures
- Data tables
- List of evaluation reports
- Procedures for protecting rights of human subjects
- Evaluation costs
- Evaluator resumés
- Evaluation organization resumé
- Members of the Evaluation Review Panel

- Attestation of the evaluation's adherence to standards of utility, feasibility, propriety, accuracy, and accountability
- Reference to the external metaevaluation, if there was one

Client response (to the summative evaluation report)

- The evaluator may invite the client to write a response to the summative evaluation report.
- If the client responds by submitting a response to the report, the evaluator would append it to the summative evaluation report, as written.
- Only the client would control the editing of her or his response to the evaluation report.

ferent segments of the evaluation's audience are likely to have differing levels of interest regarding different parts of the report. For example, persons unfamiliar with a project's background will be more interested in an explanation of why and how the project got started than will the project staff members who are already intimately acquainted with the project's origin. Also, potential adopters of the project's approach will be much more interested in the details of the project's operations and costs than will other members of the audience. On the other hand, virtually all members of the audience will be interested in the report's introduction, its findings, and its conclusions. The model outline in Table 11.6 is divided into sections to take account of this principle of organizing a report so that different segments of the audience can quickly find and study the parts of the report that most interest them.

Another noteworthy feature of the model outline is that several main sections conclude with a photographic reprise. For projects that have clearly visible processes and accomplishments, the photographic reprises can substantially increase a reader's appreciation of how the project functioned and what it achieved. For example, upon reading the summative evaluation report of one of our evaluations (of the self-help housing project described in Chapter 3), famous evaluator Professor Egon Guba remarked that he would have been skeptical about the evaluation report's claims that the project had made almost unbelievable impacts on beneficiaries had the report not contained photographs of:

- Low-income beneficiaries, including husbands and wives with no prior construction experience, constructing their own houses
- The resulting well-constructed three- and four-bedroom houses

- Each house's surrounding beautiful landscaping the participating families had developed and carefully maintained
- The participating families' obviously very happy children playing in the yards of the homes their parents had built
- The stark contrast between the 12-acre project neighborhood of 75 new homes and its surrounding poverty-stricken, run-down area

Photographic reprises won't be applicable in every evaluation, but when applicable, they can greatly enhance communication of the evaluation's findings and the audience's acceptance and appreciation of the findings.

11. Caveats Regarding Recommendations

The above final report outline contains no provision for issuing recommendations. The position of the CIPP Model is that recommendations should be issued only if they are grounded in compelling evidence that substantiates their soundness.

Typically, final evaluation reports provide evidence that only supports conclusions about the project's strengths and weaknesses, not about the strengths and weaknesses of follow-up projects or other actions that could be taken to respond to the evaluation's conclusions. Of course, the exceptions are recommending the continuation of a successful project or termination of an unsuccessful project. Other than those recommendations, a typical summative evaluation's findings would have no bearing on whether, for example, a project should be followed up by doubling funding, combining it with another approach, replacing it with an approach described in the literature, or installing it in other settings.

The CIPP Model's approach to issuing recommendations is to conduct follow-up input evaluations that systematically and empirically evaluate alternative courses of action. Through such systematic study of alternatives, evaluation clients can be properly informed about the empirically determined strengths and weaknesses of certain courses of action they might pursue. Such a follow-up input evaluation is preferable to issuing recommendations not supported by valid information on how to respond to an evaluation's conclusions. Unfortunately, all too often evaluators append to their carefully developed and vetted set of evaluation conclusions recommendations that they have not grounded in sound information. A follow-up input evaluation is a means to put forward and validly evaluate alternative recommendations for responding to an evaluation's conclusions. Of course, the client would have to approve and fund such a follow-up input evaluation.

12. Executive Summary and Briefing Materials

In reporting findings, evaluators should keep in mind that the evaluation's audience includes decision makers who are in a position not only to use findings but also to help disseminate the findings to other potential users. Such decision makers often are too busy to take the time to explain a long evaluation report to others. However, they can convey the main findings if they possess succinct materials that convey the evaluation's main findings.

Accordingly, evaluators are advised to take special care in preparing concise, clear executive summaries that the decision makers can readily digest and use in conveying evaluation findings to others. In addition, evaluators are advised to supply decision makers with briefing materials such as handouts showing key charts or checklists and PowerPoint slides for their use in presenting and leading discussions of the evaluation's findings.

13. Draft Reports to Facilitate Feedback from Reviewers

As is evident from this chapter, evaluators may issue a wide variety of formative and summative evaluation reports. Some of these will be informal evaluation reports, as in phone conversations with the client; face-to-face exchanges over lunch, for example; e-mail messages; and memos. These typically would not entail a process of drafting, reviewing, and finalizing the reported content.

Many reports, however, are formal and should undergo a process that in the end assures accuracy, clarity, and utility. The evaluator should draft such reports so that reviewers will see them as responsive to their questions, well organized, interesting, succinct, easy to read, and formatted to facilitate their critiques of the manuscript. Such reports should undergo a technically sound validation and improvement process, so that the reports' intended users will respect and accept the reported findings and act on them as appropriate.

Checklist 11.5 (at the end of this chapter) lists specific suggestions for evaluators to consider in the first part of the report validation process: the drafting of reports. The suggestions contained in the checklist are based on our experiences in conducting many project evaluations. In those evaluations, it was crucially important to format and draft formal reports to facilitate stakeholders' substantive, critical reviews. Invariably, such reviews were valuable for finalizing reports toward the goal of securing stakeholders' use of findings. We have found the checkpoints in Checklist 11.5 to be useful for drafting reports, especially extensive summative evaluation reports. (Many of the checkpoints are also applicable for finalizing reports, except for such checkpoints as those calling for double spacing, numbering lines, and placing watermarks denoting *draft* in the middle of pages.)

The checklist is a heuristic device. We do not recommend that evaluators slavishly attempt to rigidly apply every checkpoint. Instead we offer the checklist as a list of important issues to consider—and, as appropriate, address—in drafting reports. Competent reporting of evaluation findings is a creative endeavor, and different evaluators will invent and employ different approaches to reporting findings and getting their audience to attend to and make use of evaluation findings. The particular checkpoints in Checklist 11.5 comprise our attempt to share what we have learned in drafting many evaluation reports and the particular matters that we remind ourselves of in this process.

14. Obtain and Use Prerelease Reviews of Draft Reports

It is essential that evaluators make their formal evaluation reports accurate, understandable, and as useful as possible before releasing them in final form. As noted previously in this chapter, one way to achieve these ends is to engage the key client group and, as appropriate, other stakeholders, through such means as an evaluation review panel, in conducting a prerelease review of the draft report. Based on our experience, evaluators and their clients find such reviews invaluable for engaging stakeholders in the crucially important process of vetting reports and deciding to accept and apply the findings. The process for conducting a stakeholder review of a draft evaluation report includes the following steps:

- Evaluator prepares the draft report to meet requirements for utility, feasibility, propriety, accuracy, and accountability, with a heavy emphasis on clarity.
- Evaluator and client agree on the appropriateness of systematically engaging the client and stakeholders to review the draft report.
- Evaluator and client agree that the report should be reviewed, especially to identify any factual errors and issues of ambiguity and to make it as useful as possible, but not to change findings and conclusions (evaluator may do that later based on review results).
- Evaluator and client agree that review results will be used to improve and finalize the report before its release.
- Client selects a group of stakeholders to critique the draft report and subsequently to meet in a feedback workshop to systematically go over the draft report. (Typically, the group of reviewers should be broadly representative of the stakeholders, but in some cases may be narrower, e.g., the project's staff.)
- Evaluator and client agree that client or client designee will chair the feedback workshop (it is not a good idea to assign co-chairs).
- Client schedules the feedback workshop such that reviewers will have at least 10 working days to read and critique the report.
- Client mails the draft report to review panel members and stresses that they should read the report in advance of the meeting and make page-by-page marginal notes to flag any inaccuracies or areas of ambiguity.
- Evaluator drafts briefing materials that the client and other stakeholders could use in the future for informing superiors and other interested parties of the report's main contents.
- In preparing for the review session, evaluator or client provides on the conference table in front of each participant a tent-shaped placard with her or his name printed on both sides.
- Client or evaluator assigns a support staff member to make a written record of the session's main points.

- Chair conducts the review session according to an agenda, such as:
  - Chair invites each participant to introduce her- or himself.
  - Chair summarizes the workshop agenda and states the session's main goal to identify the draft report's strengths and weaknesses.
  - Chair emphasizes the importance of identifying any factual inaccuracies and areas of ambiguity that were seen in the report.
  - Chair identifies a secondary goal as reacting to briefing materials that the client and other stakeholders might use in the future to inform interested parties of the report's findings.
  - Chair cautions the group not to try to redesign the evaluation or to rewrite the findings.
  - Chair explains that participants' inputs will be recorded and considered in finalizing the report.
  - Chair explains that he or she and the evaluator will not strive to resolve disagreements between panelists during the meeting, but will accept participants' clarifications or attempts at resolution.
  - Chair and evaluator address any questions participants may still have.
  - Evaluator summarizes the report's main contents and any particular issues to be addressed.
  - Chair engages participants to give page-by-page feedback on what they found in their reviews.
  - Chair leads discussion aimed at making the report maximally useful to intended users.
  - As appropriate, chair and participants discuss possible decisions and actions that seem warranted based on the draft report.
  - Chair engages participants to react to and offer recommendations regarding draft materials the evaluator prepared for use by the client and other stakeholders in disseminating findings.
  - Chair invites each panelist to state her or his bottom-line assessment or advice for strengthening the report.
  - Evaluator states appreciation and responds to what he or she has heard.
  - Chair summarizes the meeting's results, identifies key next steps, and adjourns the meeting.

- Evaluator sends messages of appreciation to all members of the feedback session.
- Evaluator uses the review session's feedback to finalize the report.
- Evaluator also finalizes the briefing materials for client/stakeholder use in communicating the evaluation findings.
- Evaluator submits the final report and briefing materials to the client.
- Client distributes the report to right-to-know audiences (with evaluator's assistance as appropriate).
- Client uses briefing materials to inform superiors and other stakeholders about the evaluation's findings.
- Client and stakeholders use findings for program improvement, planning, and so on.

Form 11.1 (at the end of this chapter) is a sample template for planning and guiding the conduct of prerelease review sessions.

15. *Employ Effective Media in Communicating Evaluation Findings*

Based on inputs from the client group, the evaluator should employ appropriate, effective media to assist the intended users of evaluation findings to receive, understand, and apply evaluation reports. The selection and application of individual media options will depend on the type of report being delivered—for example, interim, formative reports versus a comprehensive final report; the diversity and locations of members of the audience; the project's possible state, national, or international significance; and especially the preferences of the client and other stakeholders. Checklist 11.6 (at the end of this chapter) is a checklist of media options for evaluators and their clients to consider when planning how best to deliver evaluation findings to the intended users of those findings.

As seen in Checklist 11.6, evaluators may choose from a wide range of media options to effectively get their evaluation message to the full range of intended users. We emphasize that the evaluator should review such options with the client and select the ones whose use would best secure maximum use and impact of evaluation findings.

16. Prepare Technical Documentation of Evaluation Procedures

In general, evaluators should develop technical appendices or a separate technical report to substantiate the soundness of the procedures, information, findings, and conclusions contained in a printed evaluation report. Checklist 11.7 (at the end of this chapter) is a checklist of the types of technical documentation to include in a technical appendix or separate technical report.

Ironically, although the evaluator may devote substantial time and effort to preparing an evaluation report's technical documentation, evaluation clients and other stakeholders may pay little or no attention to this backup information. The client might not even want to fund this work because they see it as relatively uninteresting and unlikely to be used.

When findings prove controversial, however, the evaluator may find it essential and useful to be able to reference solid documentation of the evaluation's technical soundness. In our past evaluation work, we have sometimes found that the mere presence of a thick, thorough, backup technical report sufficed to convince those who wanted to attack the evaluation because they didn't like its conclusions to desist from making such an attack. In some cases, such potential critics of the evaluation didn't even open the technical report when it was presented to them. We strongly advise evaluators not to skip over this important part of evaluation reporting but instead to plan, budget, and carry through in developing the appropriate technical documentation and to make it available to the client and interested members of the evaluation's audience.

17. Attest to the Evaluation's Adherence to Standards

The bottom-line requirement for program and project evaluations is that they meet professionally defined standards of sound evaluation. Evaluators employing the CIPP Model should both apply and attest to the extent to which their evaluation fulfilled the requirements of the 30 Joint Committee (2011) program evaluation standards. To fulfill the evaluation standards attestation requirement, evaluators should complete the **Evaluation Standards Attestation Form** (Form 11.2, at the end of this chapter) and append the completed form to the evaluation report. This recommendation applies especially to comprehensive final evaluation reports.

As seen in the preceding description of the evaluation standards attestation form, evaluators should conduct a kind of self-evaluation of their own evaluation. That is, they should conduct an internal, standards-based metaevaluation of their evaluation. This is one way evaluators can demonstrate accountability for the quality and utility of their work. A self-metaevaluation is an important option because clients often are reluctant to commission and fund an independent assessment of the evaluation. By appending a completed attestation of the evaluation's adherence to professional standards, the evaluator is making a positive, professional effort to provide users of an evaluation report with a standard-by-standard assessment of the evaluation against a set of professional standards.

18. Recommend and Support an External Metaevaluation

Although a self-metaevaluation has value in enhancing an evaluation's credibility, it is still only a self-assessment. Members of the evaluation audience might not fully trust the evaluator's assessment of her or his work. Accordingly, it is highly desirable that evaluators do what they can to have their evaluation evaluated by an independent party. The evaluator's responsibilities in launching an external metaevaluation are: (1) to advise the client to commission and fund an external metaevaluation and (2) if one is to be conducted, to cooperate fully with the external metaevaluator by providing access to the evaluation's materials and addressing the metaevaluators' questions.

Experience has shown that clients are unlikely to arrange for an external metaevaluation if the evaluator makes the recommendation late in the evaluation process. Experience has also shown that clients are reluctant to fund an external metaevaluation even if they are advised to do so early in the process. Nevertheless, we believe that evaluators should make significant effort—as early as possible in the evaluation process—to educate the client about the importance of commissioning an independent metaevaluation.

One particular move the evaluator can make in the interest of metaevaluation is to offer the client an opportunity to have her or his response to the evaluation appended to the final report. Of course, the evaluator should append such an assessment to the report as written and edited by the client. In introducing the client's assessment, the evaluator should make clear that it is included exactly as the client provided it. Making this move can be risky, as the client, justly or unjustly, may pan the report. However, the evaluator's willingness to invite such a client assessment is clear testimony to the evaluator's sincere interest in acting as professionally as possible in delivering findings to the evaluation audience.

If an external metaevaluation is to be conducted, the evaluator should cooperate fully with the external metaevaluator. The evaluator should especially disclose to the external metaevaluator the evaluation's particulars. These include documentation of the evaluation's guiding standards, contract, plan, staff, tools, data, reports, procedures for protecting the rights of human subjects, expenditures, and evidence of the evaluation's uses and impacts. Checklist 11.7 provides a detailed list of such particulars.

It is appropriate for an evaluator to recommend to the client that the external metaevaluation be keyed to the standards of the evaluation field. We prefer the Joint Committee (2011) *Program Evaluation Standards,* but the external metaevaluator may appropriately work from a different set of professionally developed standards, such as the U.S. Government Accountability Office's 2007 Government Auditing Standards (or the most up-to-date version). The evaluator should not choose the independent metaevaluator, as this could give the appearance of choosing an evaluator who is predisposed to give a positive metaevaluation, which could erode trust in the evaluation.

The point of all this discussion of both internal and external metaevaluation is that evaluators and their clients should keep evaluations on a high plane of professionalism. Moreover, by demonstrating that the evaluator is taking her or his own evaluation medicine and having the evaluation thoroughly vetted, he or she is making a positive, constructive move to build trustworthiness in the evaluation's findings and thus to enhance prospects for stakeholders' uses of the findings. As we have emphasized repeatedly in this book, the point of sound evaluations is to get findings used and to produce valuable impacts on improving projects, meeting accountability requirements, and preserving lessons learned for use in organizational improvement. The combination of internal and external metaevaluations

is a strong means of helping to secure valuable impacts from reported evaluation findings.

19. Provide Follow-Up Support for Use of Findings

Too often an evaluator's service ends with the delivery of the final evaluation report. In such cases, both the client group and the evaluator miss an important opportunity to work toward maximal, beneficial use of findings. Recipients of evaluation reports need to study, assess, and soundly interpret and apply the evaluation's findings. They often need a structure and assistance to do so. Competent evaluators can render valuable assistance to the client group by meeting with them to support their study and application of evaluation findings and by employing structures and procedures to foster and support sound use of findings. They may conduct follow-up focus group sessions, meet with the parent organization's board, conduct workshops with stakeholders focused on use of findings, develop a sociodrama by which stakeholders can role-play consideration and use of evaluation findings, and so forth.

If, however, evaluators are to engage meaningfully in assisting the evaluation's audience to study and apply findings, there must be advance provision and funding for such assistance in the evaluation's budget and contract. Thus, it is important for the evaluator to apprise the client of the need for such follow-up assistance at the very outset of the evaluation. At that early stage, the evaluator can project and give cost estimates for such follow-up procedures as public forums, workshops to go over findings, dramatization of evaluation findings in a sociodrama at a public gathering, and focus groups. Given that the purpose of any evaluation worth its cost is to secure informed use of evaluation findings, the client's investment in the evaluator's involvement in helping intended users apply evaluation findings is a highly cost-effective move. Doing everything feasible to get evaluation findings used is in the client's interest to demonstrate that the evaluation was worth its cost and also in the evaluator's interest in assuring that the evaluation had appropriate impacts. Certainly, the external metaevaluation should closely examine the evaluation's adequacy in supporting the client group to make effective use of findings.

20. Help Clients Identify and Retain Lessons Learned

Often, findings from a costly, sound evaluation are only used in the short term to guide decisions about the subject project and meet its accountability requirements. Although the evaluation may have produced valuable lessons that could be used outside the project, too often such lessons are set aside and forgotten. This is unfortunate because lessons learned from an evaluation may have relevance for strengthening the project's parent organization at the present or in the future, helping to focus and design future projects and evaluations, and especially avoiding mistakes of the past. The position of the CIPP Model is that organizations should set up and maintain a repository of lessons learned from past evaluations and, as the lessons prove relevant, use them to help inform ongoing organizational improvement efforts or avoid repeating past mistakes.

Project evaluators can play an important role in the identification and retention of lessons learned from project evaluations. When feasible, the evaluator should follow up the presentation of evaluation findings by helping the client group ferret out and record lessons from the evaluation that have salience for present or future efforts to strengthen organizational operations, help plan future evaluations, and, especially, help avoid repeating operations that previously failed. In addition, an evaluator with information technology qualifications could offer valuable service toward helping the client institution set up an easily accessible database for organizing, retaining, and retrieving lessons learned from evaluations. If the evaluator is to provide follow-up service regarding identification and retention of lessons learned, he or she will need to convince the client to provide for such service in the original evaluation budget and agreement.

The point of this section's discussion of lessons learned is cogently stated in the oft-repeated phrase that *those who fail to remember their history are doomed to repeat it.*

Summary

Competent reporting is indispensable to effective evaluation. The aims of evaluation reporting are to promote and assist a project's implementation through delivering timely, valid, actionable feedback to the project's staff and to inform the entire right-to-know audience about the completed project's quality and worth. Effective reporting of evaluation findings includes delivering interim, formative feedback oriented to project improvement, as well as a final, summative evaluation

report that assesses the project's value. The chapter lists and explains 20 actions of use in effectively communicating the evaluation approach and findings. The chapter supports those actions with a wide range of practical bulleted lists, checklists, and reporting formats. An essential component of competent evaluation reporting is the meaningful engagement of stakeholders throughout the evaluation process. Another essential component is the keying of evaluation reporting to relevant professional standards for evaluation. The chapter stresses the necessity to reach advance, documented agreements with the client concerning key aspects of the reporting process, including funding for the evaluator's assistance following delivery of the final report. Such follow-up support can greatly facilitate stakeholders' uses of the evaluation's findings. All aspects of evaluation reporting are to be keyed to supporting the evaluation audience's use of findings toward improving the subject project, meeting accountability requirements, and preserving lessons learned for later use.

REVIEW QUESTIONS • • • • • • • • • • •

1. What are three basic aims of competent evaluation reporting?

2. What are at least five Joint Committee (2011) program evaluation standards that are particularly useful in guiding evaluation reporting? Briefly define the relevance of each of these standards to effectively reporting evaluation findings.

3. What are at least five key provisions regarding competent evaluation reporting that should be addressed in the evaluation contract?

4. What are at least four key ways to engage stakeholders in the evaluation reporting process? Briefly define each of these ways.

5. What are the main types of formative, interim reports that an evaluator might deliver to an evaluation's audience? Briefly define each of these types of reports.

6. What is your idea of a generic outline for a summative evaluation report?

7. What are at least five key accuracy-related points to address in drafting a sound summative evaluation report?

8. What do you see as an appropriate generic outline for an executive summary?

9. What are the general contents of an evaluator's attestation of the extent to which an evaluation report met professional standards for sound evaluations?

10. What is this chapter's position and associated advice regarding whether an evaluator should include recommendations in a final, summative evaluation report?

11. After an evaluation has been completed, what are at least four techniques that an evaluator could find useful for assisting the client group to interpret and apply findings? Summarize advance agreements that are necessary for providing such follow-up assistance.

12. What are two services an evaluator might deliver to the client group regarding lessons learned from the evaluation? What preconditions are necessary for the evaluator to play this role?

13. What are this chapter's main recommendations for subjecting a final evaluation report to metaevaluation?

____	1. Client reporting role	Define with the client the role he or she will play in supporting the reporting process, especially clarifying evaluation questions, engaging project stakeholders, and fostering stakeholder use of findings.
____	2. Reporting standards	Confirm with the client the particular agreed-upon professional standards that apply to preparing, validating, and disseminating evaluation reports.
____	3. Rights of human subjects	Identify and meet the client organization's requirements to honor and protect the rights of human subjects (e.g., institutional review board criteria).
____	4. Reporting agreements	Communicate with the client and, as appropriate, other stakeholders to assure that vital aspects of the reporting process will be provided for in the evaluation's budget and contract.
____	5. Audience	With the client and others, as appropriate, confirm and further define the evaluation's intended users of evaluation findings and how they would likely use the findings.
____	6. Report planning	Secure assistance from the client and, as appropriate, other stakeholders in delineating an initial evaluation reporting plan to include report recipients, evaluation questions, stakeholder engagement strategies, the reporting venues, media, schedule, and follow-up evaluation services; throughout the evaluation communicate with the client and other project stakeholders to update the reporting plan as needed.
____	7. Contracting and budgeting	Secure advance agreements and funding for such items as follow-up evaluation assistance, editorial authority, release of findings, and provision for external metaevaluation.
____	8. Stakeholder engagement	Engage representatives of the intended users of findings and other right-to-know parties in focusing, critiquing, and using evaluation reports.
____	9. Formative evaluation reports	As appropriate, develop and deliver a succession of proactive context, input, process, and product evaluation reports.
____	10. Summative evaluation report documents	As appropriate, develop and deliver a comprehensive summative evaluation report and supporting documents: the main report, including the evaluator's standards-based attestation and, as appropriate, the client's response to the evaluation; an executive summary; the backup technical report or appendixes; and any derivative, specially tailored reports.
____	11. Caveats and a suggestion regarding recommendations	Issue recommendations only if they are supported by valid and reliable evidence of their soundness, which may require a follow-up input evaluation report.

(continued)

___	12. Executive reports and briefing material	Supply the client with an executive report and associated briefing materials for use in informing interested groups about the evaluation's main procedures and findings.
___	13. Drafting reports	Draft reports to make them responsive to audience questions, clear, and grammatically correct; format the reports to enable reviewers to quickly find sections of interest and to insert marginal notes throughout the manuscript.
___	14. Prerelease reviews of draft reports	Engage stakeholders and relevant experts—for example, a project's staff, a stakeholder review panel, and a panel of evaluation experts—to provide prerelease reviews of the draft reports; then use the reviews to correct reports for accuracy, clarity, and utility.
___	15. Effective media for communicating findings	Based on inputs from the client group, employ appropriate, effective media to assist the full range of stakeholders to receive, understand, and apply evaluation findings.
___	16. Technical documentation	Back up the final report with detailed technical documentation in an appendix or a separate technical report.
___	17. Attestation	Append to the final report the evaluator's attestation of the extent to which the evaluation met each of the agreed-upon professional standards for evaluations.
___	18. External metaevaluation	Advise the client to obtain an external metaevaluation of the final evaluation report and provide this metaevaluator—if there is one—documentation of the evaluation's guiding standards, contract, plan, staff, tools, data, reports, procedures to protect the rights of human subjects, and evidence of the evaluation's uses and impacts.
___	19. Follow-up support for use of findings	In accordance with advance agreements and funding, provide the client and other stakeholders with follow-up assistance, such as focus groups for applying the evaluation's findings.
___	20. Lessons learned	Offer to meet with the client and selected project stakeholders to help them ferret out and record lessons from the evaluation that presently or in the future would have relevance for improving the project's parent organization.

___	1. Role of the panel	Chair and evaluator should agree on the panel's role as reviewing predistributed draft materials for accuracy and clarity and confirm that the panel's role is not to offer advice concerning the evaluation's technical procedures, findings, or conclusions. The role also includes facilitating data collection and helping to communicate the evaluation's progress and findings to stakeholders.
___	2. Panel membership	Evaluator should collaborate with the client to identify and recruit members for a representative stakeholder review panel.
___	3. Panel chair	Evaluator and client should agree that the client or her or his representative will chair the panel.
___	4. Recorder	Chair should appoint a person to keep a written record of panel deliberations.
___	5. Schedule	Evaluator should ask the chair to schedule a panel meeting about two weeks following drafting of a projected report, reporting plan, or other item that has been drafted and should ask the client to stipulate the meeting's duration (e.g., 1, 2, or 3 hours, depending on the amount of material to be reviewed).
___	6. Distribution of drafts	Evaluator should distribute the draft report or other materials about 10 working days before the scheduled panel meeting and ask panelists to review and mark up the material and come to the scheduled meeting prepared to discuss issues of the report's accuracy, clarity, and utility.
___	7. Panelist seating	In preparing for the meeting, the client or her or his representative should place on a conference table, tent-shaped placards with panelist names printed on both sides.
___	8. Meeting objective	Chair should define the meeting's objective as hearing and recording panelists' critiques of the predistributed draft report or other draft evaluation materials in terms of any inaccuracies, ambiguities, and features that make use of findings difficult.
___	9. Caveat	Chair should make it clear that panelists are not expected to offer advice on the evaluation's technical approach or the substance of the report's findings and conclusions.
___	10. Protocol for exchange	Chair should instruct panelists that when desiring to speak, they should set their placard on end so the chair can recognize them; chair should state that for the sake of efficient communication, panelists should speak only when the chair calls on them.
___	11. Encouragement for full participation	Chair should emphasize that all panelists are encouraged to contribute.

(continued)

___ 12. Session record	Chair should confirm that the meeting's minutes will be recorded, distributed to participants after the meeting, and used to improve draft materials.
___ 13. Session impacts	Chair should state that panelists will see the results of their inputs in the finalized reports and other materials that will be distributed to all panelists.
___ 14. Initial briefing	Evaluator should brief panelists on the draft report or other materials to be critiqued and state key questions needing panelists' responses.
___ 15. Initial questions and answers	Before proceeding to hear panelist inputs, chair should provide panelists a brief period to pose questions for the evaluator's response.
___ 16. Panelist critiques	Chair should next devote a major part of the meeting to receiving— basically without comment—panelists' comments regarding strengths and weaknesses of the draft report or other materials, especially regarding issues of accuracy, clarity, and utility.
___ 17. Response to panelist inputs	Chair and evaluator should not criticize panelists' inputs or attempt to resolve disagreements among participants, but should dispassionately receive and record the inputs for consideration in the postmeeting finalization of draft materials.
___ 18. Panelists' bottom-line feedback	Near the meeting's end, chair should invite each panelist, at their option, to present a concise, bottom-line statement denoting her or his view of the meeting's most important message, which could be, for example, a judgment of the value of the draft report or other material, identification of a particularly irksome flaw in the report, a recommendation for strengthening future evaluation operations and reporting, key questions that should be answered in future reports, and so forth.
___ 19. Evaluator response	At the chair's invitation, the evaluator should thank panelists for their assessments, affirm that the assessments will be used in finalizing the reviewed materials, state that the finalized report or other materials will be sent to the client for agreed-upon distribution to the panel, and project when it would be useful to meet again with the panel and what materials would be reviewed.
___ 20. Adjournment	Chair should conclude the meeting by summarizing its main accomplishments, thanking all for their participation, confirming the panelists will receive minutes of the meeting and the evaluator's finalized report or other material, and projecting the panel's future involvement.

____	1. Project mission	Statement of the projected project's overall aims, for example, to improve living circumstances of low-income families in a remote Philippine Islands village
____	2. Context evaluation questions	For example: What are the characteristics of the families living in the targeted village? What are the families' most important unmet needs? How responsive are the project's draft goals to the families' assessed needs?
____	3. Environmental analysis	Description of the project's environment in such terms as values; customs; laws and court system; demographics; government agencies; political dynamics; housing; schools and universities; parks and recreation; hospitals and clinics; churches and social service organizations; police, fire, and emergency services; electrical, gas, water, and sewage treatment facilities; restaurants, department stores, and grocery stores; economy; employers and jobs; poverty and welfare rolls; crime; newspapers, radio, and TV; air pollution
____	4. Intended beneficiaries	Characterization of the intended beneficiary group in terms of such variables as age groups, family size, home ownership, educational level, aspirations, employment, gender, ethnic background, health indicators, life expectancy, welfare assistance
____	5. Needs assessment	Identification and analysis of beneficiaries' needs that are germane to setting project goals, for example, effective schools, vocational training, competent teachers, musical instruments and instruction, immunizations, transportation, clean water, electricity, food, clothing, housing, safe streets, foster care
____	6. Assets assessment	Inventory of special assets in the project's environment with relevance to the project's goals—for example, a vocational training program, a summer camp for children, the local swimming pool, a food pantry, a Habitat for Humanity house-building program, an employment service, a pertinent program of a local charitable foundation, the local Rotary and Lions Clubs, a walk-in health clinic, a free dental clinic, a military recruiting office, the local library, and/or retired professionals with relevant expertise
____	7. Funding opportunity assessment	Identification of foundation and government programs that might provide funds for the project
____	8. Relevant literature	Review of reports of similar past projects, relevant news accounts, relevant research publications, past evaluation studies, locally archived information, etc.
____	9. Stakeholder views	Gathering of stakeholder perspectives on the planned project from area residents via interviews, surveys, town hall meetings, focus groups, casual contacts, and so on
____	10. Goals assessment	Assessment of the project's goals in terms of responsiveness to assessed needs of targeted beneficiaries, clarity, layout of milestones, and feasibility

___	1. Feedback recipients	Confirm with the client the group most in need of interim evaluative feedback from both process and product evaluations.
___	2. Plan for delivering feedback	Agree with the client on protocols, intended users of findings, and a general schedule and venues for delivering interim evaluation reports.
___	3. Evaluation-oriented leadership	Confirm with the client her or his role in assuring that project staff and other stakeholders will make appropriate use of evaluation findings; for example, the client may agree to chair feedback workshops and an evaluation review panel.
___	4. Process and product evaluation questions	Regularly interact with the client and project staff to identify and update the questions to be addressed by interim process and product evaluation reports.
___	5. Documentation of project operations and achievements	Maintain printed and, as appropriate, photographic records of project events and accomplishments for use in preparing and delivering interim evaluation reports as well as helping the staff to meet accountability requirements.
___	6. Ongoing communication with the client	Maintain communication—for example, via phone calls, meetings, e-mail messages, memos—with the client and the project staff to keep them apprised of the evaluation's progress and the availability of interim findings and to keep attuned to the client group's evolving information needs.
___	7. Feedback workshops	Meet periodically with client and project staff to go over draft interim reports; receive their feedback on such reports' clarity, accuracy, and utility; secure their views on questions to be addressed in next reports; and, as appropriate, secure their assistance in gathering data for future reports.
___	8. Make all reports as useful as possible	Focus reports directly on the client group's questions; write clearly and succinctly, key findings to actions needed for project improvement; as appropriate, supplement printed reports with visual aids; and substantiate each report's technical soundness and adequate scope for assessing the project's merit and worth.
___	9. Finalize and deliver interim reports	Finalize interim evaluation reports, using client/staff feedback to make them clear and accurate, disseminate the reports to the agreed-upon recipients, and, as appropriate and feasible, meet with the client and project staff to facilitate their understanding and use of findings.

CHECKLIST 11.5. Drafting Reports

___	1. Draft notification, date, and pagination	In a footer at the bottom of each page, write *DRAFT*, the report's *date,* and the particular *page number*; also consider including a *DRAFT* watermark in the middle of each page.
___	2. Tables	Provide a detailed table of contents, also tables of tables, figures, checklists, and templates.
___	3. Focus of report	Key report to the intended audience's most important evaluative questions.
___	4. Title of report	Use a short attention-getting title that reflects the essence of the report.
___	5. Subtitle of report	Consider supplementing the report's title with an explanatory subtitle.
___	6. Type size	Use 11-point text size for main text, 14 point for main headings, and 20 point for the report's title.
___	7. Bold typeface	Put the report's title, main headings, and exhibit titles in **bold** typeface.
___	8. Type font	Use a type font that is easy to read, such as Calibri or Arial.
___	9. Margins	Use 1.5-inch margins to facilitate reviewers' insertion of marginal notes.
___	10. Spacing	Double space the text.
___	11. Line numbers	Consider numbering each line to ease reviewers' commentary on particular passages.
___	12. Active voice	Write the report in active voice; definitely avoid using passive voice.
___	13. Single-sided text	Print on a single side of each page.
___	14. Color	Draft and print in black and white to enable recipients to duplicate and distribute readable copies of the report (color may be used when the report is finalized).
___	15. Report sections	Divide body of report into logical parts—for example, Introduction, Background, Project Description, Evaluation Methods and Findings, Conclusions, and Appendix (or separate technical report).
___	16. Headings and subheadings	Within each part of the report, separate relatively discrete sections of text, using headings and subheadings to facilitate readers' quick location of particular topics of interest.
___	17. Part reprises	At the end of certain parts of the report, consider including a printed and/or visual reprise of the part's main points.
___	18. Bulleted lists and checklists	Make ample use of bulleted lists and checklists to foster and support practical applications of findings.
___	19. Illustrations of content	Summarize key areas of text in well-constructed graphs, tables, matrixes, and charts.
___	20. Pictures	Consider including pictures that make key findings vivid.

(continued)

___	21. Labels	Provide appropriate labels for inserted material, including table, checklist, figure, template, and photograph and number each one by report part and sequence within the part (e.g., Checklist 11.5).
___	22. Citations	Acknowledge with appropriate citations published material that is referenced in the report.
___	23. Endnotes	Employ endnotes rather than footnotes and list them at the back of the report.
___	24. Executive summary	Include a double-spaced, two-page executive summary at the front of the report.
___	25. Contributors	Include a page that lists the report's contributors along with the role each one played in relation to the report.
___	26. Table of contents	Include a detailed table of contents to ease readers' access to particular passages of interest.
___	27. Table of exhibits	Include detailed lists of tables, figures, checklists, templates, and photographs in the report's front matter.
___	28. Appendix	At a minimum, append brief vitas of the main evaluators, a copy or synopsis of the evaluation agreement, and the evaluator's attestation of the extent to which the evaluation met the agreed-upon evaluation standards.
___	29. Glossary	Consider including a glossary of definitions of key terms that may not be familiar to all members of the evaluation's audience.
___	30. Index	At the end of the report, include a detailed content index to facilitate location of text related to key topics.
___	31. Technical detail	Consider drafting a separate technical report to include the evaluation's log of data collection activities, instruments, data collection protocols, summaries of findings for particular data collection procedures, data tables not included in the main report, and a summary of the evaluation's costs, and so on.
___	32. Technical editing	Subject the draft main report and technical report to rigorous technical editing and correction as needed.
___	33. Assembly	Carefully consider and decide on the best and most feasible way to assemble the report (e.g., a Web-based version for downloading, a stapled manuscript, insertion in a three-ring binder, soft covers and a plastic spine); in deciding, obtain and take into account the client group's preferences, as well as the report's length.
___	34. Internal review	Conduct an internal review of the draft manuscripts and make needed corrections before distributing them to external reviewers for their assessment of the reports.

____	1. Printed formal reports	This is the standard means of recording and delivering evaluation findings; however, a printed report will sometimes be unnecessary or impractical, as when an evaluator provides informal feedback to the client, especially in response to the client's spur of the moment questions.
____	2. Memoranda	From time to time during an evaluation, the evaluator may issue memorandums to keep the client informed of the project's progress and emergent findings.
____	3. Telephone exchanges	During an evaluation, the evaluator may initiate or respond to telephone contacts with the client; while these are effective ways to apprise the client of the evaluation's progress or emergent findings with timely significance, the evaluator is well advised to follow up these exchanges by providing the client written documentation of what was presented and discussed.
____	4. E-mail exchanges	Similar to telephone exchanges, during an evaluation the evaluator may send or respond to e-mail messages to keep the client informed of the project's progress and especially pertinent recent findings.
____	5. Listserv	The evaluator may post reports on a listserv to help assure that the evaluation's full range of intended users will have timely access to evaluation findings.
____	6. Oral presentations	In addition to printed reports, the evaluator often should make face-to-face presentations of findings to the client and other members of the client group.
____	7. Slide presentations	When making oral presentations, the evaluator often should support the presentation with PowerPoint or overhead projector slides.
____	8. Videotaped presentation on compact disks	The evaluator can reach a sizable audience, many of whose members would not attend a face-to-face presentation, by videotaping the presentation, burning the presentation to a compact disk, and making the disk available to all members of the right-to-know audience.
____	9. Storage of reports on an evaluation project website	The evaluator may provide the entire evaluation audience with ready access to printed reports, videotaped presentations, slide shows, and the like, by storing them on the subject project's website or an evaluation project website.
____	10. Public forum	After releasing a printed evaluation report, the evaluator may schedule and appear at a public meeting to summarize the evaluation's findings and to respond to questions from the audience.
____	11. Op Ed pieces in newspapers	For evaluation findings that are in the public interest, for example, in the local community, the state, or nation, the evaluator may write and submit pieces for inclusion in relevant newspapers.

(continued)

___ 12. Television or radio appearances	Similar to public forums and pieces in newspapers, the evaluator may appear on a TV or radio show and address questions about the evaluation's purpose, conduct, and findings.
___ 13. Journal article	For evaluations of widespread relevance, and especially those of scientific interest, the client may authorize the evaluator to prepare an article based on the evaluation and submit it to a relevant professional journal.
___ 14. Doctoral dissertation	As seen in the literature review presented in this book's appendix, many doctoral students have reported their CIPP Model–based evaluation in their doctoral dissertation.

___	1. Evaluation tools	Interview forms, questionnaires, observation forms, content analysis protocols, and the like
___	2. Information sources	Persons/groups supplying information for the evaluation, documents reviewed and analyzed
___	3. Sample selection	Populations studied and sampling procedures employed
___	4. Rights of human subjects	Documents showing compliance with relevant rights of human subjects rules
___	5. Data collection schedule	Calendar showing what information was collected from what sources at what times
___	6. Meeting agendas	Focus group protocols, public forum protocols, feedback workshop agendas, and so on
___	7. Information storage and retrieval	Criteria for authorizing access to filed evaluation information, protocol and arrangements for accessing and storing information, persons authorized to access information, person in charge of keeping information secure, and so on
___	8. Data tables	Data tables not included in the main report
___	9. Reliability and validity of information	Procedures and evidence employed to check obtained data for reliability and validity
___	10. Analysis	Data analysis procedures and results not included in the main report
___	11. Logic model	Any project logic model not included in the main report
___	12. Evaluation cost	Record of the evaluation's expenditures in comparison to the evaluation budget
___	13. Interim reports	Listing, by date, outlet, and audience of interim evaluation reports
___	14. Evaluator resumés	Resumés for the individual evaluators and their organization
___	15. Reviewers	Listing of the persons who reviewed the draft final report
___	16. Attestation to meeting evaluation standards	Summary of the standards for sound evaluations that were invoked in planning, conducting, and reporting the evaluation plus the evaluator's attestation of the extent to which each evaluation met the standards

XYZ Evaluation Report

Meeting chair: _____

Other project representatives: _____

Lead evaluator: _____

Other evaluation team members: _____

Note taker: _____

Reviewers (representative group of report's intended users plus other stakeholders—all named on attached sheet): _____

Agenda

Chair's opening statement: Welcome, focus of session, role and importance of prerelease review of subject report, composition and role of reviewers, statement of appreciation

Participants' self-introductions (name, position, relationship to the subject project, relationship to the evaluation)

Chair's summary of the session's purposes:

- Overall, help assure that the evaluation will be accurate and maximally useful to intended users.
- Obtain each participant's assessment of the evaluation report for factual errors and ambiguities.
- Discuss ways to facilitate the report's dissemination and use.

Evaluator's summary of how the meeting's results will be used:

- Finalize the report.
- Further develop plans for disseminating the report.
- Strengthen plans to support intended users' uses of the findings.

Critique of the report:

- Evaluator's summary of the report's preparation, intended users, and intended uses.
- Page-by-page commentary on the report by all reviewers.

Plans to disseminate and foster use of findings:

- Evaluator's summary of plan for disseminating the report.
- Evaluator's summary of provisions to stimulate and support uses of the findings.
- As applicable, evaluator's distribution of draft briefing sheets for use by key users of the report.
- Review panelists' reactions and recommendations regarding plans to disseminate and secure use of the evaluation's findings.

Closing:

- Chair's invitation for each participant to make a capstone statement of what they see as the session's most important point.
- Voluntary participant-by-participant closing statements.
- Evaluator's summary of next steps.
- Chair's summary of the session's accomplishments, statement of appreciation, and adjournment.

Standard	Standard Statements	Basis for Judgments	Judgment			
			Met	Partially Met	Not Met	N/A
U1 Evaluator Credibility	Evaluations should be conducted by qualified people who establish and maintain credibility in the evaluation context.					
U2 Attention to Stakeholders	Evaluations should devote attention to the full range of individuals and groups invested in the program and affected by its evaluation.					
U3 Negotiated Purposes	Evaluation purposes should be identified and revisited based on the needs of stakeholders.					
U4 Explicit Values	Evaluations should clarify and specify the individual and cultural values underpinning the evaluation purposes, processes, and judgments.					
U5 Relevant Information	Evaluation information should serve the identified and emergent needs of intended users.					
U6 Meaningful Processes and Products	Evaluation activities, descriptions, findings, and judgments should encourage use.					
U7 Timely and Appropriate Communicating and Reporting	Evaluations should attend in a timely and ongoing way to the reporting and dissemination needs of stakeholders.					
U8 Concern for Consequences and Influence	Evaluations should promote responsible and adaptive use while guarding against unintended negative consequences and misuse.					
F1 Project Management	Evaluations should use effective project management strategies.					
F2 Human Rights and Respect	Evaluation procedures should be practical and responsive to the way the program operates.					

(continued)

Standard	Standard Statements	Basis for Judgments	Judgment			
			Met	Partially Met	Not Met	N/A
F3 Contextual Viability	Evaluations should recognize, monitor, and balance the cultural and political interests and needs of individuals and groups.					
F4 Resource Use	Evaluations should use resources effectively and efficiently.					
P1 Responsive and Inclusive Orientation	Evaluations should be responsive to stakeholders and their communities.					
P2 Formal Agreements	Evaluation agreements should be negotiated to make obligations explicit and take into account the needs, expectations, and cultural contexts of clients and other stakeholders.					
P3 Human Rights and Respect	Evaluations should be designed and conducted to protect human and legal rights and maintain the dignity of participants and other stakeholders.					
P4 Clarity and Fairness	Evaluations should be understandable and fair in addressing stakeholder needs and purposes.					
P5 Transparency and Disclosure	Evaluations should provide complete descriptions of findings, limitations, and conclusions to all stakeholders, unless doing so would violate legal and propriety obligations.					
P6 Conflicts of Interest	Evaluations should openly and honestly identify and address real or perceived conflicts of interest that may compromise the evaluation.					
P7 Fiscal Responsibility	Evaluations should account for all expended resources and comply with sound fiscal procedures and processes.					
A1 Justified Conclusions	Evaluation conclusions and decisions should be explicitly justified in the cultures and contexts where they have consequence.					

(continued)

Standard	Standard Statements	Basis for Judgments	Judgment			
			Met	Partially Met	Not Met	N/A
A2 Valid Information	Evaluation information should serve the intended purposes and support valid interpretations.					
A3 Reliable Information	Evaluation procedures should yield sufficiently dependable and consistent information for the intended use.					
A4 Explicit Program and Context Descriptions	Evaluations should document programs and their contexts with appropriate detail and scope for the evaluation purposes.					
A5 Information Management	Evaluations should employ systematic information collection, review, verification, and storage methods.					
A6 Sound Designs and Analyses	Evaluations should employ technically adequate designs and analyses that are appropriate for the evaluation purposes.					
A7 Explicit Evaluation Reasoning	Evaluation reasoning leading from information and analyses to findings, interpretations, conclusions, and judgments should be clearly and completely documented.					
A8 Communication and Reporting	Evaluation communications should have adequate scope and guard against misconceptions, biases, distortions, and errors.					
E1 Evaluation Documentation	Evaluations should fully document their negotiated purposes and implemented designs, procedures, data, and outcomes.					
E2 Internal Metaevaluation	Evaluators should use these and other applicable standards to examine the accountability of the evaluation design, procedures employed, information collected, and outcomes.					
E3 External Metaevaluation	Program evaluation sponsors, clients, evaluators, and other stakeholders should encourage the conduct of external metaevaluations using these and other applicable standards.					

CHAPTER 12

• •

Metaevaluation
Evaluating Evaluations

"Evaluators and their clients need to subject their evaluations to credible formative and summative metaevaluations."

This chapter is about metaevaluation, the process of evaluating evaluations. The main topics include metaevaluation's definition, importance, formative and summative roles, internal and external applications, need for grounding in standards, contrast with meta-analysis, main tasks, and metaevaluation checklists. The chapter also discusses client and evaluator responsibilities and qualifications needed to implement sound metaevaluations. The chapter is oriented practically to applying Stufflebeam's (2015) downloadable *Program Evaluations Metaevaluation Checklist.*

Overview

• •

Correct application of the CIPP Model includes formative and summative evaluations of context, input, process, and product evaluations through a process called *metaevaluation*. In simple terms, a metaevaluation is an evaluation of an evaluation. In more complex terms, metaevaluation of CIPP applications involves proactive, formative metaevaluation to help plan and guide context, input, process, and/or product evaluations and a retrospective summative metaevaluation to judge the totality of the completed evaluation work. Metaevaluations must be keyed to the standards of the evaluation profession.

This chapter draws upon and updates Stufflebeam's prior writings on metaevaluation: "Meta-Evaluation"

(1974, 2011), "Meta-Evaluation: An Introduction" (1978), "The Methodology of Metaevaluation" (2000c), "The Metaevaluation Imperative" (2001), Chapter 27 of Stufflebeam and Shinkfield (2007), and Chapter 25 of Stufflebeam and Coryn (2014). Whereas Stufflebeam's previous writings on metaevaluation focused on clarifying metaevaluation's concepts and theory, this chapter reprises and builds on that work but focuses on providing guidance for the practical application of metaevaluation. The chapter is keyed to Stufflebeam's (2015) Program Evaluations **Metaevaluation Checklist**, which is available for download (see the box at the end of the table of contents). The chapter is organized around nine key topics: (1) general and operational definitions of metaevaluation, (2) metaevaluation's formative and summative roles, (3) the need to ground metaevaluations in professional standards, (4) the importance of metaevaluation, (5) responsibilities for choosing and funding metaevaluations, (6) metaevaluation contrasted with meta-analysis, (7) an illustrative case, (8) metaevaluation checklists of use in planning and conducting metaevaluations, and (9) qualifications needed to conduct metaevaluations.

General and Operational Definitions of Metaevaluation

Michael Scriven (1969) introduced the term *metaevaluation* in *Educational Products Report*. However, this term's underlying concept has long been present in evaluations of evaluations across the full spectrum of professions, service areas, government programs, and nations. Such metaevaluations have helped public officials and the public adjudicate the validity of various evaluations' reported conclusions and recommendations and sometimes guided government to correct or rescind laws or regulations that were based on flawed evaluation findings. In contrast to metaevaluation's post-hoc application in judging completed evaluations, evaluators also obtain feedback from proactive, formative metaevaluations to help guide and assure the soundness of their ongoing evaluations. If a formative metaevaluation is performed well and evaluators make appropriate use of its ongoing feedback, then a subsequent summative metaevaluation is likely to judge the subject evaluation as sound and useful. Evaluators often appropriately conduct their own formative metaevaluations but may choose to engage an external metaevaluator to do so. We advise evaluation clients or funders to choose and engage an independent, external evaluator to conduct needed retrospective, summative metaevaluations.

Scriven's General Definition of Metaevaluation

In his initial explanation of metaevaluation, Scriven (1969) referred to his evaluation of a plan for evaluating educational products. Essentially, he defined a metaevaluation as any evaluation of an evaluation, evaluation system, or evaluation device. He argued that issuance of inaccurate or biased reports could seriously mislead consumers to purchase unworthy or inferior educational products and then use them to the detriment of children and youth. Thus, he stressed, the evalua-

tions of such products must themselves be evaluated as a means to help safeguard the welfare of consumers. Although Scriven initially focused the term *metaevaluation* narrowly on evaluations of educational products, the underlying concept is clearly applicable to guiding and judging evaluations across the full range of disciplines, service areas, and nations. Every evaluation study should be sound, and its soundness should be ensured and enhanced through formative metaevaluation and subsequently verified or discredited through one or more defensible summative metaevaluations. Although formative metaevaluations are vital in helping an evaluator assure her or his evaluation's quality and utility, clients, funders, and other users of the evaluation's findings are best served by an external, summative metaevaluation that independently and thoroughly assesses and judges the evaluation's procedures and findings against the standards of the evaluation field.

An Operational Definition

Operationally, we define metaevaluation as the process of delineating, collecting, reporting, and applying descriptive information and judgmental information about an evaluation's utility, feasibility, propriety, accuracy, and accountability for the purposes of helping plan and guide an evaluation and ultimately judging its strengths and weaknesses.

Metaevaluation's Formative and Summative Roles

As with any type of evaluation, metaevaluation serves formative and summative roles.

Formative metaevaluations are dedicated to helping evaluators plan and carry out sound evaluations and especially helping them identify problems in any key aspect of the evaluation and correct the problems before they compromise the evaluation. Formative metaevaluations provide the evaluator with proactive assessments of the evaluation's decisions and activities starting with the evaluation's outset and continuing throughout its execution. Such formative metaevaluation feedback is keyed to help the evaluator with such tasks as:

- Deciding whether to conduct an evaluation
- Staffing the evaluation

- Determining the evaluation's intended users and uses
- Deciding how best to engage stakeholders
- Designing, budgeting, contracting, and staffing the evaluation
- Choosing data collection tools
- Cleaning and validating data
- Improving draft reports
- Completing the final report
- Deciding how best to disseminate findings
- Deciding on ways to promote and assist uses of findings

Ongoing formative metaevaluation provides an evaluator with interim assessments of her or his work for use in keeping the evaluation headed toward a successful conclusion. Formative metaevaluation thus provides the evaluator with a valuable quality assurance tool.

Summative metaevaluations provide an evaluation's users with a retrospective assessment and judgment of a completed evaluation. Specifically, a summative metaevaluation assesses the evaluation against the contract that guided the evaluation and standards of the evaluation profession—for example, the Joint Committee's (2011) standards of utility, feasibility, propriety, accuracy, and accountability.

Both formative metaevaluation and summative metaevaluation roles may be carried out by the evaluator and/or an external metaevaluator. Table 12.1 summarizes the relationship between metaevaluation's formative and summative roles and how each may be implemented by the evaluator—as her or his own metaevaluator—and external metaevaluators.

Internal Metaevaluations

As seen in Table 12.1, evaluators should conduct their own standards-based formative and summative metaevaluations. In the internal metaevaluation's formative role, the evaluator regularly assesses the evaluation's different aspects against the evaluation field's standards for sound evaluations. He or she does so as a way to assure the evaluation's success by controlling the evaluation's quality and detecting and resolving any emergent problems in the evaluation. Ultimately, the evaluator should conduct her or his own summative metaevaluation by attesting to the evaluation's adherence, partial adherence, or lack thereof, to each of an agreed-upon set of standards for evaluations. The evaluator should append the completed attestation of the evaluation's soundness to the final evaluation report (see Chapter 11's *Evaluation Standards Attestation Form* for attesting to an evaluation's adherence to the Joint Committee [2011] *Program Evaluation Standards*).

TABLE 12.1. Framework for Internal and External Metaevaluations

Metaevaluation Roles	
Formative	**Summative**
Internal metaevaluation	
The program's evaluator systematically and continuously assesses the unfolding evaluation work—against agreed-upon standards for evaluations—and takes steps to strengthen all aspects of the evaluation, including its design, budget, contract, personnel, involvement of stakeholders, tools, procedures, data, data analysis, and draft reports.	The program's evaluator completes and appends to the final evaluation report an attestation of the extent to which the evaluation met, partially met, or failed to meet standards of utility, feasibility, propriety, accuracy, and accountability (or some other vetted set of standards for evaluations)
External metaevaluation	
An external metaevaluator—preferably selected and funded by the evaluation's client or funder to independently monitor and assess the evaluation—periodically provides the evaluator with feedback and reports that judge the evaluation's unfolding aspects against agreed-upon standards for evaluations	An external metaevaluator—selected and funded by the evaluation's client or funder to provide an independent, final assessment of the evaluation—compiles and delivers a summative report on the completed evaluation's adherence to standards of utility, feasibility, propriety, accuracy, and accountability (or some other vetted set of standards for evaluations)

External Metaevaluations

In addition to internal formative and summative metaevaluation, it is in the interests of both the evaluator and the evaluation's client and other intended users of findings to secure external formative and summative metaevaluations.

In both cases, it is preferable that the evaluation's client or funder select and fund the external metaevaluator. Ceding responsibility and authority to the client or funder for engaging external metaevaluators is an important means of assuring both the fact and the appearance of an independent metaevaluation perspective. If the evaluator chooses and funds the external metaevaluator, the metaevaluation's audience may see the ensuing metaevaluation report as overly and unduly supportive of the evaluator's work. Such an unfortunate outcome is especially likely if the evaluator's chosen metaevaluator delivers a highly favorable judgment of the subject evaluation. Thus, we emphasize that an external metaevaluation's trustworthiness and utility is best accomplished when the client or funder chooses, funds, and engages a truly independent and competent metaevaluator to deliver formative and/or summative metaevaluation services. On the matter of metaevaluation competence, it is imperative that the client select a metaevaluator who is fully knowledgeable of appropriate professional standards for evaluations and in command of the metaevaluation's needed measurement, analysis, and communication procedures.

In the external metaevaluation's formative role, the metaevaluator aims to help the evaluation succeed by periodically assessing its progress and providing the evaluator with interim reports on the evaluation's strengths and weaknesses as judged against agreed-upon standards for evaluations. Moreover, the external metaevaluator's ongoing, proactive assessment of the evaluation in progress provides a means of amassing a record of the evaluation's implementation, key strengths, problems, and corrective actions. Such a record will prove invaluable when the external metaevaluator compiles the final summative evaluation report.

In the external metaevaluation's summative role, the metaevaluator conducts an independent, retrospective, summative metaevaluation to help the evaluation's users and other interested parties judge the evaluation's overall soundness and limits of use. Preparation of the final, summative metaevaluation report depends heavily on obtaining a detailed, accurate record of the subject evaluation's design, budget, contract or memorandum of agreement, staffing, tools, procedures, implementation, interim and final reports, client group uses of findings, and the like. The main sources of this information are the evaluator, client, and, as noted above, the information amassed via a formative metaevaluation (especially an external formative metaevaluation). As with all other forms of metaevaluation, the external summative metaevaluation must be grounded in standards of the evaluation profession.

All metaevaluations—formative and summative, internal and external—should examine an evaluation's full range of important features. Among others these include:

- The evaluation's staff
- Definitions of intended users and uses
- Evaluation design
- Evaluation budget
- Contract or memorandum of agreement
- Stakeholder engagement
- Administration of the evaluation
- Data collection tools and procedures
- Data collection
- Information management
- Qualitative and quantitative information
- Data analysis
- Conclusions
- Interim reports
- Executive summary of the final report
- Final report
- Derivative, supplemental reports
- Briefing materials
- Dissemination of findings
- Client group uses of findings
- The evaluator's efforts to assist the evaluation audience's to make sound use of findings
- The evaluation's adherence to professional standards for sound evaluations

Standards for Judging Evaluations

For both formative and summative metaevaluations, we prefer that metaevaluators assess and judge evaluations against the Joint Committee (2011) *Program Evaluation Standards* of utility, feasibility, propriety, accuracy, and accountability. However, metaevaluations may appropriately be grounded in other vetted sets of standards, including the 2004 American Evaluation Association (AEA) guiding principles for evaluators (or the latest edition of these principles), the 2007 U.S. Government Accountability Office (GAO) government auditing standards (or the latest edition of these standards), and standards that were developed and validated by standards-setting bodies in countries outside North America.

Caveats in Applying Standards and Principles

In general, we advise metaevaluators and their clients to carefully select and ground metaevaluations in standards they consider appropriate. The three sets of metaevaluation standards we referenced above basically are intended for use in evaluating program evaluations in the United States. The Joint Committee *Program Evaluation Standards* specifically were developed for use in evaluating educational programs in North America. The Government Auditing Standards are intended for evaluating all types of government programs in the United States. The AEA Guiding Principles are intended for use by AEA members, or others who subscribe to the AEA Guiding Principles, in evaluating all types of programs, particularly those in North America.

None of these sets of standards is intended for universal applicability across the world. The implications of this observation are that evaluators and evaluation clients should select and apply applicable standards for use in judging and improving their evaluations; the standards produced by groups in the United States and Canada should be applied in accordance with their limited intended uses; and no one should impose a given set of standards on groups who judge them to be in any way inapplicable to their cultures and programs. Nevertheless, groups other than those intended to use a given set of standards may do so.

Basically, a **standard** is a principle that is commonly agreed to by the parties whose work will be evaluated against the standard. Such a standard should be developed and validated to reflect the group's mores and values and the canons of rigorous evaluation methodology. The standard should be systematically defined and validated by a group that represents the intended users and the relevant community of professional evaluation methodologists. Moreover, the group that develops and validates standards should clearly stipulate the boundaries and restrictions on application, so that the standards will not be imposed on groups that might find them inimical to their values and convictions concerning what criteria are and are not acceptable for judging a program in their situation.

All sets of evaluation standards are limited in their sphere of intended applicability and are not universally applicable. Each such set's intended application is bounded by such factors as the professional group that developed and adopted the standards, the disciplinary or service area of intended application, geographic boundaries for use, the relevant culture and its values and laws, and the intended time period of applicability. Some groups may object to standards reflecting values of democratic societies, especially freedoms of speech, religion, and the press, also human rights. Basically, an evaluation standard is a widely shared principle for judging evaluations that parties to an evaluation have endorsed.

Clearly, potential users of North American sets of evaluation standards should bear in mind several caveats. The standards of the Joint Committee on Standards for Educational Evaluation (1994, 2011) are focused on evaluations of education and training programs, education personnel, and students and are not designed for use in evaluating programs and other objects outside the fields of education and training. Moreover, the Joint Committee on Standards for Educational Evaluation (1981, 1994, 2011) developed these standards specifically for use in the United States and Canada and warned against the uncritical use of the standards in other nations. The committee posited that evaluators in other nations should carefully consider what standards are acceptable and functional within their cultures and should exercise caution in applying the standards of the Joint Committee on Standards for Educational Evaluation (1981, 1994, 2011) or any other set of standards developed outside their country. Experience has taught Stufflebeam, who led the Joint Committee's original 1981 development of the program evaluation standards, that there are definite problems in transferring North American standards on human rights, freedom of information, rights to privacy, and other matters covered by the Joint Committee on Standards for Educational Evaluation (1981,1994, 2011) to cultures outside the United States and Canada, especially countries with nondemocratic governance. For example, see Beywl (2000), Jang

(2000), Smith, Chircop, and Mukherjee (2000), Taut (2000), and Widmer, Landert, and Bacmann (2000).

Nevertheless, there has been a trend for evaluators in a number of countries to adapt and apply the standards of the Joint Committee on Standards for Educational Evaluation (1981, 1994, 2011) to their situations. Also, evaluators often have applied the standards of the Joint Committee on Standards for Educational Evaluation to evaluate programs outside the fields of education and training. We judge such applications to be appropriate if the evaluators and their client groups have agreed that the Joint Committee's standards are applicable to their noneducation evaluations. The Joint Committee's standards have provided a valuable service to the worldwide group of evaluators by developing useful models for consideration and possible adaptation outside the fields of education and training and outside North America. Especially instructive for other standards development efforts is the Joint Committee's systematic process for empaneling a joint committee that represents a service area's full range of interest groups and for engaging the committee through a deliberative process to reach consensus on a set of standards for sound and useful evaluation.

Evaluators who subscribe to the principles of a democratic society should not in any way set aside their values to conduct a metaevaluation in a nondemocratic society. We posit that a metaevaluator's integrity demands that evaluators walk away from any assignment that might deny the use of such propriety standards as advance contracting for evaluations, protection of participants' rights, transparency and disclosure of the evaluation's findings, and equal and fair treatment of all participants.

Although AEA's Guiding Principles for Evaluators (2004) have an American orientation, the organization's membership includes evaluators from many nations. AEA rightly espouses the position that its members should apply the Guiding Principles for Evaluators (American Evaluation Association, 2004) in guiding and assessing evaluations if they intend to claim compliance with what AEA recommends for conducting sound evaluations.

The GAO has shared its Government Auditing Standards (2007) with government accounting organizations and accountants throughout the world. Auditors in many countries have used the GAO standards at least as a model for setting and applying standards of financial accounting in government programs.

Any set of standards chosen for use in a given metaevaluation should be valid for such use. Clearly, metaevaluators can choose from alternative sets of standards for sound evaluations or they can work with their reference group to develop and validate their own standards. We have presented the standards that we prefer and employ, and we have recommended that they be applied in accordance with their stated purposes and spheres of applicability. Although these standards have been carefully developed and validated, we do not recommend them for universal use. Evaluators outside North America should carefully determine the standards that their reference groups would find professionally, ethically, and politically acceptable. These might or might not include or emulate the particular standards that have been developed and adopted for use in the United States and Canada.

The Importance of Metaevaluation

Metaevaluations, in public, professional, and institutional interests, ensure that evaluations provide sound findings and conclusions, that evaluation practices meet professional standards for evaluations and continue to improve, and that organizations administer efficient, ethical, and effective evaluation systems. Metaevaluation helps to ensure that evaluation audiences are presented with trustworthy, useful findings and conclusions, and, as appropriate, metaevaluation exposes reports that are biased, incompetent, or otherwise deficient before client group members make unwitting use of invalid findings or recommendations.

These contributions are secured by rigorously evaluating evaluations and reporting the metaevaluation findings to right-to-know audiences. As Scriven (1994) reported, even the highly respected and widely used *Consumer Reports* magazine should be independently evaluated to help readers see the limitations as well as the strengths of the many product evaluations published in the magazine. Moreover, metaevaluations are needed in all types of evaluation, including evaluations of programs, projects, products, services, budgets, expenditure reports, equipment, systems, organizations, motels, restaurants, theories, models, policies, research and evaluation designs, concerts, paintings, conferences, and personnel.

Customer reviews of services and products are an area in great need of metaevaluations. For example, when choosing a motel, it would serve customers well if the Web-based reviews reported by past customers are assessed to either assure or warn prospective customers concerning the veracity of the reviews. In this respect, it has given pause to see some word-for-word negative reviews appearing on websites for different motels. This raised the question of whether another motel was trying to steer customers away from competitive motels. On the other side, the experience of actually staying at a motel may be far below its Web-based high rating. Certainly, a motel could act on a conflict of interest by reporting inflated, unvalidated ratings to attract customers. It would be in the best interest of customers if businesses reporting customer reviews of their products or services also included on their website an up-to-date certification from an independent metaevaluator that at least a representative sample of the reported reviews had been examined for authenticity and accuracy and found to be credible. Absent such a certification, prospective customers are wise to treat Web-based ratings with a large dose of skepticism.

What Are the Risks of Not Securing Metaevaluation Feedback?

A flawed evaluation or set of ratings might yield invalid conclusions and mislead its audience. As with other professional enterprises, an evaluation can be excellent, poor, mediocre, or unjustly destructive. Owing to a host of technical, political, philosophical, psychological, conflict of interest, and organizational complications, many things can and do go wrong in evaluations. They might be flawed by unclear focus, loose and ambiguous contracts, insufficient funding, an unrealistic time limit, inappropriate criteria, weak designs, incompetent evaluators, evaluators with serious conflicts of interest, poor oversight and coordination, excessive costs, uncooperative program personnel, subterfuge or even sabotage by threatened program stakeholders, unreliable measurement tools, invalid information, recording or analysis errors, biased findings, unsupported conclusions, unsubstantiated recommendations, late reports, poorly written reports, lack of follow-up to support use of findings, censorship or withholding release of reports by the client, or corrupt or misguided use of findings. Evaluations that are conducted under severe resource and time constraints or in a restricted geographic area but are otherwise basically sound may generate valid conclusions with only highly restricted applicability. Such problems and limitations can attend evaluations

of all types and sizes, across the full range of disciplines and service areas, and in all nations.

If such deficiencies and limitations are not avoided or detected and addressed in the evaluation process, the evaluation may proceed to a flawed conclusion or unwarranted uses and thus produce deleterious impacts. If flawed reports are issued without being exposed by sound metaevaluations, evaluation audiences may make bad decisions based on the erroneous findings. Evaluations that accredit unworthy programs or institutions are a disservice to beneficiaries or other constituents. In addition, professional standards and principles for evaluations will be little more than rhetoric if they are not applied in judging and improving evaluation services and, as untasteful as this may seem, in exposing corrupt or otherwise unworthy evaluations.

So, What Does Metaevaluation Have to Offer?

With evaluation's pervasive and impactful role throughout society, it follows that evaluations themselves must be evaluated, improved as needed, and ultimately judged for quality, utility, and integrity. Just as accounting practices and reports must be subjected to **independent audits** to guard against and, as appropriate, expose fraud, waste, and abuse, evaluation practices and reports must also be evaluated and either certified as appropriate and dependable for consumer use or panned as unworthy of use. Metaevaluations based on standards of the evaluation field offer these valuable services.

Sound metaevaluations are based on vetted standards of the evaluation profession. Thus, metaevaluations reflect not the preferences of the metaevaluator but standards that have been rigorously developed and validated by representatives of the evaluation profession. It is also important to state that the cost of a metaevaluation typically is very low compared to the cost of the subject evaluation. Consequently, standards-based metaevaluations entail very cost-effective investments.

Why Is Metaevaluation Important to Evaluators?

Metaevaluation is a professional obligation of evaluators. Achieving and sustaining the status of a profession requires subjecting one's work to evaluation and using the findings to serve clients well and over time to strengthen services. This dictum pertains as much to evaluators as to accountants, architects, engineers, hotel and restaurant administrators, judges, lawyers, postal officials, policemen, fire fighters, teachers, school and university administrators, air traffic control officials, construction contractors, emergency care workers, pastors, nurses, physicians, dentists, pharmacists, psychologists, military leaders, and other service providers. It follows that evaluators should ensure that their evaluations are themselves evaluated.

Evaluators need metaevaluations to help assure and ultimately certify the soundness of their evaluations. Systematically evaluating evaluations is profoundly important because it helps evaluators detect and address problems, ensure quality in their studies, identify and address threats to the evaluation's integrity, and forthrightly reveal an evaluation's limitations. Moreover, summative metaevaluation reports help audiences to judge an evaluation's relevance, integrity, trustworthiness, cost-effectiveness, and applicability (Stufflebeam, 2001).

Apart from needing metaevaluations to ensure the quality of their evaluations, evaluators, as professionals, should use metaevaluations to provide direction for improving individual evaluations, improving evaluation approaches and tools, and earning and maintaining credibility for their services among client groups and other evaluators.

Who Else Needs Metaevaluation?

Consumers need metaevaluations to help decide whether to accept and act on evaluative conclusions about products, services, colleges, and other evaluands they are considering for use. They need metaevaluation reports to assure they are reading sound evaluation reports and using credible findings, or to expose and reject reports that are unworthy of use. Basically, cogent, defensible metaevaluations assist users in avoiding acceptance of invalid evaluative conclusions and instead making measured, wise use of sound evaluation information.

Those who may not aspire to be professional evaluators but who house and oversee evaluation systems need metaevaluations to help ensure that their institution's evaluation services are relevant, ethical, technically sound, practical, usable, timely, efficient, and worth the investment. Also, the subjects of evaluations—including program staff members, various professionals, and program beneficiaries—have the right to expect evaluations of their performance in programs to be fair and valid. Clearly, metaevaluations are in the best interests of a wide range of parties who may conduct, be served by, or be affected by evaluations (Scriven, 1969).

Responsibility and Authority for Obtaining Metaevaluations

Clients and funders as well as evaluators bear responsibility for obtaining and using sound metaevaluations. Clearly, evaluators should key their evaluations to standards of sound evaluation and should conduct both formative and summative metaevaluations. However, the evaluator has a conflict of interest in assessing her or his own evaluation.

Therefore, typically the evaluation's client or funder should commission, fund, use, and release to right-to-know audiences an independent summative assessment of the evaluation. We cannot stress this point too strongly. Far too often an independent metaevaluation has not been conducted. Or the evaluator may have engaged a highly supportive friend to conduct the metaevaluation and, in effect, deliver an overly favorable report. In our judgment, a funder or client should assume responsibility for choosing and engaging an external evaluator to conduct an independent, standards-based, summative metaevaluation. Funders and clients should not sidestep this obligation because of cost. In our experience, sound metaevaluations consume only a fraction of an evaluation's cost and can deliver findings, for the funder/client and other right-to-know audiences, whose value far outweighs the investment in the metaevaluation.

The rub is how to convince clients and funders that, beyond funding a primary evaluation, they should also commission and fund an independent metaevaluation of the subject evaluation. We lay the responsibility for making this case to the client or funder on the primary evaluator. That is, in contracting for an evaluation, the evaluator should strongly advise the client or funder to commission and fund an independent metaevaluation and should stress to the client or funder that the metaevaluation should be keyed to professional standards for sound evaluations.

The Contrast Between Metaevaluation and Meta-Analysis

To avoid confusion, it is instructive to contrast metaevaluation and meta-analysis. Although these terms refer to quite different concepts, they are often incorrectly equated. A **metaevaluation** assesses the merit and worth of a given evaluation, evaluation system, or evaluation device. A **meta-analysis** is a form of quantitative synthesis of studies that address a common research question. In program evaluation research contexts, this usually involves a treatment and control contrast or a treatment A and treatment B contrast. Across a selected set of similar studies, an investigator calculates and examines the magnitude, direction, and statistical significance of effect sizes.

Although metaevaluation and meta-analysis are different activities, metaevaluations have applications in meta-analysis studies. Metaevaluations are used first to evaluate and determine which candidate comparative studies qualify for inclusion in a defensible meta-analysis database. Also, a metaevaluation can and should be conducted to assess the merit and worth of a completed meta-analysis. The meta-analysis technique is rarely applicable in a metaevaluation, since most evaluations do not involve multiple comparative studies in a particular program area.

An Illustrative Metaevaluation Case

We turn now to an example of a metaevaluation that adhered quite closely to the preceding conceptualization of metaevaluation. The metaevaluation's special characteristics were that it was:

- Conducted by an external metaevaluation team.
- Funded by an anonymous organization that was independent of the evaluation, the metaevaluation, and the subject project's sponsors.
- Oriented to delivering both formative and summative metaevaluation reports.
- Grounded in the Joint Committee (1981) *Standards for Evaluations of Educational Programs, Projects, and Materials.*
- Periodically reviewed and assisted by a stakeholder metaevaluation review panel.
- Published in the *International Journal of Educational Research* (Finn, Stevens, Stufflebeam, & Walberg, 1997, pp. 159–173).

By describing this metaevaluation, we intend to help readers identify the tasks they need to plan and perform in conducting sound, useful metaevaluations.

Overview of the Metaevaluation

This metaevaluation assessed a Brigham Young University team's evaluation of the New York City (NYC) public school district's adaptation of the Waterford Integrated Learning System (WILS), a computer-assisted instructional approach (Miller, 1997). The subject evaluation included quantitative analysis of student outcomes from experimental and comparison schools, case studies of ten schools' applications of the WILS approach, a study to compare WILS costs with other approaches to teaching disadvantaged students, and a study to compare the different schools' implementation of the WILS approach. The metaevaluation team grounded their formative metaevaluations and summative metaevaluations in the Joint Committee Standards of utility, feasibility, propriety, and accuracy. They also formed and regularly interacted with a stakeholder review panel, especially to identify the questions that NYC school district stakeholders wanted the Utah-based evaluation team to answer. A key unique feature of the metaevaluation was that an anonymous, independent sponsor funded it, presumably to assure its immunity to any undue influence from any of the stakeholder groups.

The Project That Was Evaluated

The Utah-based Waterford Institute had developed and demonstrated the effectiveness of WILS in the Waterford private school in Utah (Becker, 1992). In light of that application's reported success, Waterford Institute projected that implementation of WILS in NYC public schools likely would produce dramatic gains in student academic achievement. The NYC version of WILS began in 1989 as a joint effort by the Fund for New York City Public Education, the New York City Board of Education, and the Waterford Institute. The NYC school district and its collaborators conducted a 4-year pilot test of the WILS approach in ten NYC public elementary schools. These schools were located in the Bronx, Brooklyn, and Manhattan. Their student bodies had high concentrations of minority students who were economically disadvantaged, which contrasted sharply with the mainly white, middle-class students who had participated in the original, Utah-based validation of the WILS approach.

The project's mission was to install and secure regular use of the integrated learning system in a selected set of elementary schools as an integral part of a school's daily instructional offerings. The project's specific goals (Miller, 1997, p. 94) were:

1. A 30–50% increase (over the previous year) in scores on the citywide standardized achievement tests in reading and mathematics after the first full year of system use.
2. An increase in students' self-esteem as a result of their increased achievement.
3. The establishment of a readily replicable educational model that could be implemented across schools with diverse populations of students and leadership styles.
4. Measurable academic improvement for a very modest increase in budget.

The WILS approach included "individualization of instruction; continuous and accurate pupil placement; acceleration of instruction; mastery learning; instructional feedback, record-keeping, and accountability; rejuvenation of faculty; demystification of computers for the faculty; 'validation' of excellence for student recruitment and fund-raising; and pricing and affordability" (Miller, 1997, p. 93). Central features of this intervention were two computer labs supported by experts in computer-assisted instruction in each of the participating schools and twice weekly in-service training for participating teachers in the WILS approach. The in-service training included becoming acquainted with the WILS courseware structure and contents, and learning how to adapt courseware to student needs, track student progress, monitor students' use of the computer labs, and integrate WILS courseware into the school's regular curriculum.

The Need to Evaluate the NYC School District's Piloting of the WILS Approach

The sound and useful evaluation of this application of WILS was crucially important to three main audiences. First, the NYC school district's leaders needed a rigorous assessment of WILS applications to help decide whether or not to continue use of WILS in the participating schools and possibly to apply the WILS approach in additional district schools. Clearly, such mainstreaming of the approach could entail expenditures in the millions of dollars and substantially influence teaching and learning for thousands of students and teachers throughout the district. Second, the creator of WILS, the Waterford Institute, needed evaluative

feedback to help assess WILS's feasibility and effectiveness for addressing the curricular needs of inner-city schools with high concentrations of low-achieving students and to identify aspects of WILS that needed to be better adapted to the needs of such schools. Finally, the educators in the participating schools needed evaluation of the use of WILS in their schools to help determine whether continued use of the approach would be in their students' best interests.

The Subject Evaluation

The evaluation of the project began in the summer of 1990 and was conducted by a four-person team. The members were Dexter Fletcher of the Institute for Defense Analyses and Harold Miller (chair), Dillon Inouye, and David Williams of Brigham Young University. Their primary audiences were the Waterford Institute—represented by Dustin Heuston—and the New York City school district.

Ultimately, the evaluation included four components: a comparative field experiment, an implementation study, a cost analysis study, and a **replication study.** The field experiment provided the evaluation's initial focus. It was conducted and reported by Dr. Harold Miller (1997, pp. 119–136). He compared gains in a host of variables for 10 WILS project schools and 20 comparison schools. This component's criterion variables included standardized achievement test scores, attitude measures, and records of students' uses of the WILS mathematics and reading courseware. Miller reported findings of eight statistical studies of a large database that was made available during the evaluation. He performed rigorous analyses to determine if the students exposed to the WILS approach performed better, especially in reading and mathematics, than students in the matched comparison schools. He probed the data extensively and systematically to ferret out any and all evidence of significant gains for the WILS approach. Overall, he reported that the results, across all eight studies, were mainly in the direction of no significant differences, with achievement in mathematics being slightly positive and better than the disappointing reading results. In discussing why the WILS approach returned findings that mainly were not statistically significant, he cited mitigating factors that matches between experimental and control schools were less than ideal and that the schools did not fully implement the WILS approach.

Drs. Williams and Miller (1997, pp. 99–117) conducted and reported an ethnographic case study in each of the ten WILS project schools. They conducted in-depth studies of each school's context and implementation of the WILS approach. They produced detailed descriptions of the project's applications based on site visits, interviews, and questionnaires. The key sources of case study information were administrators, teachers, lab managers, and in-service trainers. Each school was characterized in terms of its location, environment, demographics, school climate, and conformance to criteria for selecting project schools. Ultimately, the investigators published in-depth, highly detailed reports on two of the schools' implementation of the WILS approach. One school was chosen because it appeared to be the weakest in implementing the WILS approach. The other school was selected because the investigators judged it to be the strongest (among the ten schools) in implementing WILS. The two case study reports provide details about the environment surrounding each school, what happened in the project's computer labs and in-service training sessions, what stakeholders identified as the project's noteworthy strengths and weaknesses, and what recommendations for improving the WILS approach emanated from the interviews, questionnaires, and site visits. In contrasting the two schools' experiences, Williams and Miller reported that stakeholders' attitudes toward the project and identification of strengths in various aspects of the project were more pronounced in the school that was chosen because it appeared to be strongest in carrying out the WILS approach. The ethnographic case study investigation was descriptive and nonjudgmental. It did not refute the quantitative study's overall conclusion of noneffectiveness. Instead it illuminated how the project actually unfolded in the two targeted schools, and it recounted the judgments and recommendations given by the two schools' stakeholders for improving the WILS approach. The case study report included considerable in-depth information that the creators of WILS could consider in understanding why the project was basically unsuccessful and in better tailoring the WILS approach to inner-city school needs and circumstances. The case study findings were also germane to helping NYC school district educators decide whether or not to continue using WILS; if so, how to improve the approach's functionality and fit to school needs; and also whether to install the approach in other schools.

Drs. Inouye, Miller, and Fletcher (1997, pp. 137–152) conducted and reported evaluations of system cost and replicability. The heart of the cost study was a comparative assessment of incremental per-pupil costs of five school improvement programs: WILS; Success for All (an elementary school restructuring program for students in grades K–5); Reading Recovery (early-intervention tutoring for first-grade students at risk of failure); Writing to Read (a computer-based instructional program for elementary school students in kindergarten and first grade); and DISTAR (a highly structured reading, language, and mathematics program for elementary school students that employs the direct instruction approach).

The authors presented an analysis of costs to a school over a projected 8-year period for each of the five approaches. The totals are seen in Table 12.2. The authors were resourceful in searching the literature for cost studies on each approach. The cost evidence they found was thin for all five programs and not comparable in terms of involved grades, breakout of students, and expense categories. They presented caveats about the adequacy of the available cost information and then used what they had found. Basically, they presented costs in 1990 dollars and projected the cost for each approach over 8 years using a 4% inflation rate and an annual discount rate of 7%. As seen in Table 12.2, the projected 8-year costs varied greatly from DISTAR's low of $22,772 to Reading Recovery's $19,377,900, with WILS coming in third lowest at $836,232.

The authors also worked out and compared estimates of per-pupil costs for the five approaches, as seen in Table 12.3. We drew these figures from the authors' Table 4.6 (Inouye, Miller, & Fletcher, 1997, p. 146). Rather than breaking out WILS by the three groups of students in the authors' WILS analysis and their six breakdowns of figures for Success for All, we computed averages for those approaches for ease of communication here. The authors' estimated annual, incremental per-pupil costs ranged from DISTAR's low of $114 to Reading Recovery's high of $5,508, with WILS coming in second lowest at $229.

The authors pointed out that cost estimates alone are insufficient to guide a school's decisions about which program would best meet the needs of their students.

TABLE 12.2. Projected 8-Year Incremental Costs for Five School Improvement Programs

WILS	Success for All	Reading Recovery	Writing to Read	DISTAR
$836,232	$4,052,232	$19,377,900	$421,795	$22,772

TABLE 12.3. Average Estimated Incremental Per-Pupil Costs for Five School Improvement Programs

WILS per-pupil	Success for All	Reading Recovery	Writing to Read	DISTAR
Particulars of the approach				
Total of 685 students included in the computation	Baltimore elementary schools of 440 students in grades preK–5	Lowest-achieving 20% of first-grade students	128 students using labs in kindergarten and first grade	One class of 25 elementary school students
Per-pupil cost				
$229 (average for three groups of students)	$2,071 (average of costs across grades and categories of students)	$5,508	$412	$114

They said the schools need information about each approach's effectiveness in improving student learning. Ideally, they maintained that evaluators should provide schools with comparative cost-effectiveness assessments—not just cost comparisons—of competing programs such as the ones they studied.

In rounding out their chapter, Drs. Inouye, Miller, and Fletcher (1997, pp. 148–150) conducted and reported a replication study. They observed that their client, the Waterford Institute, had contracted with the NYC school district to have the involved project schools reliably replicate the WILS practices that had previously been installed and implemented in the Utah-based Waterford school. As a basis for understanding the largely disappointing student achievement results revealed by the field experiment, they thought it important to look hard at the extent to which the project schools had followed through on their commitments to faithfully install and implement all contracted features of the WILS approach. To assess the extent of WILS replication in the schools, the authors administered a project features compliance questionnaire to the Waterford Institute specialists who had served the project schools during 1992. The questionnaire asked those respondents to answer yes or no regarding faithful implementation of the school's compliance with particular school responsibilities that had been specified in the contract for carrying out the project. The authors reported that respondents basically said most of the 14 responsibilities had been carried out as required. The exceptions were that the schools had not complied with the requirement to have students spend 20 minutes each day applying the mathematics courseware and 20 minutes a day applying the reading courseware.

The authors also conducted a kind of simulation study to obtain teachers' judgments of the comparative

merits of WILS and five alternatives. They administered a questionnaire asking the teachers to rate WILS against: the most effective new program in which they had participated, a program that had delivered the best in-service training, a program to which they were most committed, a program that was especially time-consuming and energy-draining, and an imaginary program that would be barely acceptable. They reported that the teachers basically judged WILS favorably in comparison to these five alternatives. They reported that WILS fared best in terms of the perception of personal cost and that ratings for effectiveness, quality of training, and personal cost were generally favorable.

Inouye, Miller, and Fletcher (1997, p. 150) concluded that the project's main shortcoming was the failure of the labs to sustain a positive acceleration of students' achievement scores in mathematics and reading. They reported the following contributors to this failure: students spending too little time applying the mathematics courseware and reading courseware in the labs; inadequate match between the reading courseware and the project's standardized assessment instruments; inadequate teacher participation in in-service training; and other factors including student absenteeism and turnover, ineffective substitute teacher policies, and competing enrichment programs in the schools.

The Evaluation Team's Reflections on the WILS Project and Their Evaluation of It

After completing the quantitative study of student outcomes, the context and implementation evaluations studies, the cost study, and the replicability study, the authors reflected on the strengths and weaknesses of both the NYC school district's application of WILS and the evaluation of WILLS. Table 12.4 summarizes what they cited as the main strengths and weaknesses of both the WILS application and their evaluation of WILS. We derived this summary directly from the evaluators' retrospective assessments of the project and their evaluation. They identified a few strengths and many weaknesses of the WILS application; many strengths of the evaluation, including postevaluation impact on

the client group's planning to revise Wills; and substantial weaknesses in the attempt to conduct a comparative field experiment. We have presented the lists of strengths and weaknesses as the evaluators reported them. We turn next to a discussion of the formative and summative metaevaluations that were conducted and reported to guide the evaluation of WILS and assess its final report.

TABLE 12.4. The Evaluation Team's Reflections on the Merits of WILS and Their Evaluation of WILS

NYC Schools' Application of WILS	Evaluation of the WILS Project
Strengths	
• Schools provided space for the computer labs • Every school had a core of committed, appropriately engaged teachers • Incremental costs of WILS to a school were judged to be relatively low	• Effort to obtain all available relevant data • Delivery of findings to sponsor and participating entities • Early planning of the evaluation • Both quantitative and qualitative assessments of outcomes • Both longitudinal and school-comparison dimensions • Multiple measures, including standardized achievement tests, attitude surveys, and student records • Cost assessment • Replicability assessment • The way to effective implementation of WILS found to be much thornier than the project's leaders had assumed • Concluded with suggestions to consider in the process of adapting WILS for use in schools like those in this project • The creators of WILS already using the evaluation findings to restructure WILS for use in inner-city urban schools
Weaknesses	
• Uneven commitment to the project among participating school administrators, teachers, and paraprofessionals • Faculty resistance to technology • Some teachers' skepticism about the "new program of the month" • Lab managers' complaints about a too heavy workload • No tested evidence that WILS contributed to the acceleration of learning, even considering that WILS was in place and appeared to be in regular use • A host of competing and negative factors in the project environment likely neutralized the impact of WILS • Some teachers judged the WILS curriculum to lack compatibility with regular teaching agendas • Students spent too little time in using WILS offerings • Relatively low cost of WILS is offset by its ineffectiveness in this project • There was a considerable gulf between the implementation of WILS at the Utah-based Waterford school and its inadequate implementation in this project • The project proved naive in assuming that WILS would work equally well in accelerating students' achievement in troubled inner-city schools and in the privileged Waterford school	• No random assignment of schools to treatment and control groups • Inadequate matching of WILS schools with comparison schools • No isolation of the WILS treatment • Variable WILS treatment periods across the 10 schools • A not tight fit between the employed achievement tests and the WILS courseware

The Metaevaluation Team

The metaevaluation team included four nationally known experts: Chester E. Finn (a prominent educational policy analyst); Floraline I. Stevens (former director of the Los Angeles School District Office of Research and Evaluation and evaluator of many federal government programs); Daniel L. Stufflebeam (an expert in evaluation standards and evaluation methods); and Herbert J. Walberg (a specialist in measurement, statistics, and research design). All four had extensive experience in assessing programs in urban school districts. Dr. Dustin Heuston, chief executive of the Utah-based Waterford Institute and a main client of the evaluation of the WILS program, selected Dr. Walberg to head the metaevaluation, and, in consultation with Dr. Heuston, Dr. Walberg selected the other three metaevaluation team members. The team included three Caucasian members and one African American member.

The Metaevaluation's Audiences

The metaevaluation's most important audiences were the Utah-based evaluators, WILS project schools, involved school district offices, the central NYC Board of Education, and the Waterford Institute. Other targeted audiences included community leaders, interested parents, the national curriculum development community, providers of alternatives to the WILS approach (especially Reading Recovery), the educational research community, the metaevaluation's anonymous funder, and interested international groups.

The metaevaluation was comprised of both formative metaevaluation to help guide the evaluation and summative metaevaluation to reach bottom-line conclusions about the completed evaluation's utility, feasibility, propriety, and accuracy. In its formative role, the metaevaluation provided the evaluation team with periodic assessments of the evaluation's plans, tools, data analyses, draft reports, and stakeholder engagement. The summative metaevaluation was keyed particularly to help the subject project's stakeholders—including school board members, administrators, teachers, and educational specialists—deliberate and reach conclusions on whether to continue, revise, terminate, and ultimately institutionalize (or not) the WILS approach.

In their report, the metaevaluation team made clear that they were not responsible for the evaluation of the project and that the evaluation team was solely responsible for the evaluation. During the evaluation, the evaluation team used the metaevaluation team's formative feedback as they saw fit to strengthen their plans and activities. However, the metaevaluation team neither supervised nor conducted the project evaluation.

Funding of the Metaevaluation

A quite unique feature of this metaevaluation was that it was funded by an anonymous organization that was independent of the Utah-based evaluation team, the NYC school district, the Waterford Institute, and the metaevaluation team. The main interest of the entity that funded the metaevaluation was to assure its independence from any undue influence by the Utah-based evaluation team, the Waterford Institute, the NYC School District, and other interested parties.

The Metaevaluation Standards

The metaevaluators grounded their metaevaluation in the Joint Committee on Standards for Educational Evaluation (1981) *Standards for Evaluations of Educational Programs, Projects, and Materials*. The 30 specific standards are grouped according to four basic requirements of a sound evaluation: accuracy, propriety, feasibility, and utility. (This edition of the Joint Committee Program Evaluation Standards did not include the Evaluation Accountability standards [including Evaluation Documentation, Internal Metaevaluation, and External Metaevaluation] that are contained in the 2011 Joint Committee Program Evaluation Standards. However, the 1981 edition included a metaevaluation standard, covering both internal and external metaevaluation, within the accuracy category of standards.)

The Metaevaluation Process

The metaevaluation team met periodically in New York City with the Utah-based evaluation team to review the evaluation's plans and progress and deliver interim metaevaluation feedback. They obtained and reviewed relevant materials, including evaluation plans, evaluation instruments, data analyses, and draft reports. In addition the metaevaluation team set up and met periodically with a stakeholder review panel drawn from teacher, administrator, policymaker, and parent perspectives. The metaevaluators employed stakeholder review panel meetings to clarify stakeholders' questions and needs for information from the metaevaluation, obtain panelists' judgments of draft metaevaluation plans and reports, and record their perspectives on the utility of the WILS intervention and the educational soundness of the evolving external evaluation of this intervention. Based on their interactions with project and evaluation stakeholders and on study of evaluation materials, the evaluators provided feedback designed to help the evaluators strengthen the ongoing evaluation. In concluding their assignment, the evaluators systematically evaluated the project evaluation against the details of the 30 Joint Committee (1981) individual evaluation standards. The body of their final summative metaevaluation report included detailed assessments of the strengths and weaknesses of the evaluation's utility, feasibility, propriety, and accuracy.

Key formative metaevaluation findings were that (1) the evaluation's original, heavy orientation to using a quasi-experimental design approach was attended by severe feasibility and utility limitations, due especially to the subject project's evolving nature, the dynamic settings of the involved schools, inability to randomly assign schools to the WILS approach and a control condition, inadequate matching of WILS and control schools, and inability to hold WILS and comparison conditions constant; and (2) the comparative, quasi-experimental approach—even if it had been fully and appropriately implemented—would have produced only narrow findings that would do little to improve and adapt the WILS approach for use throughout the district. In response to the metaevaluation's interim, formative reports, the project evaluators greatly increased their conduct of in-depth, qualitative evaluation of project applications in the ten elementary schools that applied the WILS approach.

The Summative Metaevaluation Framework

Table 12.5 contains the basic framework used to complete the summative metaevaluation. This framework provided direction for assessing the strengths and weaknesses of each component of the evaluation and the overall evaluation against the 30 Joint Committee (1981) specific standards of utility, feasibility, propriety, and accuracy.

The Metaevaluation Findings

After using the framework in Table 12.5 to complete the 150 specific standards-based assessments of the evaluation's strengths and weaknesses, the metaevaluation team synthesized their findings into assessments of the utility, feasibility, propriety, and accuracy of the overall evaluation. Table 12.6 summarizes the key findings that appeared in the metaevaluation's overall report (Finn et al., 1997) in terms of the evaluation's strengths, weaknesses, and overall merit against the utility, feasibility, propriety, and accuracy standards.

In the end, the summative metaevaluation concluded that the evaluation was credibly and systematically conducted; addressed as feasible most of the Joint Committee (1981) program evaluation standards; evidenced notable strengths in all four standards areas; demonstrated significant limitations and deficiencies in the four standards areas (especially accuracy and utility); used questionable criteria and formulas to compare per-pupil costs of the WILS approach to alternative approaches, especially Reading Recovery; usefully delineated the strengths and weaknesses of the different schools' applications of WILS; and correctly concluded that the NYC school district's application of WILS had largely failed to improve students' academic achievement. Despite the deficiency in the quantitative analysis of field experiment results, the qualitative case studies produced a limited, though highly relevant, range of useful information about how WILS was carried out in the participating schools. The metaevaluation team produced the final summative metaevaluation report and presented it for use by NYC school district decision makers, the WILS project team, the participating schools, the Utah-based evaluation team, and other interested national and international parties.

Client Response to the Evaluation and Metaevaluation

A quite unique feature of this case was that the client, Dr. Dustin H. Heuston (1997, pp. 175–181) issued a response to the evaluation and metaevaluation. In general, he concluded that the evaluation proved to be valuable because it introduced a meritorious new evaluation model (metaevaluation), it exposed some serious limitations of the traditional evaluation model (especially the field experiment component), and it suggested ways of allocating future resources (e.g., adaptation of the WILS) to provide a viable solution for reading problems of disadvantaged inner-city and rural children.

In elaborating on what he termed the "new evaluation model," Heuston noted that his Institute had selected four members to serve as the outside expert panel in overseeing the evaluation, conducting regular reviews,

TABLE 12.5. The Summative Metaevaluation Framework

(U: Utility, F: Feasibility, P: Propriety, A: Accuracy)	Field Experiment	Case Studies	Cost Study	Replication Study	Overall Evaluation
U1 Stakeholder Identification					
U2 Evaluator Credibility					
U3 Information Scope and Selection					
U4 Values Identification					
U5 Report Clarity					
U6 Report Timeliness and Dissemination					
U7 Evaluation Impact					
F1 Practical Procedures					
F2 Political Viability					
F3 Cost-Effectiveness					
P1 Service Orientation					
P2 Formal Agreements					
P3 Rights of Human Subjects					
P4 Human Interactions					
P5 Complete and Fair Assessment					
P6 Disclosure of Findings					
P7 Conflict of Interest					
P8 Fiscal Responsibility					
A1 Program Documentation					
A2 Context Analysis					
A3 Described Purposes and Procedures					
A4 Defensible Information Sources					
A5 Valid Information					
A6 Reliable Information					
A7 Systematic Information					
A8 Analysis of Quantitative Information					
A9 Analysis of Qualitative Information					
A10 Justified Conclusions					
A11 Impartial Reporting					
A12 Metaevaluation					

TABLE 12.6. Summary of the Evaluation's Strengths and Weaknesses

Strengths	Weaknesses
Utility	
• Focused on basic questions of interest to the evaluation's audience • Presented a useful overview outlining WILS, where it was conducted, and who sponsored and supported it • Narrative information backed up with useful tables and figures • Presented a consistent conclusion that WILS did not produce important gains and that WILS was not fully implemented as intended • Case studies especially useful in addressing a wide range of questions of interest to the client group • Adequate stakeholder engagement • Provided a wide scope of information for the client group to consider • Identified critical competitors to WILS, attempted to compare them on incremental costs, and identified relevant caveats • Addressed the issue of replicability and associated questions • Reported statistical analyses at a level that the evaluation's audience could understand • Data probed extensively by quantitative analyses, which found that the conclusion of no effect of WILS held • Evaluators highly credible and competent • Credibility of findings enhanced by inclusion of the independently funded metaevaluators	• Completed about a year late, which did not help deter decisions to expand, possibly inappropriately, use of WILS in the school district • Provided no answers to the question of whether inadequate implementation of WILS in the project schools was only a failure of schools to honor their commitment or a manifestation of schools learning that WILS was not worth full implementation • Did not directly address stakeholders' major questions: Would WILS work without the heavy involvement of the Waterford Institute staff? Should the NYC school district board adopt WILS more widely in the district? What is necessary to adapt and integrate WILS into a school's regular program? What roles are necessary to make the program work? Was the Institute's expectation of 45 minutes a day in the lab reasonable? • Sometimes obscured the evaluation's main message that WILS failed to improve students' assessed academic achievement • Did not present clear plans for disseminating the evaluation findings—especially throughout the district • Evaluation team's lack of an expert in elementary school curriculum
Feasibility	
• Made good use of existing data • Data collection procedures shown to be reasonable and relatively unobtrusive • Secured constructive involvement of influential parties from the community • Obtained needed cooperation from a wide range of WILS project participants • Kept statistical analyses at an appropriate level of sophistication • Secured good cooperation by schools and their staffs	• Too little success in getting the NYC school district's central office to supply test data in a timely fashion
Propriety	
• Protected identities of students and teachers • Enacted effective contracting and other measures to counteract potential conflicts of interest • Balanced reporting of project strengths and weaknesses • Apparent commitment to make the full report public • Adhered to school district protocols for gathering data • No evidence of bias or censorship in the report • Presented evidence of project failure	• Interim results released prematurely, which may have misled the school district to expand use of WILS beyond the project • An unjustified undertone in the cost study suggesting that the WILS approach was effective, just not well implemented in the schools

(continued)

TABLE 12.6. *(continued)*

Strengths	Weaknesses
Accuracy	

Strengths

- Provided useful definitions of WILS and evaluation purposes
- Exposed the loose match between WILS and comparison schools
- Examined context, implementation, student outcomes, costs, and replication issues
- Examined students' use of computer labs and match between tests used and the WILS curriculum
- Discussed possibility that poor WILS effects resulted from students' insufficient time in labs and a host of uncontrolled factors
- Case studies provided clear, properly cautious, in-depth information on community, schools, labs, project implementation, possible lack of match between the WILS curriculum and the school curriculum, and the relationship of quantitative and qualitative findings
- Effectively probed quantitative data and searched for statistical interactions
- Contribution of multiple analyses to cross-checking different sets of findings
- Mainly produced properly cautious and justified conclusions

Weaknesses

- Unable to obtain timely release of needed test data from the central office
- Contradicted itself on whether the fidelity of WILS implementation was high, acceptable, or compromised
- Did not consider that full use of WILS courseware might have disserved students, especially in reading
- Silent on the issue of whether WILS could be successfully implemented without extensive support of Waterford Institute personnel
- Did not assess whether WILS implementation may have had negative side effects in areas other than math and reading
- Provided mainly a few snapshots in case studies due to limited visits and involved time spans and added only a modest amount of information on program effects, structure, and strengths and weaknesses of courseware
- Employed achievement tests that were narrow measures of student learning
- Reported dubious cost comparisons that accounted inadequately for the very different contexts of WILS and alternative intervention programs
- Failure of cost study to consider costs spread over the entire school budget, especially for the Reading Recovery option
- Not clear that all important alternative intervention programs were included in the cost study or why some apparently worthy critical competitors were excluded
- Comparable data on critical competitors in the cost study quite limited
- Failure of cost study to assess the key issue of the duration of incremental costs for every student in a school
- Replication study's failure to closely consider contextual factors, justify the selection of teachers whose implementation activities were studied, and consider the activities of teachers in the comparison schools
- Replication study's failure to consider WILS's fit to the schools' regular curriculum, its adaptability, its possible negative side effects, and its sustainability
- Replication study's failure to look at the replicability and sustainability of the alternative intervention programs
- Replication study's implication that the WILS was sound and valuable irrespective of failure to demonstrate achievement gains, but silent on the issue of whether widespread adoption of the WILS was warranted
- Replication study's failure to consider that teachers, especially reading teachers, might be justified in resisting a heavy dose of WILS
- All in all the replication study's small contribution to the overall evaluation
- No information provided to enable an assessment of the evaluation's cost-effectiveness

visiting sites, and producing their independent metae-valuation of the evaluation staff's report. He stated that direct funding of the metaevaluation by an anonymous sponsor assured the metaevaluation's independence. In his sole criticism of the metaevaluation approach, he observed that it lacked control to assure that every member did the expected work.

Heuston's (1997, p. 176) greatest reported concern was in regard to the primary evaluation of the WILS project. He faulted it for relying "on a subset of scientific method instead of following the broader goals of the full scientific method," and further said that

> according to current evaluation techniques, the project was a failure in demonstrating the effectiveness of using computer hardware and software to help children improve their reading and mathematics skills in grades 3–5. Instead of being a failure, the project is probably one of the more important in recent educational endeavors and has laid the groundwork for a fundamental breakthrough in the education of inner-city children. The Institute's concern was that current evaluation techniques were unable to recognize this.

Hueston (1997, p. 176) went on to criticize the evaluation's field experiment component for "its over-reliance on rigorous statistical techniques using the paraphernalia of control groups" and observed that "experimental efforts to improve education should be viewed as an ongoing process rather than a fixed snapshot in time." Nevertheless, he (p. 178) acknowledged that "whatever gains were achieved by the project were useless because they did not bring the weaker students up to a reasonable level of competence in mathematics and reading."

Hueston (1997, p. 178–181) then explained how the Institute would use lessons learned from the evaluation to revamp the WILS approach to better address conditions found in inner-city schools. Particularly, the Institute would pay close attention to the context of any school environment where WILS would be adapted and applied, redesign WILS for realistic implementation in such settings, focus WILS applications in inner-city schools at kindergarten and first-grade levels, make needed revisions of WILS curricular materials and software, secure funds needed for the costly adaptations of WILS, work with schools to assure employment of effective substitute teacher policies, and employ ongoing formative evaluation to guide future WILS applications. In Hueston's response to the evalu-ation and metaevaluation we see evidence that both sets of inputs met standards of utility in helping Hueston and his Institute to rethink how they could adapt WILS for use in the very challenging settings of inner-city schools.

Publication of the Evaluation and Metaevaluation

Following completion of the metaevaluation, Dr. Walberg collaborated with the Utah-based evaluation team to publish the evaluation and the metaevaluation in a special issue of the *International Journal of Education* (Harold L. Miller, Jr., Guest Editor, 27, No. 2, 1997, pp. 89–184). This journal issue's table of contents is summarized in Figure 12.1 and is presented here as an example of how an evaluator can inform a broad audience about an evaluation's design, process, and findings, and especially about perspectives by the evaluation team, metaevaluation team, and evaluation client. Such publication of an evaluation and a metaevaluation requires advance contractual agreements between the evaluator and evaluation client. It is important to reach and act on such an agreement when the evaluation findings may significantly inform program planning in other locations (e.g., national and international venues as was the case with the evaluation of the WILS NYC school district's project).

Metaevaluation Tasks Checklist

The preceding Waterford Institute Integrated Learning Systems evaluation and metaevaluation example points up main, generic tasks that should be planned and carried out in conducting a metaevaluation. Because metaevaluation is only a special type of evaluation, the tasks identified in the metaevaluation of WILS apply to evaluations in general and not just to metaevaluations.

Checklist 12.1 (at the end of this chapter) details 19 tasks for metaevaluators to consider as they plan and carry out their metaevaluation assignment. The listed tasks are derived from both the WILS metaevaluation and a range of other metaevaluations we have conducted. Our intent in presenting this checklist has been to provide a complete list of potentially relevant metaevaluation tasks. Not all the tasks would necessarily apply in every metaevaluation, and some metaevaluations might require additional tasks.

GUEST EDITOR'S PREFACE—Harold L. Miller, Jr.

CHAPTER 1. AN OVERVIEW OF THE EVALUATION
Harold L. Miller, Jr.
   The WILS and the Inservice Training Program
   The Evaluation
   Reference

CHAPTER 2. SCHOOLS AS CONTEXTS OF IMPLEMENTATION: TWO CASE STUDIES
David D. Williams and Harold L. Miller, Jr.
   Case Study: School 1
   Case Study: School 2
   Major Differences Between Schools 1 and 2
   Biography

CHAPTER 3. QUANTITATIVE ANALYSES OF STUDENT OUTCOME MEASURES
Harold L. Miller, Jr.
   The Treatment and Comparison Schools
   The Analyses
   General Summary of the Quantitative Studies
   References

CHAPTER 4. THE EVALUATION OF SYSTEM COST AND REPLICABILITY
Dillon K. Inouye, Harold L. Miller, Jr., and J. Dexter Fletcher
   The Cost of the WILS
   Success for All
   Reading Recovery
   Writing to Read
   DISTAR
   Summary of the Comparative Cost Analysis
   Analysis of System Replication Study
   References
   Biographies

CHAPTER 5. REFLECTIONS FROM THE EVALUATION
Harold L. Miller, Jr., David D. Williams, Dillon K. Inouye, and J. Dexter Fletcher
   New Hopes
   References

CHAPTER 6. A META-EVALUATION
Chester E. Finn, Jr., Floraline I. Stevens, Daniel L. Stufflebeam, and Herbert J. Walberg
   The Criteria of the Meta-Evaluation
   Findings of the Meta-Evaluation
   Final Observations
   Reference
   Biographies

(continued)

FIGURE 12.1. Summary of the table of contents for *The New York City Public Schools Integrated Learning Systems Project: Evaluation and Metaevaluation.*

CHAPTER 7. RESPONSE TO THE EVALUATION AND META-EVALUATION
Dustin H. Heuston
The New Evaluation Model
Serious Limitations of the Traditional Evaluation Model
What Was Learned and What Solutions Were Generated
References
Biography

CHAPTER 8. CONCLUDING PERSPECTIVE
Herbert J. Walberg

FIGURE 12.1. *(continued)*

Basically, the tasks in Checklist 12.1 comprise a heuristic tool for metaevaluators to use as they apply their creativity in planning and executing sound and useful metaevaluations. However, the list is only a summary of relevant metaevaluation tasks, accompanied by a brief explanation of each task. We advise readers who desire a more detailed presentation of such tasks and how to apply them to access and use Stufflebeam's (2015) downloadable Program Evaluations Metaevaluation Checklist (available online; see the box at the end of the table of contents).

Qualifications Needed to Conduct Metaevaluations

This chapter has recommended that the evaluation client assume responsibility and authority for selecting the lead metaevaluator and then communicate with the lead evaluator in choosing any additionally needed metaevaluation team members. Accordingly, clients need guidance regarding the qualifications to look for in selecting appropriately qualified metaevaluators. Drawing from the prior writings of Stufflebeam and Shinkfield (2007, pp. 653–654) and our varied experiences in conducting metaevaluations, we have prepared the Checklist of Metaevaluator Qualifications that appears in Checklist 12.2 (at the end of this chapter). We see these 19 areas of qualifications as essential to the sound conduct of metaevaluations. However, often no one individual will possess all of the listed qualifications. Consequently, in many metaevaluation assignments, the client or funder and the lead metaevaluator will need to assemble a team with the needed combination of methodological and content area expertise.

Checklist 12.2 basically identifies the 19 recommended qualifications. It does not specify how clients can reach determinations about a prospective metaevaluator on all 19 checkpoints. To apply the checkpoints, a client will need to gather from the prospective metaevaluator her or his resumé, examples of past metaevaluation plans and reports, and references that may be contacted. The client may also use the checklist as a kind of interview guide in asking the prospective metaevaluator to verbally respond to each checkpoint. In addition, the client will be wise to contact and obtain judgments of the metaevaluator's qualifications from her or his past metaevaluation clients.

Summary

This chapter serves mainly as a practical guide to commissioning, conducting, reporting, and applying metaevaluaton results. Among its practical features are identification of the Joint Committee (2011) Program Evaluation Standards (of utility, feasibility, propriety, and accuracy) as our preferred set of standards for judging evaluations. It defines and provides direction for conducting formative metaevaluations as a kind of quality assessment and assurance process to help evaluators improve their ongoing evaluations and summative metaevaluations to inform evaluation clients and other users of the soundness of a completed evaluation. The chapter describes an actual metaevaluation case that included both formative metaevaluation and summative metaevaluation of an evaluation of a computer-based program in reading and mathematics for elementary school children in ten New York City public schools. The chapter drew from this and other cases and from

Stufflebeam's (2015) downloadable Program Evaluations Metaevaluation Checklist to present a checklist for planning, conducting, and reporting metaevaluations. Among the chapter's practical features are a figure, six tables, and two checklists. Finally, the chapter is based on and substantiates the easily defensible premise that metaevaluations are very much in the interests of program funders, staffs, and beneficiaries as well as evaluators and, of course, the public at large. Metaevaluations help ensure the integrity and credibility of evaluations and are thus important to both users and producers of evaluations.

Beyond its practical orientation, the chapter defines basic concepts of metaevaluation. Metaevaluation is defined as an evaluation of an evaluation. A formative metaevaluation is an evaluation of an evaluation that assesses and is intended to help an evaluator improve her or his evaluation plan, design, implementation, and draft reports. A summative metaevaluation is an evaluation of a completed evaluation, especially in terms of its utility, feasibility, propriety, accuracy, and accountability (the five categories of the Joint Committee [2011] *Program Evaluation Standards*). The chapter explains that formative metaevaluations and summative metaevaluations may be conducted by either internal or external metaevaluators. The chapter also contrasts metaevaluation with meta-analysis, so that readers will not confuse the two concepts.

The chapter is aimed at a number of key participants in the evaluation enterprise. A primary audience includes clients of evaluations who seek summative metaevaluations to assess the extent to which evaluations of their programs are sound and useful. Harkening back to Chapter 4 on evaluation-oriented leadership, this chapter spells out a special and demanding role for evaluation clients and funders. It advises them to assume responsibility and authority for choosing and funding metaevaluators. In this regard, the chapter provides a checklist of qualifications needed to conduct sound metaevluations, advises evaluation clients and funders to use the checklist in choosing metaevaluators, and provides suggestions for applying the checklist.

The chapter is also aimed at evaluators: those who need formative metaevaluations to help strengthen their evaluation plans, operations, and draft reports and those who conduct metaevaluations. Key references and tools for evaluators and metaevaluators are Stufflebeam's downloadable (2015) Program Evaluations Metaevaluation Checklist and Chapter 27 in Stufflebeam and Coryn (2014).

REVIEW QUESTIONS • • • • • • • • • • • •

1. List at least five reasons you would give to a director of a school improvement project for justifying the expense of contracting for an independent metaevaluation of the external evaluation of that program.

2. Compare and contrast the concepts of metaevaluation and meta-analysis by (1) briefly defining each concept and (2) explaining how each of these processes may be incorporated in the other.

3. List and briefly define the essence of this chapter's nine major topics.

4. What is this chapter's basic definition of metaevaluation? List the points you would include in explaining the concept of metaevaluation to a potential client who is unfamiliar with metaevaluation.

5. Based on your understanding of this chapter, construct a checklist for designing a summative metaevaluation.

6. What advantages does a metaevaluator attain by contracting with a third party to conduct a particular metaevaluation? What do you see, if any, as disadvantages of this approach?

7. Assume a hypothetical client is considering hiring you to conduct a metaevaluation of an evaluation of a fast-food restaurant. List your qualifications to conduct the metaevaluation. Then list any important additional qualifications for this assignment that you would need but do not possess. What specific steps would you take to address any inadequacies you might have for conducting this metaevaluation, and why?

8. List at least ten things that can go wrong in an evaluation; then construct a matrix to show how certain features of a sound metaevaluation could be applied to prevent or expose these threats to the evaluation's success.

9. Develop and explain a matrix that compares and contrasts formative metaevaluation and summative metaevaluation in terms of purpose, timing, reports, and audiences.

10. Construct and explain a matrix that contrasts internal and external applications of formative metaevaluation and summative metaevaluation.

11. React to the statement that only the evaluator should choose a metaevaluator.

12. Summarize an evaluation with which you are familiar; then list at least eight features of this evaluation that should be assessed in a metaevaluation.

13. Visit *www.wmich.edu/evaluation/checklists* and review the checklists your group might use to conduct a metaevaluation of the evaluation of a fast-food restaurant. Which one or more checklists would you choose to conduct the metaevaluation? Justify your choice.

14. Refer to the evaluation standards attestation form in Chapter 11. Construct a blank copy of the form. Identify and acquire a final report from a completed evaluation. Then fill in the evaluation standards attestation form as a step toward completing a retrospective summative metaevaluation of the completed evaluation.

15. Refer to the NYC school district metaevaluation case in this chapter. Then list what you see as pros and cons of (a) that metaevaluation's funding by an independent, anonymous funder, (b) the project director's having chosen the lead metaevaluator, and (c) the publication of evaluation findings and metaevaluation findings in an international journal.

16. Develop a generic outline for reporting a completed summative metaevaluation.

SUGGESTIONS FOR FURTHER READING

American Educational Research Association, American Psychological Association, and National Council on Measurement in Education. (1999). *Standards for educational and psychological testing.* Washington, DC: American Psychological Association.

Cooksy, L. J., & Caracelli, V. J. (2005). Quality, context, and use: Issues in achieving the goals of metaevaluation. *American Journal of Evaluation, 26*(1), 31–42.

Cooksy, L. J., & Caracelli, V. J. (2009). Metaevaluation in practice: Selection and application of criteria. *Journal of MultiDisciplinary Evaluation, 6*(11), 1–15.

Datta, L.-E. (1999). CIRCE's demonstration of a close-to-ideal evaluation in a less-than-ideal world. *American Journal of Evaluation, 20*(2), 345–354.

Grasso, P. G. (1999). Meta-evaluation of an evaluation of reader focused writing for the Veterans Benefits Administration. *American Journal of Evaluation, 20*(2), 355–371.

Jang, S. (2000). The appropriateness of Joint Committee standards in non-Western settings: A case study of South Korea. In C. Russon (Ed.), *The program evaluation standards in international settings* (pp. 41–59). Kalamazoo: Western Michigan University, The Evaluation Center.

Joint Committee on Standards for Educational Evaluation. (2003). *The student evaluation standards.* Thousand Oaks, CA: Corwin Press.

Joint Committee on Standards for Educational Evaluation. (2009). *The personnel evaluation standards: How to assess systems for evaluating educators* (2nd ed.). Thousand Oaks, CA: Corwin Press.

Orris, M. J. (1989). Industrial applicability of the Joint Committee's personnel evaluation standards. Unpublished doctoral dissertation, Western Michigan University, Kalamazoo, MI.

Sanders, J. R. (1995). Standards and principles. In W. R. Shadish, D. L. Newman, M. A. Scheirer, & C. Wye (Eds.), Guiding principles for evaluators. (*New Directions for Program Evaluation,* Vol. 66, pp. 47–52). San Francisco: Jossey-Bass.

Scriven, M. (2000). The logic and methodology of checklists. Kalamazoo: Western Michigan University, Evaluation Center. Retrieved from *www.wmich.edu/evalctr/archive_checklists/papers/logic&methodology_dec07.pdf.*

Stake, R. E., & Davis, R. (1999). Summary evaluation of reader focused writing for the Veterans Benefits Administration. *American Journal of Evaluation, 20*(2), 323–344.

Stufflebeam, D. L. (2000). Guidelines for developing evaluation checklists: The checklist development checklist (CDC). Available at *www.wmich.edu/evalctr/archive_checklists/guidelines_cdc.pdf.*

Stufflebeam, D. L. (2000). Lessons in contracting for evaluations. *American Journal of Evaluation, 21*(3), 293–314.

Stufflebeam, D. L. (2001). Evaluation checklists: Practical tools for guiding and judging evaluations. *American Journal of Evaluation, 22*(1), 71–79.

Stufflebeam, D. L. (2001). Evaluation models. *New Directions for Evaluation,* 89. San Francisco: Jossey-Bass.

Stufflebeam, D. L., Jaeger, R. M., & Scriven, M. (1992, April). *A retrospective analysis of a summative evaluation of NAGB's pilot project to set achievement levels on the National Assessment of Educational Progress.* Paper presented at the annual meeting of the American Educational Research Association, San Francisco, CA.

Tasks	Comments
____ 1. Identify and meet with the metaevaluation's client.	Ideally, the client is the leader of the project being evaluated but, as a less desirable option, may be the leader of the subject evaluation.
____ 2. Select the metaevaluation team leader.	Ideally, this is the responsibility of the evaluation's client but may be done by an independent party or, as a less desirable option, the evaluator.
____ 3. Before contracting for the metaevaluation, make a preliminary investigation to develop a general perspective on the project being evaluated, the evaluation of the project, the intended metaevaluation audience, and, especially, the project stakeholders' views regarding the projected evaluation.	The evaluation team leader may do this as a part of her or his initial meeting with the metaevaluation client and, accordingly, may review documents and meet with key representatives of the project, the evaluation, and the project's stakeholders.
____ 4. Determine criteria for selecting metaevaluation team members.	Relevant criteria to consider in balancing the team members' qualifications may include expertise in the subject project's content area, quantitative and qualitative evaluation methods, evaluation standards, gender, ethnicity, policy expertise, communication expertise, and credibility to the subject project's stakeholders.
____ 5. Select the other metaevaluation team members.	The metaevaluation team leader should choose the metaevaluation team members in consultation with the evaluation's client.
____ 6. Select the standards for judging the evaluation.	Our preferred standards are the Joint Committee (2011) *Program Evaluation Standards* grouped into categories of utility, feasibility, propriety, accuracy, and accountability, with other options being the most recent edition of the U.S. GAO *Government Auditing Standards* and the most recent edition of the AEA *Guiding Principles for Evaluators*.
____ 7. Determine the evaluation questions.	Based on exchanges with the metaevaluation client, the project evaluation team, and project stakeholders, determine the, at least, initial set of evaluation questions (e.g., those pertaining to the evaluation's utility, feasibility, propriety, accuracy, and accountability).
____ 8. Develop the metaevaluation plan (including time frame, schedule, budget, and audience for metaevaluation reports) and the proposed metaevaluation contract.	The metaevaluation team leader should draft the metaevaluation plan in consultation with the other metaevaluation team leaders and the metaevaluation's client.

(continued)

Tasks	Comments
___ 9. Contract and secure funding for the metaevaluation.	In order of merit, the acceptable contracting and funding options are: a known independent party; an anonymous independent party, as was the case in the WILS metaevaluation; the evaluation's client; and (better than no metaevaluation) the evaluator.
___ 10. Establish and meet regularly with a stakeholder review panel to obtain their reviews of draft metaevaluation plans and reports.	Review panel members should reflect the various interests in the subject project, including the client, project leader and staff members, project beneficiaries, and so on.
___ 11. Collect and review pertinent available information.	Examples are the subject evaluation's budget, contract, staff resumés, provisions for stakeholder engagement, procedural plan, data collection instruments, management plan, reporting plan, and plan to support use of findings.
___ 12. Collect new information as needed.	Examples are updated evaluation plans, any new evaluation tools, feedback from the evaluation review panel, feedback from staff members of the subject project, feedback from the metaevaluation client and other intended users of findings, and interim and final evaluation reports.
___ 13. Develop a fact-based description of the subject evaluation.	Key items to document include: evaluator(s), client, subject project, guiding standards, intended uses and users of findings, time frame and budget, formative and/or summative purposes, key questions, evaluation framework, data collection procedures and tools, obtained data and information, information management, analysis and synthesis plans, reporting and follow-up assistance plans, and provisions for metaevaluation.
___ 14. As appropriate, provide the evaluators with formative metaevaluation feedback.	Such feedback should be keyed, in general, to the standards for sound evaluations and may include pointed responses to the evaluator's questions.
___ 15. Rate the evaluation's adherence to standards for sound evaluations as poor, fair, good, very good, or excellent.	We recommend rating the evaluation against the Joint Committee (2011) 30 standards (grouped according to utility, feasibility, propriety, accuracy, and accountability) by completing Part 3 of Stufflebeam's (2015) downloadable metaevaluation checklist (available online; see the box at the end of the table of contents).
___ 16. Analyze and synthesize the metaevaluation ratings.	We recommend developing summary tables for displaying ratings to include bar charts for displaying bottom-line results (of poor, fair, good, very good, or excellent) for the five categories of Joint Committee (2011) standards and specific results for each of the 30 specific evaluation standards, plus an attestation form for explaining each of the 30 ratings with a summary statement of judgment (see Part 4 of Stufflebeam's [2015] downloadable metaevaluation checklist, pp. 29–38, and the Evaluation Standards Attestation Form that appears in Chapter 11).

(continued)

Tasks	Comments
___ 17. Compile and deliver a final, summative metaevaluation report.	For example, structure it to include: title; executive summary; introduction; description of the evaluation; ratings of the evaluation; analysis, summary, and display of metaevaluation ratings; summary and conclusions; appendix (see Part 4 of Stufflebeam's [2015] downloadable metaevaluation checklist, p. 40 for a suggested detailed final metaevaluation report outline).
___ 18. As appropriate, help the client and other stakeholders interpret and apply the findings.	Consider contracting to conduct follow-up meetings with the client and other stakeholder groups to discuss findings and/ or conduct feedback workshops for client groups focused on evaluation of and use of the metaevalaution findings.
___ 19. Consider with the metaevaluation client the possibility and desirability of publishing the metaevaluation in one or more journal articles or a monograph.	As with the WILS metaevaluation, the metaevaluation could be published together with a summary of the subject evaluation and a response from the client for the evaluation and metaevaluation.

___	1. Evaluation standards	A working knowledge of vetted sets of professional standards for evaluations—particularly, the Joint Committee (2011) *Program Evaluation Standards*—together with a demonstrated ability to choose and apply standards that fit particular metaevaluation assignments
___	2. Methodological expertise	Ability to judge the evaluation's quantitative and qualitative evaluation methods
___	3. Fieldwork expertise	Facility in designing and judging field studies
___	4. Checklist expertise	Working knowledge of evaluation checklists and ability to devise specialized checklists for use in unique metaevaluation situations
___	5. Relevant content knowledge	Comprehension and preferably experience in evaluating programs like the one being evaluated
___	6. Facility in learning new program content areas	Ability to quickly learn new areas of program content
___	7. Evaluation training	Degrees or other credentials showing relevant training in the concepts, standards, methods, and checklists of evaluation and metaevaluation
___	8. Metaevaluation track record	Portfolio giving evidence of having delivered competent metaevaluation services
___	9. Ethics	Record of honesty, integrity, competence, and respect for individuals and society in general in past delivery of evaluation or metaevaluation services
___	10. Focusing metaevaluations	Skills in determining incisive initial and follow-up metaevaluation questions
___	11. Contracting	Skills in negotiating formal evaluation contracts that clarify an evaluation's client, appropriate audiences, budget, standards and methodologies to be employed, guarantees of access to needed information, and responsibility and authority for editing and distributing reports
___	12. Budgeting	Skills in building sound evaluation budgets and managing and accounting for evaluation funds
___	13. Stakeholder engagement	Record of effectively identifying and engaging stakeholders in evaluation or metaevaluation studies
___	14. Data collection	Demonstrated skills in developing rapport with those who contribute information for the evaluation and in selecting or developing needed evaluation instruments
___	15. Listening	Evidence of expertise in listening to project and evaluation stakeholders and recording and using their insights
___	16. Communication	Facility in communicating forthrightly and diplomatically with a wide range of project and evaluation stakeholders, including evidence of skills in putting at ease and having substantive exchanges with persons who might be threatened by the evaluation or intimidated by external evaluators.

(continued)

____	17. Reporting	Skills in oral and written communication, including ability to organize and write clear and engaging evaluation reports
____	18. Group process	Demonstrated ability to stimulate interest in an evaluation; generate a spirit of cooperation among an entire group toward obtaining and using valid, pertinent findings; conduct interviews; and chair group sessions
____	19. Management	Proven ability to staff, schedule, and coordinate evaluation studies

The CIPP Model in Perspective

Evaluation's Ubiquitous Nature, the Need for Systematic Program Evaluations, and the CIPP Model's Wide Range of Applications

"Evaluation is creation: hear it, you creators! Evaluating is itself the most valuable treasure of all that we value. It is only through evaluation that value exists: and without evaluation the nut of existence would be hollow. Hear it, you creators!"
—FRIEDRICH NIETZSCHE

In this appendix, we discuss the CIPP Model within the broader perspective of evaluation. We identify informal evaluation as a naturally occurring phenomenon and formal evaluation as the most basic of all disciplines. We distinguish between everyday, common, informal evaluations and the formal, systematic evaluations that are needed when stakes are high. We contrast two basic acts of evaluation, labeled description and judgment. We stress that formal program evaluations are needed across all disciplines and service areas and across national boundaries. We trace key milestones in the development and application of program evaluation, including the CIPP Model. For those readers who want to study actual applications of the CIPP Model, we have documented and provided references to about 500 CIPP-related evaluation studies, journal articles, and doctoral dissertations across nations, disciplines, and service areas.

Evaluation's Ubiquitous Nature

As its root term denotes, evaluation is a process of determining something's value (e.g., its quality, durability, cost-effectiveness, timeliness, impact, probity, fairness, attractiveness, worth, significance, safety, or credibility). As such, evaluation is ubiquitous. Throughout history, individuals and groups necessarily have conducted investigations to guide decision making and reach values-based judgments; that is, they have conducted evaluations. They could hardly do otherwise, for evaluation is a naturally occurring phenomenon. It is as natural as breathing. Whenever one attempts to assess an entity's merit or other aspect of value, they are evaluating. Irrespective of its quality, an evaluation occurs whenever a person or group selects among products or services, makes a budget, reforms city government, modifies a work plan, monitors and judges the implementation of a plan, assesses a grantee's compliance with contractual agreements, or judges a completed project. Farmers monitor and assess crop and soil conditions to decide on needs for irrigation, cultivation, and fertilization. It would be very unwise (and dangerous) for a parent to place a baby in the bathtub without testing the water's temperature, nor should an architect approve a bridge-building plan without confirming that it would more than adequately support the weight of itself and expected traffic. All of these instances entail evaluation.

Because evaluation is a ubiquitous, naturally occurring phenomenon, most evaluations are not systematic, and many do not provide a sound basis for making decisions or reaching summative conclusions. In fact, many evaluations are done on the fly, haphazardly, and sometimes with bad consequences. Consumers often buy products on impulse without carefully checking their merits. Decision-making groups frequently look at only one option, without considering other possibly superior alternatives. Also, many persons and groups that conduct their own evaluations allow their biases and conflicts of interest to cloud their judgments. Considering that invalid evaluations can lead to poor choices and bad consequences, societal groups often definitely need to engage in evaluations that are systematic, unbiased, ethical, accurate, informative, and consequential.

When the stakes are high—as in mounting a school drop-out prevention program, reforming a school district's math and science curriculum, training doctors to correctly prescribe drugs, adopting a military invasion plan, or monitoring a community development and housing project to assure its quality—evaluations must be systematic and produce valid feedback. Such evaluations must be free of bias and conflicts of interest, fair to involved and affected individuals, grounded in reliable information, timely and actionable, and culminate in sound judgments. Often, highly consequential internal, self-evaluations are not fully credible to all stakeholders and therefore should be supplemented with independent appraisals of the evaluation's quality. This book is devoted to providing readers with the systematic approach to evaluation embodied in the CIPP Model that meets the evaluation profession's requirements, as articulated in the Joint Committee on Standards for Educational Evaluation (2011) *Program Evaluation Standards*, that evaluations must be useful, feasible, ethical, accurate, and accountable.

Informal versus Formal Evaluations

We grant that many evaluations—especially those that occur on a daily basis and are not especially consequential—can appropriately be conducted in a relatively simple, informal manner and may not need to employ sophisticated data collection, analysis, and bias control procedures. Nevertheless, such informal evaluations should apply the basic logic and general standards of evaluation. As noted above, the Joint Committee (2011) standards require evaluations to be useful, feasible, ethical, accurate, and accountable.

Many sensitive evaluations necessarily are complex, costly, politically volatile, or keyed to important decisions. These evaluations typically need to employ complex, sophisticated methods, including multiple data collection procedures and complex statistical analyses. They also may need to subject the final report to an independent audit or what we label in this book as metaevaluation.

In general, investigators should key their evaluations—whether informal and relatively nonsensitive; or formal, complex, and highly important—to the evaluation field's general requirements for utility, feasibility, propriety, accuracy, and accountability. In this respect, all persons who evaluate programs need to acquire, read, and use the Joint Committee (2011) *Program Evaluation Standards*.

Two Basic Acts of Evaluation

All persons who evaluate programs necessarily engage in two main acts of a sound evaluation: description and judgment (Stake, 1967). These evaluation acts are distinctive yet complementary. Successive descriptive assessments of a program typically include such indicators as number of persons served; measured entry characteristics of program recipients; drop-out percentage; percent of stated objectives addressed, staff with college degrees, the program's schedule completed, budget expended, contracted products completed, and objectives achieved; number of visitors to the program; and number of publications citing the program. As these examples show, successive descriptive assessments of a program typically are comprised of facts about the program at particular points in time.

A judgment of the program, however, goes beyond the documented facts about the program to reach values-based conclusions about the significance of its aims; the quality of its design, execution, and results; and its overall worth compared to its costs. The judgmental process involves synthesis of the obtained descriptive evidence, comparison of the synthesized information to the program's underlying values, compilation of the bottom-line conclusions, and representation of the overall findings in a clear and useful report.

In sum, descriptive assessments are nonjudgmental and are designed and intended to be accurate and helpful to improve a program and, ultimately, to provide the basis for judging the program. The judgmental process uses the credible descriptive evidence along with values-based criteria to sum up and effectively communicate the program's value. The process of judging a program is every bit as challenging and complex as is the process of obtaining the needed descriptive evidence. This book is largely focused on helping readers to reliably and validly describe a program's characteristics and logically and rigorously reach and communicate defensible values-based judgments of its merit, worth, and significance.

Evaluation as the Most Basic of All Disciplines

Evaluation is the most fundamental of all disciplines. It is a necessary component in all other professions, as all professions need evaluation to scrutinize, improve, and excel. Evaluations are utilized to verify needs for service, assess plans for delivering service, provide ongoing information for program implementation and adjustment, make sure the implemented programs provide needed service, assess program outcomes and side effects, compare outcomes of competing programs, select programs that can best meet beneficiaries' needs, and, when called for, help terminate unworthy efforts. Programs and services can stand up to public and professional scrutiny only if they are regularly subjected to rigorous evaluation and shown to be sound. Without evaluation to help identify areas requiring development and assess extant ideas and practices, a profession or service area will become stalled and outdated and eventually will perish. With respect to assessing, assuring, and improving quality and meeting accountability requirements, all professions and service areas are dependent on evaluation. Additionally, self-evaluation aimed at improvement is an important hallmark of professionalism and the delivery of excellent services.

Evaluation is essential to society's progress and well-being. With the purpose of assessing and helping improve all aspects of society, evaluation is infused in all areas of scholarship, production, and service; and plays important roles of ensuring, maintaining, and improving products, programs, and services. In this way, it protects members of society in all aspects of interest and propels society's progress. Evaluation serves an improvement mechanism not only by stimulating and aiding efforts to strengthen enterprises, but also by preventing the funding of poor plans or terminating failing programs, thus freeing resources and time for worthy enterprises. Without evaluation, products, including poor ones, would be made in the same way year after year; without evaluation, doctors would be treating patients day in and day out the same way without gaining insights from what went right and wrong in past practices; without evaluation, ineffective education programs would be duplicated and widely implemented by school after school.

Development of Systematic Evaluation

The development of systematic evaluation in the United States can be traced back to the reform efforts in the 1800s when the federal government first employed external inspectors to evaluate public programs such as schools, hospitals, and prisons. However, the beginning of the evaluation profession is commonly dated as the middle 1960s. In this postwar period (as noted in Chapter 1), the U.S. federal government passed the Great Society legislation which mandated that funded projects be systematically evaluated. The federal government imparted large sums of money to a wide range of education and human service programs and rightfully sought to ensure rational planning, effective implementation, and public accountability. The resulting evaluations were concentrated in three strands: evaluating educational innovations such as the effectiveness of new curricula in schools; linking evaluation with resource allocation; and evaluating the Great Society program's antipoverty projects.

BOX A.1. Evaluation in History

More than 1,400 years ago, in the year 607, the emperor of China established formal proficiency evaluation of high-achieving scholars—called Ke Ju Zhi Du (科举制度)—as a way to select and appoint public officials in the Sui Dynasty (隋朝). The final stage of the evaluation, called the Palace Examination (Dian Shi 殿试), was presided over by the emperor in person and was held on the 21st day of the 4th month each year. This system lasted some 1,300 years and ended in the Qing Dynasty (清朝) in the year 1905.

As public school districts and other organizations throughout America struggled to implement the evaluation requirements, they made many mistakes, resulting in evaluation reports that were often suspect and little used. Nevertheless, over time, systematic evaluation went through a metamorphosis and emerged as a respectable area of practice oriented to helping projects succeed and meet their accountability requirements.

The commonly heard prediction in the 1960s that formalized program evaluation was a fad and soon would disappear proved false. Even without continuation of the abundant financial resources bestowed by the federal government in the 1960s and 1970s, the evaluation field has continued to grow steadily in its involvements, importance, sophistication, and stature for the past half century and gradually has developed into a distinct area of professional practice. The evaluation field now has national and state professional societies of evaluators throughout the world, annual conventions, yearbooks, encyclopedias, journals, a substantial body of literature, degree-conferring masters and doctoral programs, specialized websites, institutes and workshops, evaluation companies, a growing array of evaluation models and tools, guiding principles, and evaluation standards. Today systematic evaluation is needed and has become an integral part of the wide range of societies.

Areas of Application of Systematic Evaluation

Evaluation has been naturally woven into every fiber of human activity. It is impossible to provide an exhaustive list of objects that need evaluation because such a list would be best characterized as infinite. The following small sample of commonly evaluated objects and persons illustrates the wide range of entities that are subjected to systematic evaluation: schools, school programs, teachers, teaching methods, school administrators; sports players, sports training programs, game strategies; art works, artists, art auctions; movies, actors, movie theaters; libraries, librarians, archives, books; hospitals, physicians, patients, immunization programs, medical education programs, nurses, nursing programs; courts, lawyers, judges, laws, juvenile correction programs; universities, college students, professors, university curriculums, distance education; food, drug, other consumer products, FDA policies, disease prevention and control programs; government agencies, governors, social workers, foster care; parks and recreation programs, agricultural extension servic-

BOX A.2. Why Evaluation Is Important

Poor products, services, and policies can put society and its members at serious risk. Evaluation improves society and serves its members by providing affirmations of worth and accreditation, demanding accountability, pointing the way to improvements, and offering a basis for terminating ineffective products, services, employees, and policies.

es; soldiers, army, navy, air force, national defense; research proposals, grant proposals, inventions, theories; and many, many more. Clearly, evaluation applies to all areas of human endeavor.

An enormous number of evaluations of many sizes and scales have been conducted for various purposes in many different settings, across different disciplines and service areas such as private agencies, foundations, schools, and government agencies of all levels. For example, according to the U.S. GAO, 5,610 federal evaluations were conducted between 1973 and 1979. A nonexhaustive sample of 3,027 local mental health center evaluations was identified from the Databank of Program Evaluation at UCLA (Aaronson & Wilner, 1983). These evaluations vary in the level of the government to which they respond from the federal government to state mandates and to local project managers. Not surprisingly, countless evaluations are also widely conducted internationally (e.g., Fernandea-Ramirez & Rebolloso, 2006; Harvey, 2005).

The Widely Used CIPP Model

The evaluation profession's development has spawned a considerable body of literature concerned with evaluation's theory, methods, and applications. The CIPP Model is an integral part of this literature, owing to its being one of the first and most widely used evaluation approaches (Altschuld & Kumar, 2002). As documented in Chapter 1, this model originated in the middle 1960s to help improve and achieve greater accountability for U.S. school reform projects. Its unique place in the history of the evaluation movement was that it was created to address the limitations of the classic evaluation approaches when applied in dynamic social contexts (Stufflebeam, 1966a, 1966b, 1967, 1969, 1971a, 1971b, 2003a, 2003b, 2004, 2013, 2014; Stufflebeam et al., 1971; Stufflebeam & Shinkfield, 1985, 2007; Stufflebeam & Webster, 1988).

The CIPP Model's fundamental tenet lies in its improvement orientation. The proactive application of the CIPP framework can facilitate sound decision making and better project planning; and the retrospective use of the CIPP framework allows the investigator to continually reframe and encapsulate a program's merit, effectiveness, worth, feasibility, probity, cost, and significance. Over the years, the CIPP Model has been continuously refined and further developed, and it has evolved into an organized approach to meeting the evaluation profession's standards.

Applications of the CIPP Model

Over the past 50 years, the CIPP Model has been applied in a wide range of disciplines and service areas in the United States and many other countries. These applications have varied in size and have encompassed a wide range of organizational settings (local, state, and national) and different types of organizations (e.g., government, foundations, businesses, schools and universities), and across national borders.

A nonexhaustive search for relevant literature on the CIPP Model to support the writing of this book identified over 500 CIPP-related evaluation studies, journal articles, and doctoral dissertations across nations, disciplines, and service areas, spanning from the 1960s to the present. The model was applied in at least 150 doctoral dissertations that were completed at 88 universities and applied in 34 disciplines. Tables A.1, A.2, and A.3 present a sample of 227 evaluation studies that utilized the CIPP Model. This sample includes 93 journal articles, 74 dissertations, 52 conference presentations or reports, and 8 books, and provides a sense of the broad scope in which the CIPP Model has been employed. In this sample, the CIPP Model was applied in disciplines such as agriculture, art, aviation, business, communication, criminal justice, education, engineering, English, evaluation, government, health care, health science, language and literacy, law, law enforcement, library science, meteorology, military, music, psychology, psychotherapy, public health, religion, sociology, social work, sports and exercise, and transportation. Within each discipline, the model was applied in a wide range of service areas to address different issues.

In addition to applications, the CIPP Model has been referenced in a colossal number of publications

of all formats. Because of its extensive international usage, besides its original publications in English, the CIPP Model has been translated into Chinese, Filipino, French, German, Hebrew, Korean, Portuguese, Spanish, and Thai, and possibly other languages. It is important to note that evaluation products are rarely published; therefore, published CIPP studies represent only a small percentage of studies and evaluations that have utilized the CIPP Model. The following sections use education and health care disciplines to exemplify the CIPP Model's wide application within individual disciplines.

Applications of the CIPP Model in Education

In education settings, the CIPP evaluation model has been widely adopted and found useful in the evaluation of numerous educational programs, projects, and entities (Zhang et al., 2008, 2011). These applications span many service areas and a great variety of issues (Table A.1).

Webster and Eichelberger (1972) found that the CIPP Model provided an apt framework for their application of multiple regression to evaluate an ongoing educational program. Barnette (1977) reported that the Education Division of the Pennsylvania State University successfully applied the CIPP Model to guide organizational development of the Pennsylvania Adult Basic Education program. Felix (1979) adopted the CIPP Model to evaluate and improve instruction of school systems in Cincinnati. Nicholson (1989) recommended the use of the CIPP Model to evaluate reading instruction. Ameen (1990) described the application of the CIPP Model to Starr Commonwealth Schools, a private child-caring institution that provides a wide variety of residential and nonresidential care for emotionally disturbed and delinquent children and their families (with facilities in three locations in Michigan and Ohio, Starr Commonwealth annually provided services including residential care, specialized foster care, and outpatient child and family guidance services to over 2,000 children and families).

In more recent years, Matthews and Hudson (2001) developed guidelines for the evaluation of parent training programs within the framework of the CIPP Model. Combs and colleagues (Combs, Gibson, Hays, Saly, & Wendt, 2008) derived a course assessment and enhancement model based on the CIPP Model because of its flexibility in providing formative and summative results. A faculty development program designed to

TABLE A.1. A Sample of Research Studies in Education that Used the CIPP Evaluation Model

Service Area	Study	Type of Publication[a]	Country
Accountability models	Butcher, R. K. (1981)	Dissertation	US
Adaptive and social learning	Cadiz, M. C. (2008)	Dissertation	Philippines
Bilingual education	Gold, N. (1981)	Dissertation	US
Career development	Croom, B., Moore, C., & Armbruster, J. (2005)	Report	US
	Hecht, A. (1975)	Article	US
	Hernandez, J. (2003)	Article	US
Catholic elementary school	Liguori, J. (1980)	Dissertation	US
Character education	King, J. (2008)	Dissertation	US
Chemical engineering curriculum	Huang, C. (2000, July)	Report	Taiwan
Child care center	Cross, A. (1992)	Dissertation	US
	Ameen, C. A. (1990)	Article	US
College student leadership	Chambers, A. (1990)	Dissertation	US
College student living environments	Crimmin, N. (2008)	Dissertation	US
Compulsory education	Lai, J. (2006)	Dissertation	Taiwan
Continuing education	Barnette, J. (1977)	Report	US
Counselor education	Gavilan, M., & Ryan, C. (1979)	Report	US
Curriculum redesign	Boone, A. (2010)	Dissertation	US
Department of Education	Alford, K. (2010)	Report	US
Developmental studies programs	Jou, M. (1986)	Dissertation	US
e-learning	Armstrong, H. L., Murray, I. D., & Permvattana, R. R. (2006)	Article	US
	Chapman, D. (2006)	Article	US
	Dien, T., & Esichaikul, V. (n.d.)	Report	Vietnam
	Hooper, M. (1998)	Article	US
Early childhood education	Chavarria, M. (1985)	Dissertation	US
Education funding	Lin, C., Lee, J., & Chen, C. (2005)	Article	Taiwan
Educational administration	Gally, J. (1982)	Dissertation	US
Educational facilities construction	Bavi, R. (2005)	Dissertation	US
Educational funds	Ming-hua, C., Liang-yuan, H., Ta-chin, J., & Chu, S. (2006)	Report	Taiwan
Educational improvement programs	Ewy, R., Chase, C., & Colorado State Department of Education (1977)	Report	US
	Felix, J. (1978)	Report	US
	Felix, J. (1979)	Article	US

(continued)

TABLE A.1. *(continued)*

Service Area	Study	Type of Publication[a]	Country
Educational indicator systems	Chien, M., Lee, C., & Cheng, Y. (2007)	Article	Taiwan
Educational programs planning and evaluation	Nolin, S. (1976)	Dissertation	US
Educational technology	Kim, S., Kim, M., & Hong, J. (2010)	Book	US
	Kokoszka, K. (2009)	Dissertation	US
Elementary information education	Huang, P. (2004)	Dissertation	China
Employment and training	Combs, P., McGough, R., & Virginia Polytechnic Institute and State University (1980)	Report	US
English curriculum	Karatas, H., & Fer, S. (2009)	Article	Turkey
Extension programs	Guico, T. M., Menez, N. L., & Garcia, R. B. (n.d.)	Report	Philippines
Faculty mentoring program	Foley-Peres, K. (2005)	Dissertation	US
	Gothard, K. (2009)	Dissertation	US
Gifted and talented programs	Fortney, J. (1988)	Dissertation	US
High school retention	Kannel-Ray, N., Lacefield, W., & Zeller, P. (2008)	Article	US
Higher education	Lemon, D., & North Dakota University, G. (1986)	Report	US
Higher education reform	Hsen-Hsing. (2004)	Article	Taiwan
Inspectorate services	Alade, O. (2007)	Report	Nigeria
Junior colleges of commerce	Hsieh, W., & Hsiao, L. (2001, August)	Report	Taiwan
Learning object management	Morgado, E., Peñalvo, F., Martín, D., & Gonzalez, M. (2010)	Article	Greece
Learning readiness	Bennardo, G. (1998)	Dissertation	US
Learning society	Meng-Ching, H. (2004)	Article	Taiwan
Literature teaching	Bleakley, L. A. (1974)	Dissertation	US
Management education	Galvin, J. (1983)	Dissertation	US
Multicountry joint programs	Kundalaputra, C., Hemmings, B., & Hill, D. (2001)	Report	Thailand
Parent teacher communication	Eggeman, E. (2008)	Dissertation	US
Parent training programs	Matthews, J., & Hudson, A. (2001)	Article	US
Parental role	Martinez-Gonzalez, R., & Rodriquez-Ruiz, B. (2007)	Article	Spain
Physics program	Mishra, A., & Garg, S. (2009)	Article	India
Policy making	Bhola, H. (2000)	Article	US
Prekindergarten program	Slavenas, R., & Nowakowski, J. (1989)	Article	US
Preprimary education reform	Hamza, S. (2003)	Report	Nigeria
Principal preparation	Joseph, S. (2009)	Dissertation	US

(continued)

TABLE A.1. *(continued)*

Service Area	Study	Type of Publication[a]	Country
Professional development	Mitchem, K., Wells, D., & Wells, J. (2003)	Article	US
	Muijs, D., & Lindsay, G. (2008)	Article	England
Quality indicators	Poliandri, D., Cardone, M., Muzzioli, P., & Romiti, S. (2010)	Report	Australia, Denmark, England, Finland, France, Germany, Netherlands, New Zealand, Spain, Sweden, Switzerland, US
Reading comprehension	Conaty Burke, M. (1997)	Dissertation	US
Reading instruction	Nicholson, T. (1989)	Article	US
School counselor evaluation	Anderson, J. (1995)	Article	US
School curriculum	Lin, S. (2006)	Dissertation	Taiwan
School reform	Hodge, W. A., & Jones, J. T. (2000)	Article	US
School system evaluation	Ashburn, A. (1972)	Report	US
Science education	Lehman, J., George, M., Buchanan, P., & Rush, M. (2006)	Article	US
Secondary education	Johnson, E. M. (2003)	Dissertation	US
Secondary science program	Fidone, D. J. (1993)	Dissertation	US
Service learning	Zhang, G., Zeller, N., Griffith, R., Metcalf, D., Shea, C., Williams, J., et al. (2011b)	Article	US
Social emotional learning	Cerino, L. (2009)	Dissertation	US
Special needs program	Kelley, P. (1984)	Dissertation	US
Spelling program	Ross, G., & Middleton, M. (1980)	Report	US
Staff development	Arzoumanian, L. (1994)	Dissertation	US
	Houghton, A., & Moser, M. (2007)	Report	United Kingdom
Sustainability in higher education	Erdogan, M. (2010)	Article	Turkey
Teacher development	Kjer, M. (2009)	Dissertation	US
Teacher education	Galluzzo, G. (1983)	Report	US
	Mahmood, K. (2005)	Article	Pakistan
Teacher education module	Brouwer, N., Muller, G., & Rietdijk, H. (2007)	Article	US
Teacher evaluation	Usmani, M. (2008, December)	Report	Pakistan
Teacher induction and mentoring	Anthony, J. (2009)	Dissertation	US
Teacher training centers	Naeini, Z. (2006)	Article	Iran
Technology teacher education	Householder, D. L., & Boser, R. A. (1991)	Article	US

(continued)

TABLE A.1. *(continued)*

Service Area	Study	Type of Publication[a]	Country
Transitional education	Cleary, K. (2007)	Dissertation	US
Undergraduate programs	Horng, J., Teng, C., & Baum, T. (2009)	Article	US
Undergraduate student information literacy	Lee, J. Y. (2006)	Report	Korea
Undergraduate student needs	Fritz, S. (1996)	Dissertation	US
University academic programs	Du Toit, P. H., & Masebe, L. J. (2007)	Report	South Africa
Urban school administration	Candoli, I. C. (1976)	Article	US
Vocational education	Bowling, T. (1988)	Dissertation	US
	LaFleur, C., & El Paso Community College (1990)	Report	US
	Martinez Munoz, M. (1995)	Dissertation	Spain
Vocational schools	Kamal, D., & Salehi, K. (2006)	Article	Iran
Writing program	Church, J. R. (2008)	Dissertation	US

[a]In Tables A.1–A.3, "Article" refers to articles published in journals; "Report" includes conference proceedings, conference presentations and other reports such as those archived in the ERIC Center. Also, due to space constraints, only the names and year, rather than the full citation, are mentioned in the Study column.

support the teaching and evaluation of professionalism of medical students and residents in medicine's educational institutions was examined using the CIPP Model (Steinert, Cruess, Cruess, & Snell, 2005). Employing the CIPP Model, Armstrong and colleagues evaluated Cisco e-learning courses modified for the vision impaired (Armstrong, Murray, & Permvattana, 2006). The CIPP Model was also used as the basis for developing the Georgia School Counselor Evaluation Program (GSCEP), which was designed as a framework to be used across all systems and schools in the state of Georgia for annual evaluation purposes. The program involved an ongoing process that allowed for remediation when needed and encouraged professional growth. The evaluation program's goal was to improve support services for students in Georgia's public schools.

Over the years, some of the exemplary applications of the CIPP Model within education in the United States occurred in numerous evaluations by Bill Webster in the Dallas Independent School District; Howard Merriman in the Columbus, Ohio, School District; Gary Wegenke and his evaluators in the Des Moines, Iowa, school district; Jerry Baker in the Saginaw, Michigan, school district; Jerry Walker in the Ohio State University National Center for Research on Vocational Education; Bob Randall in the Southwest Regional Educational

Research Laboratory; Carl Candoli and his evaluators in the Lansing, Michigan, school district; Stufflebeam and colleagues in the Evaluation Centers (first at Ohio State University and subsequently at Western Michigan University); and so on. Many of the reports from these applications of CIPP were archived in ERIC centers, some appeared in dissertations, and others are archived in the Western Michigan University website (*www.wmich.edu/evaluation*).

In education settings outside of the United States, the CIPP Model has also established its widespread usefulness. The CIPP Model was used to construct Taiwan's national educational indicator systems (Chien, Lee, & Cheng, 2007). From 1998 to 2000, Taiwan's National Science Council sponsored the first comprehensive indicator project to cover all educational levels in Taiwan. A variety of research methods were used, including panel discussion, conference, Delphi technique, questionnaires, and visits to 14 international organizations and government agencies. Two educational indicator systems based on the CIPP Model were formulated: Taiwan's Educational Indicator System by educational level (TEIS by el) with 99 indicators, and Significant Indicators of Taiwan's Education (SITE) with 34 indicators. The CIPP Model was also found useful in comparative evaluations across multiple nations. Poliandri,

Cardone, Muzzioli, and Romiti (2010) explored aspects and indicators most commonly used to assess the quality of education systems in different countries through comparison of 12 national publications describing the state of educational systems: Australia, Denmark, England, Finland, France, Germany, Netherlands, New Zealand, Spain, Sweden, Switzerland, and the United States. The CIPP Model was utilized to compare the indicators. Based on the CIPP Model, a dynamic and easy-to-update electronic database for quality indicators comparison has been designed and implemented. The database enables comparisons across different countries and is available to the public; it is especially useful to researchers and scholastic decision makers.

Applications of the CIPP Model in Health Care

Even though the CIPP Model was created primarily for use in education, over the years it has been "borrowed" by virtually all disciplines. As an example, even though health care is not closely related to education, evaluation efforts aided by the CIPP Model have been pervasive in the health care field in a broad range of service areas addressing many different issues (see Table A.2).

With the CIPP Model as a framework, a method for measuring and evaluating the productivity of clinical nurse specialists was developed at an 814-bed tertiary care center, which paralleled the nursing process and was outcome oriented. The applicability of the method made it a widely useful evaluation tool for nursing managers and administrators (Anderson, McCartney, Schreiber, & Thompson, 1989). Under the direction of Mina Singh, the York-Seneca-Georgian-Durham collaborative BScN Program Evaluation Committee in Ontario developed and utilized a CIPP process evaluation (Singh, 2004). Singh noted that while the CIPP evaluation framework was applicable to any nursing evaluation program, it was practically useful for collaborative nursing programs because it allowed a full assessment of each partner in its context. Additionally, Staggers (1989) found the CIPP Model useful in the evaluation of the National Nurse Entrance Exam. Likewise, Valentine (1991) recommended use of the CIPP Model to the evaluation of nursing care. Kishchuk, O'Loughlin, Paradis, Masson, and Sacks-Silver (2009) evaluated the smoking prevention programs, and the resulting data were used to form hypotheses and recommendations for future interventions.

At the U.S. national level, Farley and Battles (2009) described the evaluation performed on the patient safety initiative operated by the Agency for Healthcare Research and Quality (AHRQ). Patient safety became a national priority in 2000, and Congress charged and funded AHRQ to improve health care safety. AHRQ funded more than 300 research projects and other activities over a 6-year period in an effort to address diverse patient safety issues and practices. A 4-year formative evaluation of the initiative using the CIPP Model, which emphasizes multiple stakeholders' interests (e.g., patients, providers, funded researchers), was completed. They monitored the progress of the patient safety initiative and provided AHRQ annual feedback that assessed each year's activities, identifying issues and offering suggestions for actions. Given the size and complexity of the initiative, the evaluation needed to examine key individual components and synthesize results across them. It also had to be responsive to changes in the initiative over time. The CIPP Model played an important guiding role and allowed the evaluators to bring together the disparate pieces to synthesize overall findings.

The CIPP Model's application in health care outside of the United States has been illustrated by Sims and Bridgman (2006). Using input and product evaluations, the progress of 12 Down syndrome and 12 multiply handicapped children attending two different therapeutic systems (Auckland Branch/outside Auckland Branches) operated by the New Zealand Society for the Intellectually Handicapped was assessed over a period of 18 months. The progress of the Auckland children was significantly better in a number of areas than for those outside Auckland. This improvement in progress was found to be primarily due to input differences that reflected the Auckland Branch's policy of service development. The most important determinants of a successful program were not staff/student ratios, time in class, or specialist assistance, all of which favored the outside Auckland groups, but the degree of structure, detail of programs and assessments, and quality of parent contact in which Auckland was found to be superior.

As in education and health care, the CIPP Model has extensive applications in virtually all disciplines, including agriculture, art, aviation, business, communication, criminal justice, engineering, English, evaluation, health science, language and literacy, law, law enforcement, library science, meteorology, military, music, psychology, psychotherapy, public health, religion, sociology, social work, sports and exercise, and transportation. Table A.3 presents a small sample of studies in each of these disciplines.

TABLE A.2. A Sample of Research Studies in Health Care That Used the CIPP Evaluation Model

Service Area	Study	Type of Publication	Country
Cancer awareness	Oliver-Vázquez, M., Sánchez-Ayéndez, M., Suárez-Pérez, E., Vélez-Almodóvar, H., & Arroyo-Calderón, Y. (2002)	Article	Puerto Rico
Child development	Burden, R. L. (1981)	Article	UK
Child inpatient intervention	Gavidia-Payne, S., Littlefield, L., Hallgren, M., Jenkins, P., & Coventry, N. (2003)	Article	Australia
Children and family health	Broome, M. (1998)	Book	US
Chronic disease	Motlagh, M. E., Kelishadi, R., Ardalan, G., Gheiratmand, R., Majdzadeh, R., & Heidarzadeh, A. (2009)	Article	Iran
Clinical nurse specialists	Anderson, E., McCartney, E., Schreiber, J., & Thompson, E. (1989)	Article	US
Clinical nursing	Schultz, A. (1991)	Dissertation	US
Dental team training	Reeves, J., & Michael, W. (1973)	Report	US
Distance learning in Obstetrics and Gynecology	Duffy, J., & McAleer, S. (2002)	Article	US
Drug addicts rehabilitation	Khuanyoung, P. (2007)	Dissertation	Thailand
Elderly health care	Duggleby, W. (2000)	Article	Japan
	Lee, T. (2000)	Article	Thailand
Family health nursing	Parfitt, B., & Cornish, F. (2007)	Article	Tajikistan
Health management	Valentine, K. (1988)	Book	US
Injury prevention	Brewin, M., & Coggan, C. (2003)	Article	New Zealand
Medical care	Asavatanabodee, P. (2010)	Article	Thailand
Medical care measures	Coyle, Y., & Battles, J. (1999)	Article	US
Medical education curriculum	El-hazmi, M., & Tekian, A. (1986)	Article	Saudi Arabia
	Frye, A., Solomon, D., Lieberman, S., & Levine, R. (2000)	Article	US
Medical training	Moorman, L. (2002)	Dissertation	US
Mental health treatment aftercare	Bostelman, S., Callan, M., Rolincik, L., & Turner, J. (1994)	Article	US
Neuro-developmental disorders	Boscardin, M. (2009, June 29)	Report	US
Nurse program entrance exam	Staggers, N. (1989)	Article	US
Nursing	Conway, J., & FitzGerald, M. (2004)	Article	US
Nursing education	Billings, D. M., & Halstead, J. A. (2005)	Book	US
	Bowen, M. (2008)	Report	US
	Hall, M. (2009)	Report	US
	Hall, M., Daly, B., & Madigan, E. (2010)	Article	US
	Kejkornkaew, S., Thanooruk, R., & Lumdubwong, A. (2008)	Article	Thailand
	Singh, M. (2004)	Article	US

(continued)

TABLE A.2. A Sample of Research Studies in Health Care That Used the CIPP Evaluation Model

Service Area	Study	Type of Publication	Country
Nursing manpower development	Othanganont, P. (2001)	Article	Thailand
Nursing quality development	Petro-Nustas, W. (1996)	Article	Jordan
Outpatient chronic care	Keyser, D., Dembosky, J., Kmetik, K., Antman, M., & Sirio, C. (2009)	Article	US
Patient safety evaluation	Farley, D., & Battles, J. (2009)	Article	US
	Farley, D., & Damberg, C. (2009)	Article	US
Radiologic technology	Scott, E. (1986)	Article	US

TABLE A.3. A Sample of Research Studies in Other Disciplines That Used the CIPP Evaluation Model

Discipline	Service Area	Study	Type of Publication	Country
Agriculture	Agricultural education	Croom, B., Moore, C., & Armbruster, J. (2005)	Report	US
	Farmer education	Kim, J. (2006)	Article	South Korea
	Food production	Osokoya, M., & Adekunle, A. (2007)	Article	Nigeria
Art	Art program	Wronski, T. (1992)	Report	US
Aviation	Aviation training	Khoury, N. (1988)	Dissertation	US
		Taylor, D. (1998)	Report	US
Business	Banking and insurance technology	Hsieh, W. (1999)	Dissertation	Taiwan
	Banking curriculum	Hsieh, W., & Liu, S. (2002)	Report	Taiwan
	Organizational training	Downing, H., Griffin, P., Humunicki, D., & Maric, Z. (2000)	Report	Australia
Communication	Technical communication programs	Battle, M. (1993)	Report	US
		Carnegie, T. A. M. (2007)	Article	US
Criminal justice	Child abuse and neglect cases	Dobbin, S., & Gatowski, S. (1998)	Report	US
Engineering	Mechanical engineering technology	Chiang, P. (1996)	Dissertation	Taiwan
English	Sign language program	Kemp, M. (1988)	Article	US
Evaluation	Accountability	Laukkanen, R. (1998)	Article	Finland
	Clinical nurse specialists	Kennedy-Malone, L. (1996, July)	Article	US
	Community college evaluation	Hekimian, S., & Florida University (1984)	Report	US
	Conceptualization of CIPP Model	Hinkle, D. E. (1971)	Dissertation	US
	Counseling program evaluation	Astramovich, R., & Coker, J. (2007)	Article	US

(continued)

TABLE A.3. *(continued)*

Discipline	Service Area	Study	Type of Publication	Country
Evaluation *(continued)*	Educational evaluation	Corley, A. (1992)	Dissertation	US
		Findlay, D. (1973)	Book	US
		Gess, D., & And, O. (1974)	Report	US
		Hinkle, D. E. (1973)	Report	US
		Webster, W., & Eichelberger, T. (1972)	Article	US
	Empowerment evaluation	Fetterman, D., Kaftarian, S., & Wandersman, A. (1996)	Book	US
	Evaluation approaches	Hui-Fang, S. (1997)	Article	Hong Kong
	Evaluation in nursing programs	Kennedy, F. (1982)	Dissertation	US
	Evaluation practices	Hebel, T. (1987)	Dissertation	US
	Evaluation simulation model	Ohara, T., & Pickard, K. (1985)	Report	US
	Extension workshops	Kelsey, K., Schnelle, M., & Bolin, P. (2005, June)	Article	US
	Impact evaluation	Grasso, J., & Ohio State University (1979)	Report	US
	Interim summative evaluation	Dodson, S. (1994)	Dissertation	US
	Operational application of CIPP Model	Randall, R. S. (1973)	Book	US
	School system evaluation	Ashburn, A. (1972)	Report	US
	STEM programs	Gullickson, A., & Hanssen, C. (2006)	Book	US
	Training programs	Norton, J. (1990)	Article	US
Health science	Distance learning in OB-GYN	Jha, V., Duffy, S., & McAleer, S. (2002)	Article	United Kingdom
	Faculty performance evaluation	Mitcham, M. (1981)	Article	US
	Health education	Shireman, J. (1991)	Dissertation	US
	Medical education	Jha, V., & Duffy, S. (2002)	Article	United Kingdom
	Residency program	Hogan, M. J. (1992)	Article	US
Language and literacy	Adult literacy	Herod, L. (2000)	Report	Canada
		Moussa, L. (1996)	Dissertation	Niger
	Language policy and planning	Piri, R. (2001)	Dissertation	Finland
Law	Juvenile offender rehabilitation	Anderson, D., & Anderson, S. (1996)	Article	US
	Juvenile protection	Nawamongkolwattana, B. (2009)	Article	Thailand
	Offender career development	Filella-Guiu, G., & Blanch-Plana, A. (2002)	Article	Spain
	Prison education	Ayers, J., University of Victoria, Canada Correctional Service, & Canadian Association for Adult Education (1981)	Report (four papers)	Canada

(continued)

TABLE A.3. *(continued)*

Discipline	Service Area	Study	Type of Publication	Country
Law enforcement	Police education and training	Conway, J. (2004)	Dissertation	Australia
Library science	Archival utility	Alegbeleye, B. (1984)	Article	Nigeria
	Library program development	Goldberg, R. (1976)	Report	US
	Library system services	Michael, M. E. (1976)	Report	US
		Michael, M., Young, A., & Illinois University (1974)	Report Report	US
	University library	Dworaczyk, W. (1998)	Dissertation	US
Meteorology	Meteorology and hydrology training	Wang, Y., & Zhi, X. (2009)	Article	China
Military	Automated instructional management system	Berkowitz, M., O'Neil, J. F., & Wagner, H. (1980)	Report	US
	Military personnel literacy program	De Vries, D. (1981)	Dissertation	US
	Military training	Berkowitz, M., & Army Research Institute for the Behavioral and Social Sciences (1980)	Report	US
Music	Music education	Ferguson, D. (2007)	Report	US
		Masear, C. (1999)	Dissertation	US
Psychology	Career counseling	Luck, M. (1990)	Dissertation	Canada
	Counseling program evaluation	Astramovich, R., & Coker, J. (2007)	Article	US
		Kooyman Kelley, D. R. (2004)	Dissertation	US
	Educational psychologists	Burden, R. (1997)	Article	UK
	Guidance program	Miller, J., & Grisdale, G. (1975)	Article	US
	School counseling and guidance	Harrison, A. (1993)	Dissertation	US
	School counselors	Anderson, J. (1995)	Article	US
	School psychological reports	Gilberg, J., & LastScholwinski, E. (1983)	Article	US
	School psychological services	Bents-Hill, C. (1991)	Dissertation	US
	Wilderness therapy for at-risk youth	Carpenter, J. (1998)	Dissertation	US
Psychotherapy	Modified STEP program	Keifer, G. (1977)	Dissertation	US
Public health	Pediatric nutrition	Shams, B., Golshiri, P., Zamani, A., & Pourabdian, S. (2008)	Article	Iran
	Smoking prevention programs	Kishchuk, N., O'Loughlin, J., Paradis, S., Masson, P., & Sacks-Silver, G. (2009)	Article	US
Religion	Christian studies	Mattox, J. (1991)	Dissertation	Mexico
	Church music	Sloan, A. (2000)	Dissertation	US
	Religious education	Demott, N. (1998)	Article	US

(continued)

TABLE A.3. *(continued)*

Discipline	Service Area	Study	Type of Publication	Country
Sociology	Family studies	Dickinson, J., & Murphy, P. (2000)	Report	Australia
	International development projects	Kuji-Shikantani, K. (1995)	Dissertation	Canada
Social work	Civil Service Training	Lin, T. (2007)	Dissertation	China
	Disability employment service	Friedenberg, J., & Ohio State University (1991)	Report	US
	Foster care	Gerson, A. (2005)	Dissertation	US
	Foster parent training	Whiting, J., Hither, P., & Koech, A. (2007)	Article	US
	Handicap support service	Kingsbury, D. (1982)	Dissertation	US
	Nutritional intervention	Green, F. (2004)	Dissertation	South Africa
	Resocialization of street children	Saripudin, D. (2010)	Article	Indonesia
	Volunteer leadership development	Cadwalader, D. (1985)	Dissertation	US
Sports and exercise	Aquatic exercises	Sanders, M. (2008)	Article	US
	Athletic training	Peer, K. (2007)	Article	US
	Olympic education program	Kellis, I., Goudas, M., Vernadakis, N., Digelidis, N., & Kioumourtzolou, E. (2007)	Article	US
Transportation	Automotive technician training	Peng, H. (1995)	Dissertation	Taiwan
	Motorcycle safety education	Ochs, R. (2001)	Dissertation	US
	Truck driver training	Sallander, C. (2007)	Dissertation	US

Applications of the CIPP Model in Doctoral Dissertations

The wide utilization of the CIPP Model in dissertation research in a full spectrum of disciplines is evidenced in the past half century in the United States and internationally. Among dissertations made publicly available, 150 doctoral dissertations in 88 universities (see Table A.4) within and outside of the United States have applied the CIPP Evaluation Model. These dissertations came from 34 disciplines (Table A.5) and addressed a wide variety of research topics in many service areas (Table A.6). These only include dissertations that are made publicly available in full text; thus, they only represent a small portion of the dissertations that applied the CIPP Evaluation Model from a limited number of countries. For example, Dr. Alex Edmonds, the director of the doctoral program of Nova University Southeastern, informed us in a written communication that many Nova doctoral students have applied the CIPP Model in their dissertations, but these dissertations are not made public. The actual number of dissertations that applied the CIPP Evaluation Model undoubtedly is much greater than 150.

These dissertation research works addressed significant issues in many disciplines, subdisciplines, and service areas. For example, mirroring the CIPP Model, Harrison (1993) provided an evaluation model that could be used by middle school counselors to evaluate counseling and guidance; this model furnishes meaningful and useful information to be used in planning a comprehensive and developmentally appropriate counseling and guidance program for early adolescence. In examining various probation classification systems utilized nationwide, Quincey (1987) proposed a probation classification model designed to serve as a model to the judicial systems and recommended the CIPP Model for generating evaluation criteria. Al-Qubbaj's dissertation (2003) utilized the CIPP Model to study the acculturation processes of Arabic children and their families in a U.S. school system, which allowed an understanding of

TABLE A.4. Universities in Which Doctoral Dissertations Applied the CIPP Evaluation Model

1. Antioch University/New England Graduate School, New Hampshire
2. Arizona State University, Arizona
3. Capella University, Minnesota
4. Catholic University of America
5. Chulalongkorn University, Thailand
6. City University of New York, New York
7. Columbia University Teachers College, New York
8. Concordia University, Canada
9. Florida International University, Florida
10. Florida State University, Florida
11. Fordham University, New York
12. Gardner-Webb University, North Carolina
13. George Mason University, Virginia
14. George Washington Univeristy, District of Columbia
15. Illinois State University, Illinois
16. Indiana University, Indiana
17. Indiana University of Pennsylvania, Pennsylvania
18. Iowa State University, Iowa
19. Johnson & Wales University, Rhode Island
20. Jyväskylän Yliopisto, Finland
21. Loyola University of Chicago, Illinois
22. Miami University, Ohio
23. Michigan State University, Michigan
24. Mississippi State University, Mississippi
25. National Sun Yat-sen University, Taiwan
26. National Yunlin University of Science and Technology, Taiwan
27. New Mexico State University, New Mexico
28. New York University, New York
29. Northern Arizona University, Arizona
30. Northern Illinois University, Illinois
31. Oklahoma State University, Oklahoma
32. Old Dominion University, Virginia
33. Oregon State University, Oregon
34. Pennsylvania State University, Pennsylvania
35. Pepperdine University, California
36. Purdue University, Indiana
37. Queen's University at Kingston, Canada
38. Southern Illinois University at Carbondale, Illinois
39. St. John's University, New York
40. Syracuse University, New York
41. Temple University, Pennsylvania
42. Tennessee State University, Tennessee
43. Texas A&M University, Texas
44. Universitat Autonoma de Barcelona, Spain
45. Université du Québec à Trois-Rivières, Canada
46. University of Alberta, Canada
47. Universitat Autonoma de Barcelona, Spain
48. University of California at Santa Barbara, California
49. University of Delaware, Delaware
50. University of Florida, Florida
51. University of Georgia, Georgia
52. University of Houston, Texas
53. University of Idaho, Idaho
54. University of Iowa, Iowa
55. University of Jos, Nigeria
56. University of Kansas, Kansas
57. University of Kentucky, Kentucky
58. University of La Verne, California
59. University of Maryland College Park, Maryland
60. University of Massachusetts Amherst, Massachusetts
61. University of Michigan, Michigan
62. University of Minnesota, Minnesota
63. University of Nebraska at Omaha, Nebraska
64. University of Nevada, Reno, Nevada
65. University of New Brunswick, Canada
66. University of North Carolina at Chapel Hill, North Carolina
67. University of North Carolina at Greensboro, North Carolina
68. University of North Texas, Texas
69. University of Ottawa, Canada
70. University of Pretoria, South Africa
71. University of Puerto Rico, Puerto Rico
72. University of Rochester, New York
73. University of San Diego, California
74. University of Sarasota, Florida
75. University of Southern California, California
76. University of Southern Queensland
77. University of Tennessee, Tennessee
78. University of Texas at Austin, Texas
79. University of the Philippines Los Baños, Science and Technology, The Philippines
80. University of Toledo, Ohio
81. University of Toronto, Canada
82. University of Tulsa, Oklahoma
83. University of Washington, Washington
84. Virginia Commonwealth University, Virginia
85. Virginia Polytechnic Institute and State University, Virginia
86. Walden University, Minnesota
87. Wayne State University, Michigan
88. Western Michigan University, Michigan
89. Wilmington College, Delaware

TABLE A.5. Disciplines in Which Doctoral Dissertations Applied the CIPP Evaluation Model

1. Agriculture	13. Economics	25. Music
2. Anthropology	14. Education	26. Psychology
3. Architecture	15. English	27. Psychotherapy
4. Aviation	16. Engineering	28. Public safety
5. Behavioral sciences	17. Evaluation	29. Religion
6. Biology	18. Health care	30. Social security administration
7. Botany	19. Health sciences	31. Social work
8. Business	20. Language and literature	32. Sociology
9. Chemistry	21. Law	33. Sports
10. Cosmetology	22. Law enforcement	34. Transportation
11. Criminology	23. Library and information science	
12. Dentistry	24. Military	

how the Arabic language and culture affected both the students and their families within the home and public school arenas. Anthony's dissertation study (2009), which used the CIPP evaluation model with a formative approach, evaluated a beginning teacher induction and mentor program in a rural, county school system in western North Carolina and its effectiveness in the retention of teachers. Instructive information was systematically gathered about the conditions that necessitated the program, procedures, and practices used by the system to provide support and assistance to beginning teachers, whether or not established processes were being followed. Also studied was the impact of the program on beginning teacher retention.

Outside the United States, Peng (1995) employed the CIPP Model to develop an effective inservice training program for teachers in vocational senior high schools across Taiwan. Using the CIPP Model, Nyandindi (1995) evaluated the primary school oral health education program in Tanzania. Applying the CIPP Evaluation Model as a framework, Boonprakob (1994) developed and evaluated a curriculum model for teaching science in secondary schools in Thailand.

International Applications of the CIPP Model

As described previously, the CIPP Model's wide applications have crossed the U.S. national border and spread into many other countries. In the approximately 500 identified studies, the CIPP Model has been applied in at least 38 other countries and regions: Australia, Brazil, Canada, China, Denmark, England, Finland, France, Germany, Greece, Hong Kong, India, Indonesia, Iran, Israel, Japan, Jordan, Mexico, Netherlands, New Zealand, Niger, Nigeria, Pakistan, Palestine, Philippines, Saudi Arabia, Slovenia, South Africa, South Korea, Spain, Sweden, Switzerland, Taiwan, Tajikistan, Thailand, Turkey, United Kingdom, and Vietnam.

The CIPP Model's applications outside of the United States also cover many disciplines and service areas and target diverse programs. For example, the CIPP Model was employed to evaluate the Methodist Church archives of Nigeria and to examine whether archives satisfy the immediate tangible needs of its users (Alegbeleye, 1984). Upon the successful completion of the evaluation effort, the CIPP Model was recommended to evaluate the performance and immediate utility of archives.

A cross-sectional, descriptive study was conducted utilizing the CIPP Model to evaluate the one-year performance outcome of Community Medical Care Unit (CMU) in Mahasarakham Hospital, Thailand (Asavatanabodee, 2010). The target population was divided into two groups: (1) the executive committee of Mahasarakham Hospital, including one director, five vice directors, and 16 CMU paramedical personnel and public health administrators; and (2) 281 randomized people in the service area of CMU, Mahasarakham Hospital. The evaluation of context, input, and output was ranked highly useful in both groups, while the process ranking was moderate in the first group and high in the other group. Based on the evaluation results, the study recommended explicit policies, improvement in behavioral service, an appropriate workload, an adequate parking lot, and a network sharing of hospital data bank contents. The study's results provided useful data for improving and developing community health care service in Thailand's urban areas.

TABLE A.6. Research Topics and Service Areas Investigated in Doctoral Dissertations That Applied the CIPP Evaluation Model

- Academic guidance counseling
- Academic mentoring
- Adult education
- Aircraft maintenance
- Athletic academic support
- Automotive technician training
- Aviation training
- Banking
- Bilingual education
- Business education
- Career counseling
- Catholic school
- Chapter 1 school
- Character education
- Chemical engineering
- Chemistry education
- Child care
- Christian education
- Christian studies
- Church
- Citizenship education
- Civil engineering
- Clinics
- Communicable disease
- Community college education
- Community colleges
- Community counseling
- Community service
- Compulsory Education Advisory Group
- Continuing education
- Cosmetology training
- Counseling
- Cultural anthropology
- Curriculum development
- Curriculum evaluation
- Dental care
- Developmental psychology
- Doctoral program development
- Dropout prevention
- Educational administration
- Educational evaluation
- Educational leadership
- Educational policy
- Educational sociology
- Educational software development
- Educational technology
- Elementary education
- Elementary schools
- Employment supports
- Entrepreneurship
- Evaluation

- Faculty development
- Fellowship
- Foreign language
- Forestry, wildlife, and range sciences
- Foster care
- Gifted education
- Health care management
- Health education
- High school education
- Higher education
- Hockey coaching
- Home economics
- Housing
- Human resources development
- Industrial engineering
- Industrial technical education
- Industry training
- Information systems
- Inservice training
- Instructional materials
- Instructional media
- Insurance
- International law
- International relations
- Judicial systems
- Juvenile court probation program
- Labor relations
- Language arts
- Language policy
- Leadership preparation
- Learning enrichment program
- Library
- Literacy
- Management education
- Mechanical engineering
- Medical training
- Mentoring
- Middle school education
- Military
- Minority and ethnic groups
- Motorcycle safety administration
- Multicultural counseling
- Multicultural education
- Music education
- Nursing
- Nursing education
- Nutrition education
- Nutritional intervention
- Occupational psychology
- Oral health

- Philanthropic grant making
- Philanthropic organization
- Physical education
- Police education and training
- Postliteracy programs
- Preschool education
- Principal preparation
- Probation classification
- Psychotherapy
- Public administration
- Reading instruction
- Rehabilitation therapy
- Religious education
- Religious school
- Rural development
- School administration
- School facility
- School finance
- School leadership
- School psychological services
- School–university partnership
- Science education
- Secondary education
- Service learning
- Small business
- Social emotional learning
- Social security administration
- Social structure
- Social work
- Special education
- Sports medicine
- Staff development
- STEP program
- String program
- Summer school
- Teacher assistance program
- Teacher competency program
- Teacher development
- Teacher education
- Teacher induction
- Teacher qualification
- Teacher retention
- Teaching
- Teaching assistant training
- Theological education
- Values education
- Vocational education
- Welfare services
- Wellness program
- Women's studies

A qualitative evaluation of the implementation of family health nursing in Tajikistan was reported by Parfitt and Cornish (2007). Using the CIPP Model, they successfully evaluated this program's progress and identified factors that helped or hindered its implementation. Similarly, Othanganont (2001) described a CIPP Model–guided evaluation of the Thai-Lao collaborating nursing manpower development project involving 309 nurses. The study recommended that a periodic supervisory activity be implemented to enhance the instruction of trainers, that 2-year and 4-year continuation programs for bachelor's degrees in nursing be developed, and that a nursing education master's-degree program be initially obtained from neighboring countries.

Osokoya and Adekunle (2007) recounted an evaluation of enrollees of the Leventis Foundation (Nigeria) Agricultural Schools established to train youths to develop their state and their nation in the area of food production. Aided by the CIPP Model, the evaluators assessed the trainability of a sample of 247 enrollees in the three operating schools by using questionnaires, structured interviews, and observations as data collection techniques.

In Spain, a Filella-Guiu and Blanch-Plana (2002) study described the evaluation results of PORO, a three-level occupational guidance program designed to improve offenders' job-finding possibilities and to reduce reoffending after imprisonment. The program was carried out at a Catalan prison, and the CIPP Model was used to evaluate the program's efficiency, effectiveness, and impact. The evaluation outcomes yielded many practical suggestions for prison population career development.

The impact of inpatient intervention provided by a child mental health unit in Victoria, Australia, was assessed on a number of key child and family variables (Gavidia-Payne, Littlefield, Hallgren, Jenkins, & Coventry, 2003). A total of 29 parents, 42 teachers, and 37 referrers provided reports on a series of child, parent, and family functioning measures. Significant improvements in child behavior and functioning, parenting competency and efficacy, parenting practices, and reduced parental depression were observed over time, based on the data gathered from systematic evaluation guided by the CIPP Model.

Iran's assessment of national child growth showed that a high percentage of the country's children were afflicted by stunted growth (Shams et al., 2008). A community-based field trial was then rendered on 74 pairs of mothers and children less than 3 years of age.

A model was designed for increasing the mothers' participation, and a group of mothers volunteered and were instructed in growth monitoring and child nutrition. The program was evaluated by use of the CIPP Model regarding the effect of mothers' participation in improving growth and nutrition of children. The results revealed that enhancing the mothers' participation resulted in considerable improvement of their knowledge and practice concerning children's growth and nutrition. Additionally, individual and social capabilities of the mothers, including their self-confidence, were increased. The program's sustainability and transportability were also evaluated using the CIPP Model.

Saripudin (2010) evaluated the resocialization program of street children at open houses in Bandung, Indonesia, by focusing on the CIPP Model's input, process, and product components. Systematic random sampling was used to select respondents from 16 open houses in Bandung. The sample of the study was 522 people: 36 administrators/managers, 132 facilitators, and 354 street children. The data, collected through questionnaires, interviews, and observations, revealed that the resocialization program of street children at open houses in Bandung had a number of weaknesses that needed to be addressed. The study suggested that to reach the goal of the street children resocialization program at open houses, the improvement efforts from everyone who was responsible should be integrated.

In this section, we have reported on instances of the CIPP Model's applications, but not on their quality, as determined by credible audits or metaevaluations. Nevertheless, the fact that many applications of the CIPP Model made it through dissertation processes and that some made it through juried publication processes attest to their quality.

Summary and Conclusions

This chapter has noted the ubiquity of evaluation; stressed the need for systematic evaluation; outlined the development of the evaluation field; distinguished between informal and formal evaluation; and explained and contrasted two of evaluation's main acts: description and judgment. The chapter also noted the role of the CIPP Evaluation Model in the evaluation field's development and provided detailed background information on the model's applications. The historical overview shows that the evaluation discipline has developed rapidly and substantially since the 1960s.

The documentation of uses of the CIPP Model shows that the model has been one of the core elements in the evaluation discipline's development and that it has been widely applied across the full range of disciplines and service areas and in many nations. Truly, the need for systematic evaluation is pervasive, and the CIPP Model has been widely applied to help meet this need.

Formal, systematic evaluation is needed in all human endeavors, as evaluation provides a method for accountability and offers the opportunity for improvement and growth. Evaluation is the most fundamental of all disciplines, for all disciplines need evaluation to improve and advance. Evaluations are utilized to identify needs, to choose approaches, to examine program implementation, to assess outcomes, to compare competing programs, and to help eliminate unworthy programs. It serves as an improvement mechanism for society by identifying needs for intervention, affirming worth and accreditation, demanding accountability, initiating improvements, and instigating reasonable terminations. As such, evaluation plays an indispensable role in society's progress and well-being. Today evaluation is recognized as a distinct area of professional practice. Innumerable evaluations have been conducted in the United States and internationally.

The results of a survey of the members of the American Society for Training and Development revealed that the CIPP Model was preferred over other evaluation models (Galvin, 1983b). A comparative analysis of several evaluation approaches showed that the CIPP Model is one of the most useful evaluation approaches for program directors and teachers, providing them with a clear record-keeping framework regarding school programs (Hui-Fang, 1997).

Glossary

accountability The ability to account for the use of resources, execution of planned activities, and achievement of outcomes.

accuracy standards Standards that in combination require an evaluation's procedures, data, conclusions, and reports to be unbiased, valid, reliable, and of sufficient scope to address the targeted questions.

Advocate Teams Technique A technique for use in input evaluations whereby teams—usually in isolation from each other—develop competing proposals for meeting targeted needs or achieving stated objectives, and an independent team evaluates the alternative proposals against established criteria. The client then selects the most promising proposal for implementation or may assign another team to converge the best features of the competing proposals into the needed action plan.

Agency for Healthcare Research and Quality (AHRQ) A part of the United States Department of Health and Human Services which supports research and is designed to improve the outcomes and quality of health care.

analysis of covariance (ANCOVA) A general linear model that blends ANOVA and regression. ANCOVA evaluates whether population means of a dependent variable (DV) are equal across levels of a categorical independent variable (IV), often called a treatment, while statistically controlling for the effects of other continuous variables that are not of primary interest, known as covariates (CV) or nuisance variables. Mathematically, ANCOVA decomposes the variance in the DV into variance explained by the CV(s), variance explained by the categorical IV, and residual variance. Intuitively, ANCOVA can be thought of as "adjusting" the DV by the group means of the CV(s).

analysis of variance (ANOVA) A collection of statistical models, developed by Ronald Fisher, used to analyze the differences among group means and their associated procedures.

anonymity, provision for An evaluator's actions to honor her or his commitments to certain persons involved in an evaluation—for example, as program beneficiaries, program staff, respondents to data requests—that their identities will not be revealed or made identifiable in any aspect of the evaluation, including reports, feedback sessions, database, and publications.

assets Grants, expertise, facilities, media, services, and the like, that could be accessed and used to help fulfill a program's purpose.

background check A systematic investigation of background factors—such as criminal history, past job performance, and credit records—that an evaluator or program director may obtain and consider in the process of recruiting and selecting such evaluation or program participants as staff members and program beneficiaries.

beneficiaries Persons to be served by a program.

"buying a contract" The unethical practice of knowingly submitting an overly low bid to win a competitive contract (or grant) and then as the program unfolds informing the funder of the original miscalculation and requesting the additional required funds.

case study A characterization and in-depth depiction, thick description, analysis, and assessment of a particular program or other entity, as it unfolds or how it occurred in the past. The case study's focus is on illuminating the case holistically but also in terms of such particulars as its boundaries, involved persons, history, structure, workings, and outcomes.

checklist A list of items—such as tasks or criteria—to consider when designing, budgeting, contracting, conducting, reporting, or assessing a program, evaluation, or other enterprise.

chi-square test A statistical examination that tests whether the distribution of one measured event differs by more than chance from the distribution of another measured event. Chi-square can be used to distinguish between the expected outcome and the actual occurrence of an event.

CIPP Evaluation Model An extensively defined and illustrated approach to formatively and summatively assessing the context, inputs, process, and products of a program or other entity.

clinical investigation An in-depth, heavily qualitative and often diagnostic inquiry into the workings and problems of a program or other entity.

cluster random sampling A sampling technique in which groups of individuals are randomly selected, in contrast to the usual sampling technique of directly selecting individuals.

coding The process of organizing qualitative data into chunks or segments of text and assigning meaning to the information.

community development An organized process for working with a community to assess its needs, problems, and assets; clarify its mission; plan and carry out improvement efforts in such areas as housing, education, infrastructure, safety, jobs, welfare, and health; and evaluate and strengthen its progress.

conclusion An evaluation's final interpretations of findings and bottom-line judgments.

confidence interval A range of values so defined that there is a specified probability that the interval has a predetermined probability of spanning a given parameter.

confidentiality Arrangements and actions to ensure that information about an individual is kept private and secure and is not revealed to any unauthorized person.

conflict of interest A past experience, association, commitment, or orientation that could bias or have the appearance of biasing one's judgment or decision about a program or other matter irrespective of the relevant evidence. Because everyone has conflicts of interest, evaluators are charged to openly reveal any conflict of interest that could or might be perceived to affect their judgment of a program and take steps to assure that the real or potential conflict does not interfere with or taint any aspect of their evaluation service.

construct validity The appropriateness of inferences made on the basis of observations because the test measures one or more dimensions of a theory or trait.

Consuelo Foundation A charitable foundation, based in Hawaii, that is devoted to meeting the needs of disadvantaged children and women in Hawaii and the Philippines.

content analysis Systematic examination of the contents of a set of written materials.

content validity In psychometrics, content validity (also known as logical validity) refers to the extent to which a measure represents all facets of a given construct. For example, a depression scale may lack content validity if it assesses the affective dimension of depression but fails to take into account the behavioral dimension.

context evaluation An evaluation involving the systematic assessment of needs, problems, assets, and opportunities to help decision makers set defensible goals and priorities and help relevant users judge goals, priorities, and outcomes.

contingency fund A section of a budget that sets aside an amount of money to be used if needed to cover unanticipated legitimate expenses.

contract A legally enforceable set of agreements.

control group The group of subjects in a comparative experimental study that does not receive the experimental treatment but whose outcome measures are compared to those of the experimental group.

convenience sample A sampling technique in which a group of individuals are chosen because they are conveniently available for study.

cooperative agreement An arrangement in which the evaluator and funder collaborate in conducting an evaluation.

correlation The extent of relation between two variables.

cost analysis Documentation and breaking out of a program's costs in such terms as its line items, task areas, or time periods.

cost-effectiveness The extent to which an entity produces equal or better outcomes than one or more competitors that cost about the same; or the extent to which the entity produces the same outcomes as competitors but at less cost.

cost-plus contract A formal evaluation agreement that includes the funds required to conduct an evaluation assignment, plus an additional agreed-on charge for the evaluator's services that falls outside the sphere of the contracted evaluation.

cost plus a fee contract The type of cost-plus contract that includes a charge to help sustain the evaluation organization.

cost plus a grant contract The type of cost-plus contract that includes funds to support activities outside the scope of the evaluation assignment, such as research, stipends for graduate students, or staff attendance at a professional meeting.

cost plus a profit contract The type of cost-plus contract that allows the evaluation organization to make a profit on the evaluation.

cost-reimbursable contract An agreement that the evaluator will account for, report, and be reimbursed for actual evaluation project expenditures, usually up to a certain budgetary ceiling.

covariate A variable used in an analysis of covariance to adjust the scores on the dependent variable.

covert observations Observations in which the researcher's identity and task or intention are kept secret from those being studied.

credibility Trustworthiness based, for example, on an excellent track record, educational credentials, practical orientation, reputation, cultural competence, honesty, communication skills, and professionalism.

criteria Explicit variables and interpretation rules for use in assessing and judging a program or other entity.

cross-break (or contingency) table A two-way analysis showing the distribution of one variable (such as heights) in rows and another (such as weights) in columns, used to study the association between the two variables.

(data) cleaning A systematic process of proofing and correcting data to ensure its accuracy.

data mining Examination of the contents of a database or other set of data to address particular questions of interest.

decision makers Persons—such as policymakers, board members, administrators, teachers, military officers, business owners, physicians, and nurses—who have the authority and responsibility to make choices in their spheres of operation.

defensible purpose A desired end that has been legitimately defined and that is consistent with a guiding philosophy, code of ethics, set of professional standards, institutional mission, organizational policies, school district curriculum, or national constitution, for example.

Delphi technique The consensus-building technique in which a panel of stakeholders read advance position papers posing alternative policies (or other types of options), work through successive rounds of rating the alternatives, and ultimately attempt to reach consensus on a preferred set of the considered options.

demographic analysis Investigation of statistical data on a population, especially to determine the central tendencies and dispersion of such variables as age, income, ethnicity, housing, education, employment, and marital status.

description A written account to delineate and make vivid the distinctive nature, inner workings, and impacts of a program or other entity.

descriptive statistics Indexes used to characterize a group, especially means, medians, modes, and standard deviations.

design A defined set of specific procedures to ensure that a given enterprise will meet specified technical requirements; be carried out efficiently; and achieve its objectives.

discriminant function analysis A statistical method used to identify and combine predictor variables into a function that maximally explains observed differences on a dependent variable between two groups.

distribution A systematic grouping of data into classes or categories according to the frequency of occurrence of each successive value. The distribution may be presented in either a numerical table or a graph. A "normal distribution" would look similar to a bell shape and is referred to as a "bell curve." A skewed distribution would peak at either end of the scale and taper off at the opposite end.

diagnostic test The process of determining by examination the nature and circumstances of the problems and associated conditions that are contributing to a defective program or other problematic entity or to the failure to meet the needs of a targeted group of beneficiaries.

document review The evaluation procedure by which an evaluator obtains, examines, and extracts data—from a set of files or other source of documents—for use in addressing particular evaluation questions.

effect parameter analysis An analysis procedure for identifying and assessing a program's effects.

effectiveness The extent to which a program or other entity produces the intended results.

environmental analysis Systematic collection and assessment of information in a program's context, such as population characteristics, related programs and services, educational and cultural offerings, housing stock, parks and recreation, boys and girls clubs, fraternal organizations, restaurants, churches, businesses, food and clothing stores, welfare programs, social service organizations, area economics, jobs, employment rate, health services, local governance, the area power structure, political dynamics, fire and police services, transportation, theaters, utilities, air and water quality, crime statistics, homeless people, tax base and tax rates, infrastructure, and the needs of the target population.

epidemiological study A retroactive, in-depth examination of an epidemic disease to identify causal agents and thereby pave the way for finding a solution to stop the epidemic.

equivalent-forms method A technique for measuring reliability in which two different but equivalent forms of an instrument are administered during the same time period to carefully matched or randomized groups of individuals, or a single group. In either case, the two sets of scores are analyzed to produce an equivalent forms estimation of the instrument's reliability, which is indicated by the extent of correlation between the two sets of measures.

ESEA: Titles I and III Elementary and Secondary Education Act of 1965, which provided federal funds under Title I to help schools address the needs of disadvantaged children and under Title III to help schools develop innovative approaches to improving teaching and learning.

ethical standards Codes of probity for guiding the behavior of evaluators.

evaluand The object of an evaluation, especially a program, project, or organization.

evaluation The assessment of something's value, especially in terms of its merit, worth, and significance.

evaluation accountability standards Three standards labeled Evaluation Documentation, Internal Metaevaluation, and External Metaevaluation that comprise the final subset of standards in the Joint Committee on Standards for Educational Evaluation (2011) *Program Evaluation Standards.*

evaluation boundaries Defined limits for an evaluation in such terms as the study's geographic area and time frame.

evaluation budget A detailed estimate of financial and associated resources required to implement the full range of projected evaluation tasks within a given time period. This budget should ensure that the study can be carried out as designed and convince the sponsor that the study is affordable and feasible, and will be conducted at a high level of quality, professionalism, and utility.

evaluation client The person who requested the evaluation and who, among others, will use the evaluation's results for some purpose, such as program improvement or accountability to a funder.

evaluation contract A legally enforceable, written set of agreements between the evaluator and funder concerning the evaluation's tasks, both parties' responsibilities for conducting the evaluation, the conditions and schedule for payments, and provisions for reviewing and, if needed, renegotiating the contract.

evaluation database The arrangements, rules, and facilities for organizing, storing, and retrieving the evaluation's quantitative and qualitative information.

evaluation design A defined set of specific procedures to ensure that an evaluation will meet the standards of sound evaluation; be carried out efficiently; validly appraise the subject program's merit and worth; and effectively report its findings.

evaluation documentation standard The Joint Committee on Standards for Educational Evaluation (2011) *Program Evaluation Standards* standard that requires evaluations to be fully documented in terms of their negotiated purposes and implemented designs, procedures, data, and outcomes.

evaluation expertise Demonstrated ability to carry out the full range of tasks in an evaluation, especially designing, budgeting, and contracting evaluations; involving stakeholders; collecting, organizing, analyzing, and synthesizing information; producing and delivering oral, graphic, and printed reports; facilitating the use of evaluation findings; delivering evaluation training; and conducting standards-based metaevaluations.

evaluation listserv A computerized, regularly updated repository of information related to an ongoing evaluation that is accessible by interested parties that enroll in the service.

evaluation memorandum of agreement Written agreements for the conduct of an evaluation between an evaluator and a client (often an official in the evaluator's organization) that are relatively informal and usually not legally binding.

evaluation mission An organization's formal written statement of (1) requirements to systematically evaluate specified organizational facets and (2) the evaluation's intended benefits.

evaluation newsletter An evaluator's periodic dissemination of a brief newsletter—usually via a dedicated computer website—to keep an evaluation's interested parties informed about the ongoing evaluation's recent and projected activities, available reports, needs for stakeholder involvement, and the evaluation's updated schedule.

evaluation planning grant In the context of projecting a relatively long-term evaluation, an evaluator may secure a short-term grant for the purpose of becoming acquainted with the subject program and its environment, identifying and developing rapport with at least representatives of the full range of stakeholders, clarifying evaluation questions and information requirements, and crafting a responsive and functional evaluation design.

evaluation profession The body of trained evaluators who practice competent evaluation, define and regularly improve standards and methods of sound evaluation, regularly record significant historical milestones in the evaluation field, conduct and report research on evaluation, and maintain and improve their evaluation competencies through continuing evaluation education.

evaluation stakeholder review panel A panel of evaluation stakeholders—typically chaired by the evaluation's client—who provide the evaluator with timely reviews of draft reporting plans and reports and who may facilitate the evaluator's collection of data.

evaluation standard A principle commonly agreed to by experts in the conduct and use of evaluation used to guide an evaluation and judge its quality and value.

evaluation technical report An appendix to a final evaluation report or a separate, back-up report that includes such items as evaluation instruments, data tables, documentations of the evaluation's cost, evaluators' resumés, and a completed evaluation standards attestation form.

evaluation uses Applications of findings that include, especially, guiding the planning and execution of programs or other entities, maintaining quality control, summing up a program's merit and worth, and meeting accountability needs.

evaluation-oriented client An evaluation client who embodies and carries out the role of evaluation-oriented leader.

evaluation-oriented leader An administrator or other decision maker who has mastered and regularly and effectively exercises the concept of evaluation-oriented leadership.

evaluation-oriented leadership That brand of leadership in which an administrator or other decision maker learns and embraces the standards of sound evaluation; learns effective approaches for meeting the

standards; acquires the skills to carry out client responsibilities in evaluations; takes the initiative in obtaining needed evaluation services; requires evaluators to deliver defensible, useful evaluations; facilitates the evaluation process; helps assure that contracted evaluations are accurate, ethical, cost-effective, useful, and accountable; and exercises leadership in helping stakeholders understand, value, and apply sound evaluation findings.

Evaluation Standards Attestation Form A form for an evaluator to complete and append to a final evaluation report that documents the evaluator's self-assessment of the extent that the evaluation met, partially met, or did not meet the requirements of each of the 30 standards appearing in the Joint Committee on Standards for Educational Evaluation (2011) *Program Evaluation Standards*.

evaluation transparency The evaluator's acts to document and make available to all right-to-know parties information on all important aspects of an evaluation, including its standards, design, costs, contract, staff, involvement of stakeholders, data collection instruments, data analysis procedures, reports, technical appendixes, impacts, and metaevaluation findings.

evaluative criteria Explicit variables and interpretation rules for examining and judging a program or other entity, including, for example, its definition of beneficiaries, focus on beneficiaries' needs, defensible plan, quality of execution, impacts, cost-effectiveness, sustainability, and transferability.

evaluator The person with ultimate authority and responsibility for carrying out and reporting an evaluation in accordance with the standards of the evaluation field.

experimental design A structure for rigorously determining the effects of a program or other intervention. The evaluator employs random assignment or matching procedures to assign subjects or organizations to experimental or control groups, administers a treatment to the experimental group, contrasts outcomes for the comparison groups, and makes inferences about the intervention's effects.

expert review panel A panel of experts engaged to review various aspects of a program or other entity.

external metaevaluation Evaluation of an evaluation that is conducted and reported by an independent metaevaluator.

external validity The extent to which the results of a study can be generalized to other settings.

factor analysis A statistical method for interpreting correlations between scores from a single test or a number of tests by identifying a relatively small number of relatively independent dimensions that can be used to obtain factor scores on individuals. A factor describes the area within which individuals respond consistently, in contrast to how they score on other dimensions. Examples of names for factors that might be assigned based on a factor analysis of the correlations between the items on a comprehensive educational achievement test could include vocabulary, knowledge, comprehension, application, and speed of reading.

fairness The extent to which an evaluation treats all parties to an evaluation in an even-handed, impartial, unbiased, honest, and just manner.

feasibility standards Evaluation standards that require evaluation procedures to be efficient, relatively easy to implement, adequately funded, politically viable, and cost-effective.

Feedback Workshop Checklist An ordered list of checkpoints—created by Arlen Gullickson and Daniel Stufflebeam—for planning and conducting feedback workshops.

feedback workshop technique A method for systematically conveying draft interim findings to a program's leaders and staff (and possibly other designated stakeholders), guiding their discussion of findings, obtaining their critical reactions to draft plans, reports, and other materials, assisting their use of findings, and using their feedback to update or strengthen evaluation plans, reports, and other materials.

fiscal viability The state of an evaluation or other entity in which the entity possesses sufficient resources to fulfill its mission.

fixed-price contract A contractual agreement that a contracted enterprise will receive a fixed amount of funds for carrying out the assignment. For example, the evaluator would receive and retain only the set amount of funds for the evaluation assignment irrespective of whether the evaluation work turned out to cost more or less than the set amount.

focus group A method in which the evaluator or a trained facilitator engages a small, representative group of stakeholders to study an evaluation report and deliberate about practical ways to apply the evaluation's findings.

focusing an evaluation An evaluation's initial stage of determining and clarifying the program or other entity to be evaluated; identifying the intended users and uses of findings; agreeing on the use of an evaluation model or general evaluation approach and on the standards for guiding and assessing the evaluation; determining the key evaluation questions, needed information, and required reports; clarifying the evaluation's time frame and any budgetary limitations; determining the evaluation's staffing and resource needs; examining the study's political context, potential barriers, and required protocols; and agreeing on metaevaluation arrangements.

formal evaluation An evaluation that is designed and systematically executed to meet professional standards of utility, feasibility, propriety, accuracy, and accountability.

formative evaluation Evaluation keyed to helping a program or other entity succeed by such actions as assessing needs, problems, assets, and opportunities to assist goal-setting; identifying and assessing alternative program approaches to inform program planning; documenting and assessing program implementation to help strengthen program activities; and measuring and reporting interim outcomes to help strengthen the overall effort.

formative metaevaluation A metaevaluation keyed to helping an evaluation succeed by providing proactive feedback on the evaluation's adherence to standards of sound evaluation; more specifically, evaluating and providing feedback on initial evaluation plans; documenting, monitoring, and providing feedback on the implementation of evaluation plans; and assessing and offering feedback on draft evaluation reports.

formative reports Reports providing proactive feedback for use in strengthening ongoing program decisions and operations.

Friedman two-way analysis of variance A nonparametric statistical test used to detect differences between treatments across multiple test attempts.

goal-free evaluation An evaluation in which the evaluator is kept ignorant of a program's goals so that he or she can uncover the full range of program outcomes regardless of what was intended. The goal-free evaluator searches for what actually is occurring in a program and for all of the program's effects, and examines processes and outcomes against assessed needs of intended beneficiaries.

goal-free evaluation manual A manual prepared by a contracted goal-free evaluator to include the projected goal-free inquiry approach, the safeguards against keying the study to stated program goals, the standards to be met by the goal-free evaluation, the intended sources of information, the procedures and tools for conducting the study, the protocols for collecting information, the plan for determining the needs of intended beneficiaries, the plan for assessing goal-free outcomes against assessed needs, and the projected timing and nature of goal-free evaluation reports.

goal-free evaluator An evaluator—preferably with training in qualitative as well as quantitative methods—who conducts goal-free evaluations.

grant An award of funds to support an investigator to conduct an evaluation or other project that serves the investigator's professional interests (but not necessarily those of the grantor) and is of some social value.

graph A visual presentation of numeric data. Examples include histograms, boxplots, line graphs, bar graphs, scatterplots, and stem-and-leaf plots.

hearings Meetings in which interested parties are invited to express their opinions and judgments about some entity, such as a program, evaluation, or evaluation report.

historical analysis The process of interpreting a program's current status, issues, accomplishments, strengths, weaknesses, significance, and overall value by retrieving and studying relevant historical documents and interviewing persons with relevant knowledge of the program's antecedents.

impacts A program's assessed influence and effects.

importance An evaluative criterion denoting a program's level of significance, consequence, standing, distinction, or widespread relevance.

improvement orientation An orientation to evaluation that sees evaluation's purpose as not only to prove, but also—and more importantly—to improve.

independent evaluation audit A commissioned, standards-based—usually post-hoc—examination and judgment of an evaluation's data, methods, tools, and reports by an external/third-party metaevaluation expert.

independent metaevaluation A commissioned, standards-based examination and judgment of an evaluation's data, methods, tools, and reports by an external/third-party metaevaluation expert. Such metaevaluations are summative and conducted following the completion of an evaluation but may also be formative to help guide an evaluation throughout its implementation.

indirect costs Those costs incurred to address needs—such as security, utilities, custodial services, administrative oversight, and accounting—that span projects, programs, and other operations in a contracted enterprise's parent organization and that cannot be readily and specifically partitioned to determine associated direct costs for the contracted enterprise.

inferential statistics A form of research design and data analysis used to reach defensible inferences about a population based on measures taken from a randomized or otherwise representative sample of the population.

informal interview A relatively free-form, naturally occurring approach to asking questions and obtaining responses from an interviewee; this approach resembles a casual conversation and does not follow an established protocol.

information analysis A process of inspecting, cleaning, transforming, and modeling data with the goal of describing characteristics and patterns, high-lighting useful information, suggesting conclusions, and supporting decision making.

information collection The process of systemati-cally gathering and validating information on variables that are relevant to answering stated evaluation ques-tions and fully judging a program's value.

information synthesis The process of connecting an evaluation's value base, information, and analyses into a unified set of conclusions.

input evaluation Evaluation in which the evaluator assesses alternative program strategies, competing ac-tion and staffing plans, and associated budgets to de-termine their differential feasibility and potential cost-effectiveness in meeting targeted needs and achieving goals.

institutional sustainability fee A category of funds in a cost plus a fee budget to support organizational purposes beyond those of the contracted evaluation, such as administration, advisory groups, and proposal development.

institutionalizing evaluation A process whereby an organization defines, sets policy for, installs, and regularly operates and uses results from an evaluation system. Such a system is relatively permanent and rou-tinely funded in the organization.

interaction effect The differing effects of a treat-ment or other independent variable on the outcome measures of two or more subgroups. For example, girls may respond quite differently from boys to a certain educational intervention, in which case it would be mis-leading to only look at and make inferences about the combined outcome.

internal consistency methods Statistical strategies for determining how well items on a test measure the same construct or idea. An example is the split-half procedure.

internal metaevaluation An organization's standards-based evaluations of its evaluations that may be conducted by the organization's evaluation shop or by the staff members of the subject evaluation. Such internal self-assessments usually culminate, at least, in a written attestation of the extent to which the evalua-tion met, partially met, or did not meet each standard in a set of professional standards for evaluations, such as the 30 standards contained in the Joint Committee on Standards for Educational Evaluation (2011) *Program Evaluation Standards.*

internal validity The truthfulness of inferences about whether two or more variables have a causal re-lationship.

interrater reliability A measure of reliability in which the scores given by different raters are assessed for consistency.

interval data Data in which values can be placed on a scale of differing degrees, with the distances between scale points being equal and there being no exact zero value on the scale (e.g., measures of ambient tempera-ture).

interview A formal meeting between an evaluator and one or more key informants in which the evalua-tor obtains and documents responses to questions con-cerning such matters as the enterprise's background, structure, operations, accomplishments, problems, strengths, weaknesses, or overall value.

Joint Committee on Standards for Educational Evaluation A committee established in 1975 by the American Educational Research Association, American Psychological Association, and the National Council on Measurement in Education to develop standards for educational evaluations. The committee has continued in this work, is currently sponsored by 15 professional societies, and has issued standards for evaluations of programs, projects, materials, personnel, and students.

judgment A conclusion based on a set of values or standards plus examination of an entity's strengths and weaknesses.

justified conclusion A conclusion that is substantiat-ed by valid information, sound logic, plausible assump-tions, and the evidence-based rejection of alternative interpretations.

Ke Aka Ho'ona A Hawaiian phrase meaning "the Spirit of Consuelo," which is the title of a self-help housing project conducted on Hawaii's Waianae Coast.

key informants Persons who are highly knowledgeable about a program and therefore important sources of information for evaluating the program.

Kruskal–Wallis one-way analysis of variance A rank-based statistical test used to determine if there is a statistically significant difference between scores of two or more groups on a continuous or ordinal dependent variable.

kurtosis An indication of the "peakness" of a distribution.

legality The extent to which an evaluation is conducted and reported in accordance with applicable laws and statutes.

line-item cost categories Common main items in a budget, for example, personnel, travel, consultants, supplies, equipment, services, and indirect costs.

literature review A structured process of searching for, selecting, analyzing, and extracting information from documents with relevance to a study's objectives and then using the information in the process of describing and judging the subject program.

logic of evaluation The four main evaluative acts of scoring, ranking, grading, and apportioning, as identified by Michael Scriven.

logic model A graphic representation—for example, in the form of a network or matrix, typically supported by a narrative explanation—that depicts the interrelationships between an enterprise's aims, tasks, resources, schedule, milestones, and intended outcomes.

logistic regression A statistical method for analyzing a dataset in which there are one or more independent variables that determine an outcome.

main effect Result obtained on a primary outcome variable of interest (in contrast to a "simple effect" that is revealed as a consequence of a statistically significant interaction, e.g., an effect on a subgroup of the studied sample).

mainstreaming of evaluation Institution of policies and processes by which an organization articulates, staffs, funds, and spreads use of systematic evaluation throughout the organization's horizontal and vertical levels, such that all aspects that are vital to fulfilling the organization's mission are regularly reviewed, assisted, strengthened, and held to accountability standards.

Mann–Whitney *U* Test A nonparametric test of the null hypothesis that two samples come from the same population against an alternative hypothesis. It is useful when the sample size is small and the data distribution is unclear.

mean A measure of central tendency, which represents the arithmetic average computed by summing all the values in the dataset and dividing the sum by the number of data values.

measures of central tendency Statistics that describe the center of a dataset, especially means and medians.

measures of dispersion or variability Statistics that describe the amount of difference and spread in a dataset (e.g., range, variance, and standard deviation).

median A measure of central tendency, which represents the middle score or the point between two adjacent scores in the middle of a distribution when all data points are arranged in ascending order.

merit Excellence of an entity as evidenced by its intrinsic qualities or performance.

meta-analysis A form of quantitative analysis of a set of studies that address a common research question. In program evaluation research contexts, this usually involves a treatment and control contrast or a treatment A and treatment B contrast. Across a selected set of similar studies, an investigator calculates and examines the magnitude, direction, and statistical significance of effect sizes.

metaevaluation An evaluation of an evaluation. Operationally, a metaevaluation is the process of defining, collecting, reporting, and applying descriptive information and judgmental information about an evaluation's utility, feasibility, propriety, accuracy, and accountability for purposes of helping plan and guide an evaluation and ultimately judging its strengths and weaknesses.

Metaevaluation Checklist Daniel Stufflebeam's 2015 edition of his checklist for clients and metaevaluators used in conducting standards-based assessments of evaluations.

mission statement An organization's formal written statement of its main objectives.

mode A measure of central tendency, which represents the score with the highest frequency in a dataset.

modular budget A budget in which the evaluator breaks out costs for main budget modules, including line items, tasks, and time periods.

multiple logistic regression A statistical classification method that generalizes logistic regression to multiclass problems.

multiple regression A statistical test that uses the correlation of each of several predictor variables and their intercorrelations to estimate the value of a dependent variable.

multivariate analysis of variance (MANOVA) An analysis of variance (ANOVA) test with several dependent variables.

naturalistic observation A method in which an observer watches a group in their natural setting and without manipulating any variables simply observes and documents what naturally occurs.

need Something that is essential for attaining or maintaining a satisfactory mode of existence; those things that are necessary or useful for fulfilling a defensible purpose.

needs assessment A study to determine deficiencies in the well-being or performance of targeted beneficiaries, or in the resources and services needed to prevent beneficiaries from suffering bad consequences. Uncovering such outcome and treatment needs provides a basis for setting goals and determining criteria for judging a program's outcomes.

nominal data Data in which the values merely name the category to which the object under study belongs (e.g., U.S. citizen or Canadian citizen).

nonparametric test A statistical test that makes no assumptions about the parameters of a population distribution from which samples were drawn.

nonparticipant observation An observation approach in which the researcher observes and documents processes without participating in the processes or interacting with the subjects being observed.

nonprobability sampling Sampling in which participants are not selected randomly, but on some other basis, such as those who are conveniently available, chosen in some systematic way (such as every third person in a list), interested to be heard, and so on. Such nonrandomly selected samples may be unrepresentative and biased in unknown ways.

nonresponse error A bias that occurs when selected individuals who choose not to participate differ from those who do choose to participate in a study.

objective measurement An impartial measurement that is not affected by bias or opinion.

objectivist epistemology An ideology that proposes reason as the basis of all knowledge and that posits that all knowledge can be obtained only through reasoning.

objectivist orientation An emphasis on concrete solutions rather than subjective thoughts or feelings unique to an individual.

observation technique A research method that involves collecting and analyzing data through watching others, directly or indirectly, in a natural or planned environment.

observer bias The influence of the observer's expectations of what will be seen in the information that he or she notices and records.

observer effect The fact that being observed will influence the setting under observation and subjects' responses.

opportunities Advantageous circumstances, especially including funding programs that could be used to help fulfill targeted needs.

ordinal data Data in which the values can be ordered to reflect various degrees or amounts, but the intervals between values are not necessarily equal (e.g., ranking of refrigerators).

overt observations Observations in which the researcher is open about his/her intentions and those being studied are aware of the researcher's role.

p-**value** The level of marginal significance within a statistical hypothesis test, representing the probability of the occurrence of a given event.

parametric test A statistical test that makes assumptions about the parameters of the population distribution from which samples were drawn.

participant observation An observation method in which the observer takes part in the situation being observed and fully participates in the activities being observed.

path analysis A form of multiple regression that provides estimates of the magnitude and significance of hypothesized causal connections between sets of variables.

peakness The degree to which a dataset's distribution comes to a point, or remains flat, at the top. This is measured through kurtosis.

Pearson's *r* A measure of the linear correlation between two variables, ranging from –1 to +1, which represents the strength and direction of the relationship between two variables.

photographic reprises Photographic records placed at the end of main sections of an evaluation report that are designed to help readers appreciate the section's main findings. Examples include pictures at the end of a context evaluation section that make vivid, relevant environmental circumstances, such as dilapidated schools or shuttered business establishments; at the end of a process evaluation section, photos of project participants building their own houses; or at the end of a product evaluation section, photos of a program's graduates at work in their newly acquired jobs.

pilot trial A small-scale, initial experiment or set of observations undertaken to decide how and whether to launch a full-scale project.

point-of-entry issue The decision situation an evaluator faces when deciding where to begin an evaluation assignment. In the case of the CIPP Model, the evaluator and evaluation client need to determine if the evaluation should follow the sequence of context, input, process, and product evaluations or, instead, should start by first conducting one of the latter types of evaluation. In this decision process, the evaluator should be responsive to the client group's most important evaluation questions and should take into account the nature and extent of already available relevant information.

political sensitivity Avoiding vocabulary or actions that may be considered offensive, discriminatory, or judgmental, typically in regards to gender or race.

political viability The probability of a political policy or program creating a long-lasting impact.

post-hoc test A test run after a significant result is found through a one-way ANOVA (i.e., a significant difference between group means), which confirm where differences occurred between groups.

principal component analysis (PCA) A statistical procedure that converts a set of observations of possibly correlated variables into a set of values of linearly uncorrelated variables called principal components.

probability sampling A sampling technique in which participants are randomly selected in order to make inferences about a population based on the information gathered from the sample.

problem An undesirable condition to be corrected.

Problem-Solving Inventory An inventory developed by Heppner and Petersen in 1982 to assess perceived problem-solving abilities. Using confirmatory factor analysis, results supported a bilevel model of PSI scores with a sample of 164 Mexican American students. Findings support the cultural validity of PSI scores with Mexican Americans and enhance the generalizability with culturally diverse samples.

process control A series of assessments ensuring that a process is predictable, stable, and consistently operating at the target level of performance within normal variation.

process evaluation Evaluation in which the evaluator assesses the implementation of program plans, first to help staff carry out activities and thereafter to help a broader range of users judge program implementation. Through documentation of processes and reporting on progress to appropriate program staff members and other interested parties, the evaluator makes a judgment about the extent to which planned activities are being (or were) carried out on schedule, as planned, and efficiently.

product evaluation In the context, input, process, and product (CIPP) model, evaluation in which the evaluator identifies and assesses outcomes—intended and unintended, short term and long term—to help staff keep an enterprise focused on achieving agreed-on, important outcomes and ultimately to help relevant users gauge the success of the effort in meeting targeted needs. In assessments of consumer products, this term refers to evaluation of such tangible products as computers, automobiles, and cameras. In consumer product evaluations, it is important to identify and validate criteria of merit; weight them according to their relative importance; assess the product on each criterion; and, where possible, reach an overall conclusion.

program evaluation In general, an evaluation that assesses a program's value. Specifically, it is the systematic process of delineating, obtaining, reporting, and applying descriptive and judgmental information about a program's quality, cost-effectiveness, feasibility, safety, legality, sustainability, transferability, fairness, importance, and so on. The result of an evaluation process is an evaluation as product (i.e., an evaluation report for intended uses by intended users).

Program Evaluation and Review Technique (PERT) A networking tool used to identify, sequence, schedule, and monitor the tasks required to complete a project.

Program Evaluation Standards A 2011 set of standards developed by the Joint Committee on Standards for Educational Evaluation and approved by the American National Standards Institute. The 30 standards are grouped according to the five essential attributes of a sound evaluation: utility, feasibility, propriety, accuracy, and evaluation accountability.

project antecedents subreport An early section of an evaluation report that explains why and how a program was started and what persons and groups were instrumental in its initiation.

project implementation subreport A section in an evaluation report that provides a detailed, factual description of how a project was actually carried out.

project profile technique A procedure whereby the evaluator develops an initial profile of a project's aims, staff, and procedures; periodically updates the profile to keep the client and other interested parties apprised of the project's evolution; and ultimately files a comprehensive profile of the project at its conclusion. The final profile serves as an invaluable source of information about how the project started, evolved, and concluded.

project results subreport A section near the end of an evaluation report that reviews the evaluation's design; presents findings in relation to the client group's questions; addresses any additional questions that are essential to assessing the project's merit and worth; and culminates in judgments of the subject project's quality, value, and significance.

propriety standards Evaluation standards requiring that evaluation be conducted legally, ethically, and with due regard for the welfare of the affected parties, including beneficiaries as well as service providers.

psychometrics The science of measuring an individual's mental characteristics, traits, capacities, and processes.

public forum A place that is available for general, public use for speech-related purposes.

purposive sample A sampling technique in which individuals are selected because they have some special qualification or characteristic.

qualitative analysis The process of compiling, analyzing, and interpreting qualitative information to answer particular questions about a program.

quality The standard of something as measured against others of a similar kind.

quality assurance The maintenance of a desired level of quality in a service, or product, typically through fine attention through every stage in the process.

quality control or assurance A system of maintaining standards by testing the output against the specification.

qualtrics A Web-based tool for creating and conducting online surveys.

quantitative analysis Analysis involving a wide range of concepts and techniques for using quantitative information to describe a program and to study and communicate its effects. The process involves compiling, exploring, validating, organizing, summarizing, analyzing, synthesizing, and interpreting quantitative information. Quantitative analysis techniques include descriptive, inferential, and nonparametric statistical techniques, among many others.

quartile rank Any of the three points that divide a serially ranked distribution into four parts, each of which contains one-fourth of the scores.

random measurement error An inconsistency in an individual's score based on purely chance happenings.

randomized true experiment An experimental design used to establish cause-and-effect relationships in which there is at least one experimental group, at least one control group, and random assignment into each group.

range A measure of variability that measures the difference between the largest and smallest values in a dataset.

rating scale A set of categories designed to elicit information about a quantitative or qualitative attribute.

ratio data Data in which values are placed on a ratio scale: one with an exact zero point and equal intervals between scale points (e.g., measures of weight).

reach to intended beneficiaries An assessment, in the product evaluation section of the CIPP Model, of the extent to which a project actually served the full set of intended beneficiaries.

records analysis An evaluator's acquisition and examination of an organization's existing records for use in addressing an evaluation's questions.

regression analysis A statistical process for estimating the relationships among variables.

relativist epistemology A concept of inquiry oriented to a pluralistic, flexible, holistic, subjective, constructivist approach. No final, authoritative conclusion is sought. Beauty is in the eye of the beholder.

reliability A condition that is achieved when the information obtained is free from internal contradictions and when repeated information collection episodes yield, as expected, the same answers.

replication study The repetition of a study using the same methods with different subjects and different experimenters.

resident observer A variation of the travelling observer technique in which one researcher completes evaluations at a single site rather than multiple sites.

responsive evaluation Also known as stakeholder-centered evaluation; a relativistic social agenda and advocacy approach whereby the evaluator interacts with stakeholders (often a diverse group) to support and help develop, administer, and improve a program in a nondirective, counseling manner. An evaluator using this approach employs descriptive and judgmental information to examine a program's background, rationale, transactions, standards, and outcomes. Special features of this approach are searching for side effects, representing the inputs and judgments of diverse stakeholders, and issuing holistic reports.

RFP Request for Proposal; a public or direct mail request for evaluation.

rights of human subjects All human research subjects have certain rights which include: informed consent; treatment as autonomous agents; protection from physical, mental, and emotional harm; access to information regarding research; and protection of privacy and well-being. Human subjects are also entitled to the right to end participation at any time and the right to safeguard integrity.

safety A concern for keeping a program's participants free from danger that is manifested in assessments of the risks associated with implementing and operating the program.

sampling The process of selecting a number of individuals from a population in the hopes that the sample will be representative of the population from which it was chosen.

scenario A postulated sequence or development of events.

secondary data analysis The use of existing data, collected for a previous study, in order to pursue a research interest distinct from the original work.

self-assessment device A test used to evaluate one's personal abilities, failings, or feelings.

Self-Efficacy Scale A scale used to assess a general sense of perceived self-efficacy (one's belief in one's ability to succeed), with the aim of predicting coping with daily hassles and adapting after experiencing stressful life events.

semistructured interview An interview that follows a series of questions but is also open to adding new questions as the interview progresses based on the respondent's answers.

side effects A secondary, typically undesirable effect of a drug or medical treatment.

sign test A test used to test the null hypothesis that the median of a distribution is equal to some value.

significance A concept referring to a program's potential influence, importance, and visibility.

significance test A statistical analysis used to determine whether a null hypothesis should be rejected or retained.

simple effect The effect of one independent variable within one level of a second independent variable.

simple random sampling A sampling process in which each member of the population has an equal and independent chance of being selected.

site visit An evaluation of verbal, written, and visual evidence of an institution by an external team.

skewness An indication of a distribution's lack of symmetry.

Spearman's correlation A nonparametric statistical test that measures the strength of an association between two ranked variables.

split-half method A technique for measuring reliability in which two halves of a test are scored separately for each person.

SPSS Statistical Package for the Social Sciences; a statistical software program that can perform highly complex data manipulation and analysis with simple instructions.

staff-kept diary A record kept by staff members of project observations and outcomes.

stakeholder engagement procedures The process by which an organization involves people who may be affected by the decisions it makes or can influence the implementation of its decisions.

stakeholder interviews A dialogue between stakeholders and evaluators used to gauge program success and implementation of program goals.

stakeholders Those who are the intended users of an evaluation's findings, others who may be affected by the evaluation, and those expected to contribute to the evaluation. These persons are appropriately engaged in helping affirm foundational values, define evaluation questions, clarify evaluative criteria, contribute needed information, interpret findings, and assess evaluation reports.

standard deviation A measure of variability that is the positive square root of a distribution's variance and that is used to assess distances of individual observations from the mean.

(standard professionally endorsed) principles of sound evaluation The authoritative criteria for guiding and judging evaluations, which prevent bias and enhance credibility when used correctly. These standards deal with the independence of the audit organization and individual auditors; the exercise of sound professional judgment in conducting and reporting audits, exercising quality control, and engaging in external peer reviews; the competence and continuing education of audit staff; and provisions for quality control to provide reasonable assurance of compliance with applicable auditing standards.

statistical conclusion validity The correctness of inferences regarding covariation between two or more variables. In program evaluation, statistical conclusion validity assesses inferences about the cause-and-effect relationship between program implementation and observed outcomes, as well as the strength of said relationship.

statistical interaction A situation in which the simultaneous influence of two variables on a third variable is not additive. In other words, an interaction involves the relationship among three or more variables.

statistical significance A number that expresses the probability that the result of a given experiment or study could have occurred purely by chance.

steering committee A committee that decides the priorities or order of business of an organization and manages the general course of its operations.

stratified random sampling A sampling method in which the population is separated into discrete, non-overlapping groups called strata, and a simple random sample is then chosen from each stratum.

structural equation modeling Statistical tests used to test a conceptual or theoretical model.

structured interview A formal interview that follows a strict series of questions designed to elicit specific answers from respondents.

summative evaluation Evaluation that helps consumers decide whether a product or service—refined through development and formative evaluation—is a better buy than other alternatives. In general terms, summative evaluation typically occurs following the development of a product, completion of a program, or end of a service cycle. The evaluator draws together and supplements previous information and provides an overall judgment of the evaluand's value.

summative metaevaluation The judgment of an evaluation's strengths, weaknesses, merit, and worth.

survey A series of questions that, when answered, provide a comprehensive view of a condition or situation.

sustainability The ability to continue a defined behavior indefinitely.

symmetry The degree to which the two sides of a dataset's distribution are equal to, or reflect, one another. This is measured through skewness.

system analysis A problem-solving technique that decomposes a system into its individual pieces to study how well the pieces work and interact to achieve their purpose.

systematic measurement error An inconsistency in an individual's score based on some characteristic of the person or the test that is unrelated to the construct being measured.

systematic sample A sampling technique in which every nth person in a population is selected.

t-test A statistical examination used to determine if there is a significant difference between the means of two groups.

test item analysis A process that examines student responses to individual questions in order to assess the quality of those items individually, as well as the test as a whole.

test–retest method A technique for measuring reliability, which involves administering the same test twice to the same group and then correlating the two sets of scores.

thematic analysis A process of pinpointing, examining, and recording patterns within data, which are important to the description of a phenomenon.

town hall meeting An informal public meeting, function, or event.

track record The past achievements or performance of a person, organization, or product.

transferability The degree to which the results of qualitative research can be generalized, or transferred, to other contexts or settings.

transportability The degree to which causal effects learned in experimental studies can be transferred to a new population.

traveling observer A preprogrammed investigator, working on site, who investigates and characterizes how staff members are carrying out a project. Subsequently, this observer reports findings to other evaluation team members and assists them in planning follow-up site visits.

traveling observer technique A procedure developed by the Evaluation Center at Western Michigan University that directly addresses process evaluation data requirements while also yielding information that is useful in context, input, and product evaluations.

Traveling Observer Handbook A collection of information that a traveling observer gathers. Information included in the handbook can include observer credentials, evaluation credentials, contact information, professional behavior protocols, data collection procedures, daily logs, self-assessments, and observer budget.

trend analysis A method of analysis that involves comparison of data over a series of time in order to identify patterns and predict future outcomes.

utility standards A set of evaluation standards stating that an evaluation should serve the information needs of its intended users.

utilization A form of eclectic evaluation developed by Michael Patton that is geared toward ensuring that evaluations have an impact. The utilization-focused evaluator guides the evaluation process in collaboration with an identified group of priority users, placing focus squarely on their intended uses of the evaluation.

validation The process of compiling and examining evidence to assess the precision and relevance of a data collection instrument, evaluation procedure, or complete set of evaluation findings for answering given evaluation questions. Validity resides not in any instrument, procedure, or completed evaluation report, but in its use in generating sound inferences and conclusions.

validity A property that refers to the appropriateness, correctness, meaningfulness, and usefulness of the inferences a researcher makes based on the data collected.

values Defensible guiding principles or ideals that should be used to determine an evaluand's standing. A value might be one out of a number of ideals held by a society, group, or individual. As the root term in evaluation, *value* is central to determining the criteria for use in judging programs or other entities.

values-based conclusions Evaluation conclusions based on a set of guiding principles or ideals held by a society, group, or individuals.

variable manipulating experiment A research design in which an independent variable is manipulated or changed in the hopes of finding a similar change in a dependent variable.

variance A measure of variability, which is the square of the standard deviation and measures how much the values in a dataset differ from the mean.

vision A mental image of what the future will or could be like.

visiting investigator A person from an outside organization who observes and assesses the effectiveness of a program.

webinar A seminar conducted over the Internet.

working poor Working people whose incomes fall below a given poverty line.

worth A program's combination of excellence, service, and cost-effectiveness in an area of clear need, within a specified context.

References

Aaronson, N. K., & Wilner, D. M. (1983). Evaluation and outcome research in community mental health centers. *Evaluation Review, 7,* 303–320.

Agresti, A., & Finlay, B. (1997). *Statistical methods for the social sciences* (3rd ed.). Upper Saddle River, NJ: Prentice-Hall.

Alegbeleye, B. (1984). The application of the CIPP Model to archival planning. *Archives and Manuscripts, 12*(2), 136–146.

Alkin, M. C. (2004). *Evaluation roots: Tracing theorists' views and influences.* Thousand Oaks, CA: Sage.

Alkin, M. C. (2013). *Evaluation roots: Tracing theorists' views and influences* (2nd ed.). Thousand Oaks, CA: Sage.

Al-Qubbaj, K. (2003). *The process of acculturation among Arabic children and their families in the United States: Some educational considerations* (Publication No. AAT 3115660). Unpublished doctoral dissertation, New Mexico State University, Las Cruces.

Altschuld, J., & Kumar, D. (2002). *Innovations in science education and technology. Evaluation of science and technology education at the dawn of the new millennium.* New York: Kluwer Academic/Plenum Press.

Alvarez Hernandez, J. (2003). Preliminary evaluation of the educational program for career and vocational development, "Making up my mind. . . ." *Electronic Journal of Research in Educational Psychology, 1*(2), 115–138.

Ameen, C. A. (1990). Use of the Joint Committee standards: Benefits gained and lessons learned. *American Journal of Evaluation, 11*(33), 33–38.

American Evaluation Association. (2004). Guiding principles for evaluators. Available at *www.eval.org/Publications/GuidingPrinciples.asp.*

Anderson, E., McCartney, E., Schreiber, J., & Thompson, E. (1989). Productivity measurement for clinical nurse specialist. *Clinical Nurse Specialist, 3*(2), 80–84.

Anthony, J. B. (2009). *Teacher retention: Program evaluation of a beginning teacher and mentor program* (Publication No. AAT 3354873). Unpublished doctoral dissertation. Gardner-Webb University, Bolling Springs, NC.

Armstrong, H. L., Murray, I. D., & Permvattana, R. R. (2006, July). *Evaluating Cisco e-learning courses modified for the vision impaired.* Paper presented at the Seventh International Conference on Information Technology Based Higher Education and Training, Sydney, NSW, Australia.

Arzoumanian, L. (1994). *Increasing community college child development associate (CDA) advisor skills in recording observations as a component of a competency-based assessment.* (ERIC Document Reproduction Service No. ED367506)

Asavatanabodee, P. (2010). The evaluation of primary care unit of Mahasarakham Hospital. *Journal of the Medical Association of Thailand, 93*(2), 239–244.

Ash, S., & Clayton, P. (2004). The articulated learning: An approach to guided reflection and assessment. *Innovative Higher Education, 29*(2), 137–154.

Baker-Boosmara, M., Guevara, J., & Balfour, D. (2006). From service to solidarity: Evaluation and recommendations for international service-learning. *Journal of Public Affairs Education, 12*(4), 479–500.

Bamberger, M., Rugh, J., & Mabry, L. (2012). *Real world*

evaluation: Working under budget, time, data, and political constraints (2nd ed.). Thousand Oaks, CA: Sage.

Banta, W. T. (1999). What's new in assessment? *Assessment Update, 11*(5), 3–11.

Barnette, J. (1977). The role of evaluation in organizational development. Evaluation in support of the Pennsylvania ABE Improvement Program. Retrieved from *http://jproxy.lib.ecu.edu/login?url=http://search.ebscohost.com/login.aspx?direct=true&db=eric&AN=ED152824&site=ehost-live.*

Becker, H. J. (1992). Computer-based integrated learning systems in the elementary and middle grades: A critical review and synthesis of evaluation reports. *Journal of Educational Computing Research, 8,* 1–41.

Beywl, W. (2000). Standards for evaluation: On the way to guiding principles in German evaluation. In C. Russon (Ed.), *The program evaluation standards in international settings* (pp. 60–67). Kalamazoo: Western Michigan University, The Evaluation Center.

Bickman, L., & Rog, D. J. (2009). *Handbook of applied social research methods* (2nd ed.). Thousand Oaks, CA: Sage.

Birks, M., Chapman, Y., & Francis, K. (2008). Memoing in qualitative research: Probing data and processes. *Journal of Research in Nursing, 13*(1), 68–75.

Bogdan, R., & Biklen, S. K. (1992). *Qualitative research for education: An introduction to theory and methods.* Boston: Allyn & Bacon.

Boonprakob, M. (1994). *The development of a curriculum model for teaching science in secondary schools in Thailand* (Publication No. AAT 9510421). Unpublished doctoral dissertation, Illinois State University, Normal, IL.

Bordelon, T. (2006). A qualitative approach to developing an instrument for assessing MSW students' group work performance. *Social Work with Groups, 29*(4), 75–91.

Borenstein, M., Hedges, L. V., Higgins, J. P. T., & Rothstein, H. R. (2009). *Introduction to meta-analysis.* West Sussex, UK: Wiley.

Borges, N., & Hartung, P. (2007). Service-learning in medical education: Project description and evaluation. *International Journal of Teaching and Learning in Higher Education, 19*(1), 1–7.

Brennan, R. L. (2001). *Generalizability theory.* New York: Springer-Verlag.

Bringle, R., & Kremer, J. (1993). Evaluation of an intergenerational service-learning project for undergraduates. *Educational Gerontology, 19*(5), 407–416.

Brinkerhoff, R. O. (2003). *The success case method: Find out quickly what's working and what's not.* San Francisco: Berrett-Koehler.

Burke, C. (1980). The reading interview. In B. P. Farr & D. J. Strickler (Eds.), *Reading comprehension: Resource guide* (pp. 82–108). Bloomington: School of Education, Indiana University.

Butin, D. (2003). Of what use is it?: Multiple conceptualizations of service-learning within education. *Teachers College Record, 105*(9), 1674–1692.

Butler-Kisber, L. (2010). *Qualitative inquiry: Thematic, narrative and arts-informed perspectives.* London: Sage.

Campbell, D. T., & Stanley, J. C. (1963). Experimental and quasi-experimental designs for research on teaching. In N. L. Gage (Ed.), *Handbook of research on teaching* (pp. 171–246). Chicago: Rand McNally.

Candoli, I. C., Cullen, K., & Stufflebeam, D. L. (1997). *Superintendent performance evaluation: Current practice and directions for improvement.* Norwell, MA: Kluwer.

Chenail, R. (2010). Getting specific about qualitative research generalizability. *Journal of Ethnographic and Qualitative Research, 5,* 1–11.

Chien, M., Lee, C., & Cheng, Y. (2007). The construction of Taiwan's educational indicator systems: Experiences and implications. *Educational Research for Policy and Practice, 6*(3), 249–259.

Clandinin, D. J., & Connelly, R. M. (2000). *Narrative inquiry: Experience and story in qualitative research.* San Francisco: Jossey-Bass.

Clary, E. G., Snyder, M., Ridge, R. D., Copeland, J., Stukas, A. A., Haugen, J., et al. (1998). Understanding and assessing the motivation of volunteers: A functional approach. *Journal of Personality and Social Psychology, 74,* 1516–1530.

Clay, M. M. (1993). *An observation survey of early literacy achievement.* Portsmouth, NH: Heinemann.

Cohen, J. W. (1988). *Statistical power analysis for the behavioral sciences* (2nd ed.). Hillsdale, NJ: Erlbaum.

Combs, K. L., Gibson, S. K., Hays, J. M., Saly, J., & Wendt, J. T. (2008). Enhancing curriculum and delivery: Linking assessment to learning objectives. *Assessment and Evaluation in Higher Education, 33*(1), 87–102.

Consuelo Zobel Alger Foundation. (1999). *1999 annual report: A decade of vision and hope.* Honolulu, HI: Author.

Cook, D. L., & Stufflebeam, D. L. (1967). Estimating test norms from variable size item and examinee samples. *Educational and Psychological Measurement, 27,* 601–610.

Cook, T. D., & Campbell, D. T. (1979). *Quasi-experimentation: Design and analysis issues for field settings.* Chicago: Rand McNally.

Corbin, J. M., & Strauss, A. (2007). *Basics of qualitative research: Techniques and procedures for developing grounded theory* (3rd ed.). Thousand Oaks, CA: Sage.

Creswell, J. W. (2013). *Qualitative inquiry and research design: Choosing among five approaches* (3rd ed.). Thousand Oaks, CA: Sage.

Creswell, J. W. (2014). *Research design: Qualitative, quantitative, and mixed methods approaches* (4th ed.). Thousand Oaks, CA: Sage.

Crocker, L., & Algina, J. (2008). *Introduction to classical and modern test theory.* Mason, OH: Cengage Learning.

Cronbach, L. J. (1963). Course improvement through evaluation. *Teachers College Record, 64,* 672–683.

Cronbach, L. J., Gleser, G. C., Nanda, H., & Rajaratnam, N. (1972). *The dependability of behavioral measures.* Hoboken, NJ: Wiley.

Davey, J. W., Gugiu, P. C., & Coryn, C. L. S. (2010). Quantitative methods for estimating the reliability of qualitative data. *Journal of MultiDisciplinary Evaluation, 6*(13), 140–162.

Davidson, E. J. (2005). *Evaluation methodology basics: The nuts and bolts of sound evaluation.* Thousand Oaks, CA: Sage.

Davis, K., Hodson, P., Zhang, G., Boswell, B., & Decker, J. (2010). Providing physical activity for students with intellectual disabilities: The motivate, adapt, and play (MAP) program. *Journal of Physical Education, Recreation and Dance, 81*(5), 23–28.

Davis, K., Zhang, G., & Hodson, P. (2011). Promoting health-related fitness for elementary students with intellectual disabilities through a specifically designed activity program. *Journal of Policy and Practice in Intellectual Disabilities, 8*(2), 77–84.

Davis, K., Zhang, G., Hodson, P., Boswell, B. B., & Decker, J. T. (2010). A close look at the fitness level of elementary students with intellectual disabilities. *Sport Science Review, 19*(3–4), 77–92.

de Ayala, R. J. (2009). *The theory and practice of item response theory.* New York: Guilford Press.

Denzin, N. K., & Lincoln, Y. S. (Eds.). (2011) *The Sage handbook of qualitative research* (4th ed.). Thousand Oaks, CA: Sage.

Dillman, D. A., Smyth, J. D., & Christian, L. M. (2009). *Internet, mail, and mixed-mode surveys: The tailored design method* (3rd ed.). Hoboken, NJ: Wiley.

Driscoll, A., Gelmon, S., Holland, B., Kerrigan, S., Spring, A., Grosvold, K., et al. (1998). *Assessing the impact of service learning: A workbook of strategies and methods* (2nd ed.). (ERIC Document Reproduction Service No. ED432949)

Driscoll, A., Holland, B., Gelmon, S., & Kerrigan, S. (1996). An assessment model for service-learning: Comprehensive case studies of impact on faculty, students, community, and institution. *Michigan Journal of Community Service Learning, 3,* 66–71.

Edmonds, W. A., & Kennedy, T. D. (2013). *An applied reference guide to research designs: Quantitative, qualitative, and mixed methods.* Thousand Oaks, CA: Sage.

Eisner, E. W. (1983). Educational connoisseurship and criticism: Their form and functions in educational evaluation. In G. F. Madaus, M. Scriven, & D. L. Stufflebeam (Eds.), *Evaluation models: Viewpoints on educational and human services evaluation* (pp. 335–348). Norwell, MA: Kluwer.

Embretson, S. E., & Reise, S. P. (2000). *Item response theory for psychologists.* Mahwah, NJ: Erlbaum.

Evaluation. (n.d.). Online etymology dictionary. Retrieved January 15, 2011, from *http://dictionary.reference.com/browse/evaluation.*

Evers, J. (1980). *A field study of goal-based and goal-free evaluation techniques.* Unpublished doctoral dissertation, Western Michigan University, Kalamazoo, MI.

Eyler, J., & Giles, D. E. (1999). *Where's the learning in service-learning?* San Francisco: Jossey-Bass.

Farley, D. O., & Battles, J. B. (2009). Evaluation of the AHRQ Patient Safety Initiative: Framework and approach. *Health Services Research, 44*(2, Pt. 2), 628–645.

Felix, J. L. (1979). Research and evaluation to improve instruction: The Cincinnati strategy. *Educational Evaluation and Policy Analysis, 1*(2), 57–62.

Felten, P., Gilchrist, L. Z., & Darby, A. (2006). Emotion and learning: Feeling our way toward a new theory of reflection in service-learning. *Michigan Journal of Community Service-Learning, 12*(2), 38–46.

Fernandea-Ramirez, B., & Rebolloso, E. (2006). Evaluation in Spain: Concepts, contexts, and networks. *Journal of MultiDisciplinary Evaluation, 5,* 134–152.

Fetterman, D. M. (1998). *Ethnography: Step-by-step* (2nd ed.). Thousand Oaks, CA: Sage.

Fetterman, D. M. (2010). *Ethnography: Step-by-step* (3rd ed.). Thousand Oaks, CA: Sage.

Fielding, N. G., & Lee, R. M. (1998). *Using computers in qualitative research.* Thousand Oaks, CA: Sage.

Filella-Guiu, G., & Blanch-Plana, A. (2002). Imprisonment and career development: An evaluation of a guidance programme for job finding. *Journal of Career Development, 29*(1), 55–68.

Finn, C. E., Stevens, F. I., Stufflebeam, D. L., & Walberg, H. J. (1997). A meta-evaluation. *International Journal of Educational Research, 27*(2), 159–174.

Fitzpatrick, J. L., Sanders, J. R., & Worthen, B. R. (2011). *Program evaluation: Alternative approaches and practical guidelines* (4th ed.). Upper Saddle River, NJ: Pearson.

Fonteyn, M., Vettese, M., Lancaster, D., & Bauer-Wu, S. (2008). Developing a codebook to guide content analysis of expressive writing transcripts. *Applied Nursing Research, 21,* 165–168.

Fraenkel, J. R., & Wallen, N. E. (2011). *How to design and evaluate research in education* (8th ed.). New York: McGraw-Hill.

Fraenkel, J. R., Wallen, N. E., & Hyun, H. H. (2015). *How to design and evaluate research in education* (9th ed.). New York: McGraw-Hill.

Freund, J. E., & Simon, G. A. (1997). *Modern elementary statistics* (9th ed.). Upper Saddle River, NJ: Prentice-Hall.

Gally, J. (1984). *The evaluation component.* Paper presented at the annual conference of the American Educational Research Association, New Orleans, LA.

Galvin, J. (1983a). *Evaluating management education: Models and attitudes of training specialists.* Unpublished doctoral dissertation, Northern Illinois University, DeKalb, IL.

Galvin, J. C. (1983b). What can trainers learn from educators about evaluating management training? *Training and Development Journal, 37*(8), 52–57.

Gavidia-Payne, S., Littlefield, L., Hallgren, M., Jenkins, P., & Coventry, N. (2003). Outcome evaluation of a statewide child inpatient mental health unit. *Australian and New Zealand Journal of Psychiatry, 37*(2), 204–211.

Gelmon, S. B. (2000a, Fall). Challenges in assessing service-learning. *Michigan Journal of Community Service-Learning, Special Issue,* pp. 84–90.

Gelmon, S. (2000b). How do we know that our work makes a difference? Assessment strategies for service-learning and civic engagement. *Metropolitan Universities: An International Forum, 11*(2), 28–39.

George, T. R. (2000). *Solar water systems benefit the working poor in three different ways: A case study of Consuelo Foundation's self-help housing initiative in Waianae, Oahu.* Paper presented at the Energy Efficiency Policy Symposium, Honolulu, HI. Retrieved from *www.hawaii. gov/dbedt/ert/symposium/george.pdf.*

Glass, G. V., Wilson, V. L., & Gottman, J. M. (2008). *Design and analysis of time-series experiments.* Charlotte, NC: Information Age.

Golafshani, N. (2003). Understanding reliability and validity in qualitative research. *The Qualitative Report, 8*(4), 597–607.

Granger, A., Grierson, J., Quirino, T. R., & Romano, L. (1965). *Training in planning, monitoring, and evaluation for agricultural research management: Manual 4—Evaluation.* The Hague, The Netherlands: International Service for National Agricultural Research.

Griffith, R., Zeller, N., & Zhang, G. (2010). Connecting, listening, and learning to teach. *Community Works Journal.* Retrieved from *http://communityworksjournal.org.*

Griffith, R., & Zhang, G. (2013). Service learning in teacher preparation: Returns on the investment. *The Educational Forum, 77*(3), 256–276.

Griffith, R., Zhang, G., Metcalf, D., & Heilmann, J. (2008, December). *Reaching out to RTI students: Service learning projects in undergraduate methods courses.* Paper presented at the 2008 National Reading Conference, Orlando, FL.

Grissom, R. J., & Kim, J. J. (2005). *Effect sizes for research: A broad practical approach.* Mahwah, NJ: Erlbaum.

Guba, E. G. (1966, October). *A study of Title III Activities; report on evaluation* [Mimeo]. Bloomington: National Institute for the Study of Educational Change, Indiana University.

Guba, E. G. (1978). *Toward a methodology of naturalistic inquiry in educational evaluation.* Los Angeles: University of California, Center for the Study of Evaluation.

Guba, E. G., & Stufflebeam, D. L. (1968). Evaluation: The process of stimulating, aiding, and abetting insightful action. In R. Ingle & W. Gephart (Eds.), *Problems in the training of educational researchers.* Bloomington, IN: Phi Delta Kappa.

Guilford, J. P. (1936). *Psychometric methods.* New York: McGraw-Hill.

Gullickson, A., & Stufflebeam, D. (2001). *Feedback Workshop Checklist.* Kalamazoo: Western Michigan University, The Evaluation Center. Available at *www.wmich.edu/ evalctr/checklists.*

Hamm, D., Dowell, D., & Houck, J. (1998). Service learning as a strategy to prepare teacher candidates for contemporary diverse classrooms. *Higher Education, 112*(2), 196–204.

Hammond, R. L. (1972). *Evaluation at the local level.* Tucson, AZ: EPIC Evaluation Center.

Hancock, G. R., & Mueller, R. O. (2010). *The reviewer's guide to quantitative methods in the social sciences.* New York: Routledge.

Harrison, A. (1993). *An evaluation model for middle school counseling and guidance.* Unpublished doctoral dissertation, Old Dominion University, Norfolk, VA.

Harvey, L. (2005). A history and critique of quality evaluation in the UK. *Quality Assurance in Education, 13*(4), 263–276.

Heuston, D. H. (1997). Response to the evaluation and meta-evaluation. In H. L. Miller (Ed.), The New York City public schools integrated learning systems project: Evaluation and meta-evaluation [Special issue]. *International Journal of Educational Research, 27*(2), 175–181.

Holland, B. (2001). A comprehensive model for assessing service-learning and community-university partnerships. *New Directions for Higher Education, 114,* 51–60.

Hopkins, K. D., & Glass, G. V. (1978). *Basic statistics for the behavioral sciences.* Upper Saddle River, NJ: Prentice Hall.

Hosmer, D. W., & Lemeshow, S. (2000). *Applied logistic regression* (2nd ed.). New York: Wiley.

House, E. R., & Howe, K. R. (2000). Deliberative democratic evaluation. In K. E. Ryan & L. DeStefano (Eds.), *Evaluation as a democratic process: Promoting inclusion, dialogue, and deliberation* (New Directions for Evaluation, No. 85, pp. 3–12). San Francisco: Jossey-Bass.

House, E. R., Rivers, W., & Stufflebeam, D. L. (1974). A counter-response to Kearney, Donovan, and Fisher. *Phi Delta Kappan, 56,* 19.

Hui-Fang, S. (1997). A comparative analysis of alternative evaluation approaches. *Journal of Education and Psychology, 20*(2), 203–216.

Inouye, D. K., Miller, H. L., Jr., & Fletcher, J. D. (1997). The evaluation of system cost and replicability. In H. L. Miller (Ed.), The New York City public schools integrated learning systems project: Evaluation and meta-evaluation [Special issue]. *International Journal of Educational Research, 27*(2), 137–138.

Jaeger, R. M. (1990). *Statistics: A spectator sport* (2nd ed.). Thousand Oaks, CA: Sage.

Jang, S. (2000). The appropriateness of Joint Committee standards in non-Western settings: A case study of South Korea. In C. Russon (Ed.), *The program evaluation standards in international settings* (pp. 41–59). Kalamazoo: Western Michigan University, The Evaluation Center.

Johnson, R. B., & Christensen, L. B. (2000). *Educational research: Quantitative and qualitative approaches.* Boston: Allyn & Bacon.

Joint Committee on Standards for Educational Evaluation. (1981). *Standards for evaluations of educational programs, projects, and materials.* New York: McGraw-Hill.

Joint Committee on Standards for Educational Evaluation. (1994). *The program evaluation standards: How to assess evaluations of educational programs* (2nd ed.). Thousand Oaks, CA: Sage.

Joint Committee on Standards for Educational Evaluation. (2011). *The program evaluation standards: A guide for evaluators and evaluation users* (3rd ed.). Thousand Oaks, CA: Sage.

Karayan, S., & Gathercoal, P. (2005). Assessing service-learning in teacher education. *Teacher Education Quarterly, 32*(3), 79–92.

Kezar, A. (2002). Assessing community service-learning. *About Campus, 7*(2), 14–20.

Kishchuk, N., O'Loughlin, J., Paradis, S., Masson, P., & Sacks-Silver, G. (2009). Illuminating negative results in evaluation of smoking prevention programs. *Journal of School Health, 60*(9), 448–451.

Kline, R. B. (2008). *Becoming a behavioral science researcher: A guide to producing research that matters.* New York: Guilford Press.

Koliba, C. J., Campbell, E. K., & Shapiro, C. (2006). The practice of service-learning in local school-community contexts. *Educational Policy, 20*(5), 683–717.

Kraft, R., & Krug, J. (1994). *Building community: Service-learning in the academic disciplines.* Denver: Colorado Campus Compact.

Krueger, R., & Casey, M. (2009). *Focus groups: A practical guide for applied research* (4th ed.). Los Angeles: Sage.

LaCompte, M. D., & Goetz, J. P. (1982). Problems of reliability and validity in ethnographic research. *Review of Educational Research, 52*, 31–60.

Leninger, M. (Ed.). (1985). *Qualitative research methods in nursing.* Orlando, FL: Grune & Stratton.

Leslie, L., & Caldwell, J. (2006). *Qualitative Reading Inventory–4.* Boston: Pearson.

Lincoln, Y. S., & Guba, E. G. (1985). *Naturalistic inquiry.* Beverly Hills, CA: Sage.

Mabry, J. B. (1998). Pedagogical variations in service-learning and student outcomes: How time, contact, and refection matter. *Michigan Journal of Community Service Learning, 5*, 32–47.

Madaus, G. F., & Stufflebeam, D. L. (1989). *Educational evaluation: Classic works of Ralph W. Tyler.* Boston: Kluwer Academic.

Mann, H. B., & Whitney, D. R. (1947). On a test of whether one of two random variables is stochastically larger than the other. *Annals of Mathematical Statistics, 18*(1), 50–60.

Marchel, C. (2004). Evaluating reflection and sociocultural awareness in service learning classes. *Teaching of Psychology, 31*(2), 120–123.

Margolis, E., & Pauwels, L. (Eds.). (2011). *The Sage handbook of visual research methods.* Thousand Oaks, CA: Sage.

Matthews, J. M., & Hudson, A. M. (2001). Guidelines for evaluating parent training programs. *Family Relations, 50*(1), 77–86.

Meredith, M. D., & Welk, G. J. (2010). *FITNESSGRAM & ACTIVITYGRAM Test Administration Manual.* Champaign, IL: Human Kinetics.

McKenna, M. C., & Kear, D. J. (1990). Measuring attitude toward reading: A new tool for teachers. *The Reading Teacher, 43*(8), 626–639.

Miles, M. B., & Huberman, A. M. (1984). *Qualitative data analysis: An expanded sourcebook* (2nd ed.). Thousand Oaks, CA: Sage.

Miller, H. L. (Ed.). (1997). The New York City public schools integrated learning systems project: Evaluation and meta-evaluation [Special issue]. *International Journal of Educational Research, 27*(2).

Moore, D. T. (1999). Behind the wizard's curtain: A challenge to the true believer. *National Society for Experiential Education Quarterly, 25*(1), 23–27.

Morris, M. (2003). Ethical considerations in evaluation. In T. Kellaghan & D. L. Stufflebeam (Eds.), *International handbook of education evaluation* (pp. 303–328). Norwell, MA: Kluwer.

Morse, J. M. (1991). Approaches to qualitative-quantitative methodological triangulation. *Nursing Research, 40*, 120–123.

Moustakas, C. (1994). *Phenomenological research methods.* Thousand Oaks, CA: Sage.

Myers, J. L., & Well, A. D. (2003). *Research design and statistical analysis* (2nd ed.). Mahwah, NJ: Erlbaum.

National Youth Leadership Council. (2008). K–12 service-learning standards for quality practice. Retrieved April 30, 2010, from *www.nylc.org/pages-resourcecenter-downloads-K_12_Service_Learning_Standards_for_Quality_Practice?emoid=14:803.*

Nevo, D. (1974). *Evaluation priorities of students, teachers, and principals.* Unpublished doctoral dissertation, The Ohio State University, Columbus, OH.

Nicholson, T. (1989). Using the CIPP Model to evaluate reading instruction. *Journal of Reading, 32*(40), 312–318.

Nyandindi, U. S. (1995). *Evaluation of a school oral health programme in Tanzania: An ecological perspective* (Publication No. AAT C489393). Unpublished doctoral dissertation, University of Jyväskylä, Jyväskylä, Finland.

Osokoya, M., & Adekunle, A. (2007). Evaluating the trainability of enrollees of the Leventis Foundation (Nigeria) agricultural schools' programs. *Australian Journal of Adult Learning, 47*(1), 111–135.

Othanganont, P. (2001). Evaluation of the Thai–Lao collaborating nursing manpower development project using the Context Input Process Product Model. *Nursing and Health Sciences, 3*(2), 63–68.

Owens, T. R., & Stufflebeam, D. L. (1964). An experimental comparison of item sampling and examinee sampling for estimating test norms. *Journal of Educational Measurement, 6*(2), 75–83.

Padilla, M., & Zhang, G. (2011). Estimating internal consistency using Bayesian methods. *Journal of Modern Applied Statistical Methods, 10*(1), 277–286.

Pallant, J. (2010). *SPSS Survival Manual: A step by step guide to data analysis using the SPSS program.* Berkshire, UK: Open University Press.

Parfitt, B., & Cornish, F. (2007). Implementing family health nursing in Tajikistan: From policy to practice in primary health care reform. *Social Science and Medicine, 65*(8), 1720–1729.

Patton, M. Q. (2002). *Qualitative evaluation and research methods* (3rd ed.). Thousand Oaks, CA: Sage.

Patton, M. Q. (2008). *Utilization-focused evaluation* (4th ed.). Thousand Oaks, CA: Sage.

Peng, H. (1995). *Design and evaluation of an inservice model for vocational high school automotive electronic technology teachers in Taiwan* (Publication No. AAT 9543496). Unpublished doctoral dissertation, Florida International University, Miami, FL.

Peterson, T. (2004). Assessing performance in problem-based service-learning projects. *New Directions for Teaching and Learning, 100,* 55–63.

Poliandri, D., Cardone, M., Muzzioli, P., & Romiti, S. (2010). Dynamic database for quality indicators comparison in education [Working paper]. Retrieved from *www.eric.ed.gov/PDFS/ED510974.pdf.*

Pritchard, I. (2002). Community service and service-learning in America: The state of the art. In A. Furco & S. H. Billig (Eds.), *Service-learning: The essence of the pedagogy* (pp. 3–19). Stamford, CT: Information Age.

Provus, M. N. (1969). *Discrepancy evaluation model.* Pittsburgh, PA: Pittsburgh Public Schools.

Quincey, R. D. (1987). Probation workload activities management system (PWAMS): An alternative approach in judicial systems (Publication No. AAT 8727282). Unpublished doctoral dissertation, University of La Verne, La Verne, CA.

Raudenbush, S. W., & Bryk, A. S. (2002). *Hierarchical linear models: Applications and data analysis methods* (2nd ed.). Thousand Oaks, CA: Sage.

Reeb, R. N., Katsuyama, R. M., Sammon, J. A., & Yoder, D. S. (1998). The community service self-efficacy scale: Evidence of reliability construct validity, and pragmatic utility. *Michigan Journal of Community Service Learning, 5,* 48–57.

Reinhard, D. (1972). *Methodology development for input evaluation using advocate and design teams.* Unpublished doctoral dissertation, The Ohio State University, Columbus, OH.

Rosenberg, M. (1965). *Society and the adolescent self-image.* Princeton, NJ: Princeton University Press.

Rossi, P. H., Lipsey, M. W., & Freeman, H. E. (2004). *Evaluation: A systematic approach* (7th ed.). Thousand Oaks, CA: Sage.

Rossman, G. B., & Rallis, S. F. (1998). *Learning in the field: An introduction to qualitative research.* Thousand Oaks, CA: Sage.

Sanders, J. R., & Stufflebeam, D. L. (1978, January–February). *School without schools: Columbus, Ohio's educational response to the energy crisis of 1977* (Case studies in science education, Booklet VIII). Champaign, IL: CIRCE.

Saripudin, D. (2010). Resocialization program evaluation of street children. *International Journal for Educational Studies, 2*(2), 185–196.

Scriven, M. S. (1967). The methodology of evaluation. In *Perspectives of curriculum evaluation.* Skokie, IL: Rand McNally.

Scriven, M. (1969). An introduction to meta-evaluation. *Educational Products Report, 2*(5), 36–38.

Scriven, M. S. (1973). Goal-free evaluation. In E. R. House (Ed.), *School evaluation: The politics and process* (pp. 319–328). Berkeley, CA: McCutchan.

Scriven, M. (1994). Product evaluation: The state of the art. *Evaluation Practice, 15,* 45–62.

Scriven, M. S. (2007). *Key Evaluation Checklist (KEC).* Kalamazoo: Western Michigan University, The Evaluation Center. Retrieved from *www.wmich.edu/evalctr/archive_checklists/kec_feb07.pdf.*

Shadish, W. R. (2010). Campbell and Rubin: A primer and comparison of their approaches to causal inference in field settings. *Psychological Methods, 15,* 3–17.

Shaffer, J. P. (1980). Control of directional errors with stagewise multiple test procedures. *Annuals of Statistics, 8,* 1342–1347.

Shams, B., Golshiri, P., Zamani, A. R., & Pourabdian, S. (2008). Mothers' participation in improving growth and nutrition of the children: A model for community participation. *Iranian Journal of Public Health, 37*(2), 24–31.

Sheskin, D. J. (2007). *Handbook of parametric and nonparametric statistical procedures* (4th ed.). Boca Raton, FL: Chapman & Hall/CRC.

Shinkfield, A. J., & Stufflebeam, D. L. (1995). *Teacher evaluation: Guide to effective practice.* Boston: Kluwer.

Sims, M., & Bridgman, G. (2006). Evaluation of progress using the context input and product model. *Child: Care, Health and Development, 10*(6), 359–379.

Singh, M. (2004). Evaluation framework for nursing education. *International Journal of Nursing, 1*(1), 1–16.

Smith, E. R., & Tyler, R. W. (1942). *Appraising and recording student progress.* New York: Harper.

Smith, N. L., Chircop, S., & Mukherjee, P. (2000). Considerations on the development of culturally relevant evaluation standards. In C. Russon (Ed.), *The program evaluation standards in international settings* (pp. 29–40). Kalamazoo: Western Michigan University, The Evaluation Center.

Staggers, N. (1989). Electronic mail basics. *Journal of Nursing Administration, 19*(10), 31–35.

Stake, R. E. (1967). The countenance of educational evaluation. *Teachers College Record, 68,* 523–540.

Stake, R. E. (1976). A theoretical statement of responsive evaluation. *Studies in Educational Evaluation, 2,* 19–22.

Stake, R. (1983). Program evaluation, particularly responsive evaluation. In G. Madaus, M. Scriven, & D. Stufflebeam (Eds.), *Evaluation models* (pp. 287–310). Boston: Kluwer-Nijhoff.

Stake, R. E. (1995). *The art of case study research.* Thousand Oaks, CA: Sage.

Steinert, Y., Cruess, S., Cruess, R., & Snell, L. (2005). Faculty development for teaching and evaluating professionalism: From program design to curriculum change. *Medical Education, 39*(2), 127–136.

Steinke, P., & Buresh, S. (2002). Cognitive outcomes of service-learning: Reviewing the past and glimpsing the future. *Michigan Journal of Community Service Learning, 8*(2), 5–14.

Straus, A. (1987). *Qualitative analysis for social scientists.* Cambridge, UK: Cambridge University Press.

Stufflebeam, D. L. (1966a). A depth study of the evaluation requirement. *Theory into Practice, 5*(3), 121–133.

Stufflebeam, D. L. (1966b, January). *Evaluation under Title I of the Elementary and Secondary Education Act of 1967.* Address delivered at the Title I Evaluation Conference sponsored by the Michigan State Department of Education, Lansing, MI.

Stufflebeam, D. L. (1967a). *Applying PERT to a test development project.* Paper presented at the annual conference of the American Educational Research Association, Chicago, IL.

Stufflebeam, D. L. (1967b). The use and abuse of evaluation in Title III. *Theory into Practice, 6,* 126–133.

Stufflebeam, D. L. (1968, January). *Evaluation as enlightenment for decision-making.* Paper presented at the Association for Supervision and Curriculum Development Conference on Assessment Theory, Sarasota, FL.

Stufflebeam, D. L. (1969). Evaluation as enlightenment for decision making. In A. Walcott (Ed.), *Improving educational assessment and an inventory of measures of affective behavior* (pp. 41–73). Washington, DC: Association for Supervision and Curriculum Development.

Stufflebeam, D. L. (1971a). The relevance of the CIPP evaluation model for educational accountability. *Journal of Research and Development in Education, 5*(1), 19–25.

Stufflebeam, D. L. (1971b). The use of experimental design in educational evaluation. *Journal of Educational Measurement, 8*(4), 267–274.

Stufflebeam, D. L. (1974). *Meta-evaluation* (Occasional Paper Series No. 3). Kalamazoo: Western Michigan University, The Evaluation Center.

Stufflebeam, D. L. (1978). Metaevaluation: An overview. *Evaluation and the Health Professions, 1*(2), 146–163.

Stufflebeam, D. L. (1982). Institutional self-evaluation. In *International encyclopedia of educational research.* Oxford, UK: Pergamon.

Stufflebeam, D. L. (1983). The CIPP Model for program evaluation. In G. F. Madaus, M. Scriven, & D. L. Stufflebeam (Eds.), *Evaluation models: Viewpoints on educational and human services evaluation* (pp. 117–141). Norwell, MA: Kluwer.

Stufflebeam, D. L. (1985). Stufflebeam's improvement-oriented evaluation. In D. L. Stufflebeam & A. J. Shinkfield, *Systematic evaluation* (pp. 151–207). Norwell, MA: Kluwer.

Stufflebeam, D. L. (1997). *Strategies for institutionalizing evaluation: Revisited* (Occasional Paper Series No. 18). Kalamazoo: Western Michigan University, The Evaluation Center.

Stufflebeam, D. L. (2000a). The CIPP Model for evaluation. In D. L. Stufflebeam, G. F. Madaus, & T. Kellaghan (Eds.), *Evaluation models* (2nd ed., pp. 279–317). Boston: Kluwer Academic.

Stufflebeam, D. L. (2000b). Lessons in contracting for evaluations. *American Journal of Evaluation, 22*(1), 71–79.

Stufflebeam, D. L. (2000c). The methodology of metaevaluation. In D. L. Stufflebeam, G. F. Madaus, & T. Kellaghan (Eds.), *Evaluation models: Viewpoints on educational and human services evaluation* (2nd ed., pp. 457–496). Norwell, MA: Kluwer.

Stufflebeam, D. L. (2001). The metaevaluation imperative. *American Journal of Evaluation, 22*(2), 183–209.

Stufflebeam, D. L. (2002). CIPP Evaluation Model Checklist. Available at *www.wmich.edu/evalctr/checklists.*

Stufflebeam, D. L. (2003a). The CIPP Model for evaluation. In T. Kellaghan & D. L. Stufflebeam (Eds.), *The international handbook of educational evaluation* (pp. 31–62). Boston: Kluwer.

Stufflebeam, D. L. (2003b). Institutionalizing evaluation in schools. In T. Kellaghan & D. L. Stufflebeam (Eds.), *The international handbook of educational evaluation* (pp. 775–806). Boston: Kluwer.

Stufflebeam, D. L. (2004). The 21st-century CIPP Model: Origins, development, and use. In M. C. Alkin (Ed.), *Evaluation roots* (pp. 245–266). Thousand Oaks, CA: Sage.

Stufflebeam, D. L. (2005). CIPP Model (context, input, process, product). In S. Mathison (Ed.), *Encyclopedia of evaluation* (pp. 61–66). Thousand Oaks, CA: Sage.

Stufflebeam, D. L. (2013). The 21st-century CIPP Model: Origins, development, and use. In M. C. Alkin (Ed.), *Evaluation roots* (2nd ed., pp. 243–260). Thousand Oaks, CA: Sage.

Stufflebeam, D. L. (2014). Daniel Stufflebeam's CIPP Model for evaluation: An improvement and accountability-oriented approach. In D. L. Stufflebeam, & C. L. S. Coryn (Eds.), *Evaluation theory, models, and applications* (2nd ed., pp. 309–340). San Francisco: Jossey-Bass.

Stufflebeam, D. L. (2015). Program Evaluations Metaevaluation Checklist. Available at *www.wmich.edu/evaluation/checklists.* (Also available on The Guilford Press website; see the box at the end of the table of contents.)

Stufflebeam, D. L., & Coryn, C. L. S. (2014). *Evaluation*

theory, models, and applications. San Francisco: Jossey-Bass.

Stufflebeam, D. L., Foley, W. J., Gephart, W. J., Guba, E. G., Hammond, R. L., Merriman, H. O., et al. (1971). *Educational evaluation and decision making.* Itasca, IL: Peacock.

Stufflebeam, D. L., Gullickson, A., & Wingate, L. (2002). *The spirit of Consuelo: An evaluation of Ke Aka Ho'ona.* Kalamazoo: Western Michigan University, The Evaluation Center.

Stufflebeam, D. L., Jaeger, R. M., & Scriven, M. S. (1992, April). *A retrospective analysis of a summative evaluation of NAGB's pilot project to set achievement levels on the National Assessment of Educational Progress.* Paper presented at the annual conference of the American Educational Research Association, San Francisco, CA.

Stufflebeam, D. L., & Shinkfield, A. J. (1985). *Systematic evaluation: A self-instructional guide to theory and practice.* Norwell, MA: Kluwer.

Stufflebeam, D. L., & Shinkfield, A. J. (2007). *Evaluation theory, models, and applications.* San Francisco: Jossey-Bass.

Stufflebeam, D. L., & Webster, W. J. (1988). Evaluation as an administrative function. In N. Boyan (Ed.), *Handbook of research on educational administration* (pp. 569–601). White Plains, NY: Longman.

Taut, S. (2000). Cross-cultural transferability of the program evaluation standards. In C. Russon (Ed.), *The program evaluation standards in international settings* (pp. 5–28). Kalamazoo: Western Michigan University, The Evaluation Center.

Tesch, R. (1990). *Qualitative research: Analysis types and software tools.* New York: Falmer.

Thomas, G. (2011). A typology for the case study in social science following a review of definition, discourse and structure. *Qualitative Inquiry 17*(6), 511–521.

Troppe, M. (Ed.). (1995). Foreword. In M. Troppe (Ed.), *Connecting cognition and action: Evaluation of student performance in service-learning courses.* Providence, RI: Campus Compact.

Tyler, R. W. (1932). *Service studies in higher education.* Columbus: Bureau of Educational Research and Services, Ohio State University.

Tyler, R. W. (1942). General statement on evaluation. *Journal of Educational Research, 36,* 492–501.

U.S. Government Accountability Office. (2007). *Government auditing standards* (GAO-07-731G). Washington, DC: U.S. Government Printing Office.

Valentine, K. (1991). Comprehensive assessment of caring and its relationship to outcome measures. *Journal of Nursing Care Quality, 5*(2), 59–68.

Wang, Y., & Zhi, X. (2009). An evaluation system for the online training programs in meteorology and hydrology. *International Educational Studies, 2*(4), 45–48.

Webster, W. J. (1975, March). *The organization and functions of research and evaluation in large urban school districts.* Paper presented at the annual conference of the American Educational Research Association, Washington, DC.

Webster, W. J., & Eichelberger, T. (1972). A use of the regression model in educational evaluation. *Journal of Experimental Education, 40*(3), 91–96.

Widmer, T., Landert, C., & Bacmann, N. (2000). Evaluation standards recommended by the Swiss Evaluation Society (SEVAL). In C. Russon (Ed.), *The program evaluation standards in international settings* (pp. 81–102). Kalamazoo: Western Michigan University, The Evaluation Center.

Wiersma, W., & Jurs, S. G. (2005). *Research methods in education: An introduction* (8th ed.). Needham Heights, MA: Allyn & Bacon.

Williams, D. D., & Miller, H. L., Jr. (1997). School contexts of implementation: Two case studies. In H. L. Miller, Jr. (Ed.), The New York City public schools integrated learning systems project: Evaluation and meta-evaluation [Special issue]. *International Journal of Educational Research, 27*(2), 99–117.

Winer, B. J. (1962). *Statistical principles in experimental design.* New York: McGraw-Hill.

Winnick, J. P., & Short, F. X. (1999). *The Brockport physical fitness test manual.* Champaign, IL: Human Kinetics.

Wolcott, H. T. (1994). *Transforming qualitative data: Description, analysis, and interpretation.* Thousand Oaks, CA: Sage.

Wolcott, H. T. (1999). *Ethnography: A way of seeing.* Walnut Creek, CA: AltaMira.

Wolcott, H. T. (2001). *Writing up qualitative research* (2nd ed.). Thousand Oaks, CA: Sage.

Yin, R. K. (2014). *Case study research: Design and methods* (5th ed.). Thousand Oaks, CA: Sage.

Zeller, N., Griffith, R., & Zhang, G. (2009, July). *The passage from otherness: How service learning can change preservice teachers' attitudes toward diverse populations.* Paper presented at the 2009 Assessment Institute, Indianapolis, IN.

Zeller, N., Griffith, R., Zhang, G., & Klenke, J. (2009, June). *From stranger to friend: The effect of service learning on pre-service teachers' attitudes toward diverse populations.* Paper presented at the 21st Annual Ethnographic and Qualitative Research Conference, Cedarville, OH.

Zeller, N., Griffith, R., Zhang, G., & Klenke, J. (2010). From stranger to friend: The effect of service learning on preservice teachers' attitudes towards diverse populations. *Journal of Language and Literacy Education, 6*(2), 34–50.

Zhang, G., & Algina, J. (2008). Coverage performance of the non-central F-based and percentile bootstrap confidence intervals for root mean square standardized effect size in one-way fixed-effects ANOVA. *Journal of Modern Applied Statistical Methods, 7*(1), 56–76.

Zhang, G., & Algina, J. (2011). A robust root mean square standardized effect size and its confidence intervals in one-way fixed-effects ANOVA. *Journal of Modern Applied Statistical Methods, 10*(1), 77–96.

Zhang, G., Bolker, B. M., Bruna, E. M., Christman, M. C., Kitajima, K., Martcheva, M. N., et al. (2010, April). *No boundaries: Preparing tomorrow's leading scientists by transcending traditional disciplinary borders with the Integrative Graduate Education and Research Traineeship Program.* Paper presented at the annual conference of the American Educational Research Association, Denver, CO.

Zhang, G., Griffith, R., Metcalf, D., Zeller, N., Misulis, K., Shea, D., et al. (2009, April). *Assessing service and learning of a service-learning program in teacher education using mixed-methods research.* Paper presented at the annual conference of the American Education Research Association, San Diego, CA.

Zhang, G., Williams, S., & Majewski, D. (2014, April). *A multi-level evaluation of an academic support program for college students with learning differences.* Paper presented at the annual conference of the American Education Research Association, Philadelphia, PA.

Zhang, G., Zeller, N., Griffith, R., Metcalf, D., Shea, C., Williams, J., et al. (2010, October). *Using the CIPP Model as a comprehensive framework to guide the planning, implementation, and assessment of service-learning programs.* Paper presented at the annual conference of the 2010 National Evaluation Institute, Williamsburg, VA.

Zhang, G., Zeller, N., Griffith, R., Metcalf, D., Williams, J., Shea, C., et al. (2011a, April). *An effective framework to guide the planning, implementation and assessment of service-learning programs: The CIPP Evaluation Model.* Paper presented at the annual conference of the American Education Research Association, New Orleans, LA.

Zhang, G., Zeller, N., Griffith, R., Metcalf, D., Williams, J., Shea, C., et al. (2011b). Using the Context, Input, Process, and Product Evaluation Model (CIPP) as a comprehensive framework to guide the planning, implementation, and assessment of service-learning programs. *Journal of Higher Education Outreach and Engagement, 15*(4), 57–84.

Zhang, G., Zeller, N., Shea, C., Griffith, R., Metcalf, D., Misulis, K., et al. (2008, October). A 360° assessment of the multidimensional effects of a service-learning program in teacher education using mixed-methods research. Paper presented at the Eighth International Research Conference on Service-Learning and Community Engagement, New Orleans, LA.

Zhang, G., Zeller, N., Shea, C., Griffith, R., Misulis, K., Metcalf, D., et al. (2013). Toward a better understanding: A 360° assessment of a service-learning program in teacher education using Stufflebeam's CIPP Model. In V. M. Jagla, J. A. Erickson, & A. Tinkler (Eds.), *Transforming teacher education through service learning* (pp. 211–231). Charlotte, NC: Information Age.

Author Index

Subject Index

Page numbers in *italic* indicate figures or tables

About the Authors

Daniel L. Stufflebeam, PhD, is Distinguished University Professor Emeritus at Western Michigan University (WMU). He founded and directed The Evaluation Center at The Ohio State University and moved it to WMU, where he directed it until 2002. He also designed the WMU Interdisciplinary PhD Program in Evaluation. The developer of the CIPP Evaluation Model, Dr. Stufflebeam led development of the General Educational Development Tests (GED) and other standardized tests; founded the Joint Committee on Standards for Educational Evaluation and was principal author of the Committee's original standards; and designed and directed the national Center for Research on Educational Accountability and Teacher Evaluation. He led development of many evaluation systems and has lectured, advised, and conducted evaluations in more than 20 countries. The author of 21 books and about 100 journal articles and book chapters (appearing in eight languages), Dr. Stufflebeam is a recipient of the Paul F. Lazarsfeld Evaluation Theory Award from the American Evaluation Association, among numerous other honors.

Guili Zhang, PhD, is Professor and Interim Chair of the Department of Special Education, Foundations, and Research at East Carolina University and Guest Professor at the Institute of International and Comparative Education at Beijing Normal University in China. Dr. Zhang has presented and published extensively on evaluation. She currently serves as Chair of the Assessment in Higher Education topical interest group and the Quantitative Methods topical interest group of the American Evaluation Association. Internationally, she serves as an expert advisor to China's Ministry of Education and the Beijing Faculty Development Center for Higher Education. Dr. Zhang is a recipient of awards including the Benjamin J. Dasher Best Paper Award from the Frontiers in Education conference, the Best Paper Award from the American Society for Engineering Education, and the Edward C. Pomeroy Award for Outstanding Contribution to Teacher Education from the American Association of Colleges for Teacher Education.